A Text Book of

PHARMACOGNOSY AND PHYTOCHEMISTRY - I

As Per PCI Regulations

SECOND YEAR B. PHARM., SEMESTER IV

Dr. Kuntal Das
Professor
Dept. of Pharmacognosy and Natural Product Chemistry
Krupanidhi College of Pharmacy,
#12/1, Chikka Bellandur, Varthur, Hobli,
Bangalore-35, Karnataka

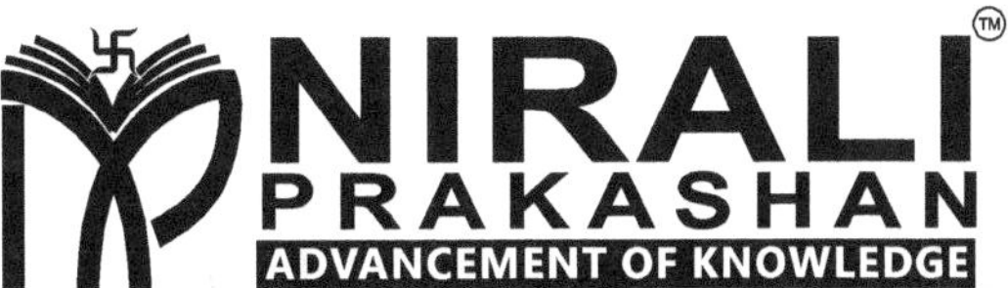

N4357

Pharmacognosy and Phytochemistry I　　　　　　　ISBN 978-93-88706-36-0

Second Edition : February 2020

©　　　　:　**Author**

Published By :

NIRALI PRAKASHAN

Abhyudaya Pragati, 1312, Shivaji Nagar,
Off J.M. Road, PUNE – 411005
Tel - (020) 25512336/37/39, Fax - (020) 25511379
Email : niralipune@pragationline.com

> ## DISTRIBUTION CENTRES

PUNE

Nirali Prakashan　:　119, Budhwar Peth, Jogeshwari Mandir Lane, Pune 411002, Maharashtra
Tel : (020) 2445 2044, 66022708
Email : bookorder@pragationline.com, niralilocal@pragationline.com

Nirali Prakashan　:　S. No. 28/27, Dhyari, Near Pari Company, Pune 411041
Tel : (020) 24690204 Fax : (020) 24690316
Email : dhyari@pragationline.com, bookorder@pragationline.com

MUMBAI

Nirali Prakashan　:　385, S.V.P. Road, Rasdhara Co-op. Hsg. Society Ltd.,
Girgaum, Mumbai 400004, Maharashtra
Tel : (022) 2385 6339 / 2386 9976, Fax : (022) 2386 9976
Email : niralimumbai@pragationline.com

> ## DISTRIBUTION BRANCHES

JALGAON

Nirali Prakashan　:　34, V. V. Golani Market, Navi Peth, Jalgaon 425001,
Maharashtra, Tel : (0257) 222 0395, Mob : 94234 91860
Email : niralijalgoan@pragationline.com

KOLHAPUR

Nirali Prakashan　:　New Mahadvar Road, Kedar Plaza, 1st Floor Opp. IDBI Bank
Kolhapur 416 012, Maharashtra. Mob : 9850046155
Email : niralikolhapur@pragationline.com

NAGPUR

Nirali Prakashan　:　Above Maratha Mandir, Shop No. 3, First Floor,
Rani Jhanshi Square, Sitabuldi, Nagpur 440012, Maharashtra
Tel : (0712) 254 7129; Email : niralinagpur@pragationline.com

DELHI

Nirali Prakashan　:　4593/15, Basement, Agarwal Lane, Ansari Road, Daryaganj
Near Times of India Building, New Delhi 110002 Mob : 08505972553
Email : niralidelhi@pragationline.com

BANGALURU

Nirali Prakashan　:　Maitri Ground Floor, Jaya Apartments, No. 99, 6th Cross, 6th Main,
Malleswaram, Bengaluru 560003, Karnataka; Mob : 9449043034
Email: niralibangalore@pragationline.com

Other Branches : Hyderabad, Chennai

niralipune@pragationline.com | www.pragationline.com
Also find us on [f] www.facebook.com/niralibooks

Dedicated to

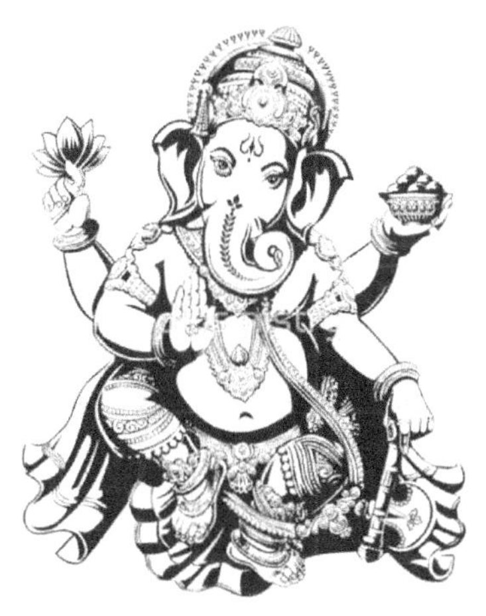

My beloved
Parents, Wife and Son

Preface

This is the first edition and first time the attempt has been made to write a Pharmacognosy & Phytochemistry-I text book as per the new syllabus prescribed by Pharmacy Council of India for semester-4. There are many text books on Pharmacognosy already available in market by famous authors. Most of the information in this book has presented in a very simple manner, with more tables, figures and wherever necessary with diagrams. The aim of this book is a made easy for understandable to the student. This book is as per the revised syllabus prescribed by the Pharmacy Council of India under Regulations 6, 7 & 8 of the Bachelor of Pharmacy (B. Pharm.) course regulations 2014 in 2016 and amended from 2017 onwards throughout India under same uniform syllabus. As per the norms, the book is compiled with semester wise syllabus in which Pharmacognosy & Phytochemistry-I is under semester-IV.

Semester - IV, Pharmacognosy & Phytochemistry-I subject is divided into five sub-units.

Unit – I: This sub-topic has discussed history, scope, linkage with other branches and modern application of Pharmacognosy. Discussed about crude drugs along with their classifications, various sources etc. Furthermore quality control of herbal drugs in terms of adulteration, substitution, their types and how adulterants are detected through various drug evaluation techniques (special emphasis has given for quantitative measurement through microscopic evaluation using camera lucida), described in detail in this unit.

Unit – II, deals with detail study on cultivation, collection, processing and storage conditions for natural originated drugs. Cultivation is the most important agrotechnology through which supply of raw materials are important for drug development. Hence as per Good Agricultural Practice, cultivation carried out by considering various factors and role of plant hormones. Thereafter crop improvement of crop production and varieties through genetical modification especially polyploidy, mutation and hybridization techniques are discussed. Furthermore conservation of medicinal and aromatic plants are very important for the existing of various plant species which are also discussed in this unit.

Unit – III, discussed about the alternate method for cultivation of herbal plants i.e. *in-vitro* technique. It is also known as plant cell and tissue culture which is carried out in artificial medium under aseptic laboratory conditions. Hence detail historical development of plant tissue culture, types of cultures, nutritional requirements, growth and their maintenance are explained detail in this unit. Edible vaccines as well as applications of plant tissue culture in Pharmacognosy are also discussed.

Unit – IV: This part has discussed about the role of Pharmacognosy in allopathy and with various traditional systems of medicine namely, Ayurveda, Unani, Siddha, Homeopathy and Chinese systems of medicine. Thereafter importance of plant secondary metabolites are discussed in terms of definition, classification, properties and test for identification of Alkaloids, Glycosides, Flavonoids, Tannins, Volatile oil and Resins.

Unit – V: This unit explained about study of biological source, chemical nature and uses of drugs of natural origin containing plant fibres and various plant primary metabolites. General introduction, detailed study with respect to chemistry, sources, preparation, evaluation, preservation, storage, therapeutic used and commercial utility as Pharmaceutical aids are also explained with special topics such as carbohydrate, proteins, enzymes, lipids etc. Furthermore important drugs procured from marine sources are discussed in detail in this unit.

It is hoped that all the units will provide up to date knowledge to all the students with the detail information by systemic manners described in this book.

I am forced to publish this first edition of my book with better hope to gain the popularity by the students and readers throughout the country. Any criticism and suggestions from the readers are always welcome. In the future editions, such suggestions will be incorporated and other mistakes will be rectified.

It is my great privilege to acknowledge the help from all the published books and websites from the internet for completing this book. My sincere and heartiest gramercy to Dr. Raman Dang, Registrar of DPSRU New Delhi, for his valuable suggestions and positive motivation. My sincere thanks and respect to Chairman Sir, Prof Suresh Nagpal, vice chairperson madam, directors present principal Dr. Amit Kumar Das, all my teaching, non teaching staffs, of my college for their active co-operation and encouragement.

I felt no word to express sense of indebtedness to my parents, Mrs. Kalyani Das and Dr. Dilip Kumar Das (Emeritus Fellow UGC), whose silent blessings, encouragement, and helping me to put my best foot forward in all my endeavors of chasing my dreams in life.

My special and sincere thanks to my wife Mrs. Sangita Das and son Master Niladri Das for their inspiration to pursue the work in all the situations.

Lastly but not the least, I thank to M/S Nirali Prakashan publishers for kind publication of the book with much care.

Prof. Kuntal Das

(Ph.D, FIC, FAELS, FICS)

Syllabus

Unit - I : 10 Hours

Introduction to Pharmacognosy
(a) Definition, History, Scope and Development of Pharmacognosy.
(b) Sources of Drugs: Plants, Animals, Marine and Tissue Culture.
(c) Organized Drugs, Unorganized Drugs (Dried Latex, Dried Juices, Dried Extracts, Gums and Mucilages, Oleoresins and Oleo-Gum-Resins).

Classification of Drugs: Alphabetical, Morphological, Taxonomical, Chemical, Pharmacological, Chemo and Sero Taxonomical Classification of Drugs.

Quality Control of Drugs of Natural Origin: Adulteration of Drugs of Natural Origin. Evaluation by Organoleptic, Microscopic, Physical, Chemical and Biological Methods and Properties.

Quantitative Microscopy of Crude Drugs including Lycopodium Spore Method, Leaf Constants, Camera Lucida and Diagrams of Microscopic Objects to scale with Camera Lucida.

Unit - II : 10 Hours

Cultivation, Collection, Processing and Storage of Drugs of Natural Origin
Cultivation and Collection of Drugs of Natural Origin
Factors influencing Cultivation of Medicinal Plants
Plant Hormones and their Applications
Polyploidy, Mutation and Hybridization with reference to Medicinal Plants
Conservation of Medicinal Plants.

Unit - III : 07 Hours

Plant Tissue Culture
Historical Development of Plant Tissue Culture, Types of Cultures, Nutritional Requirements, Growth and their Maintenance. Applications of Plant Tissue Culture in Pharmacognosy. Edible Vaccines.

Unit - IV : 10 Hours

Role of Pharmacognosy in Various Systems of Medicines.
Role of Pharmacognosy in Allopathy and Traditional Systems of Medicine namely, Ayurveda, Unani, Siddha, Homeopathy and Chinese Systems of Medicine.

Introduction to Secondary Metabolites: Definition, Classification, Properties and Tests for Identification of Alkaloids, Glycosides, Flavonoids, Tannins, Volatile oil and Resins.

Unit V : 08 Hours

Study of Biological Source, Chemical Nature and Uses of Drugs of Natural Origin containing following drugs:
Plant Products:
Fibers - Cotton, Jute, Hemp.
Hallucinogens, Teratogens, Natural allergens.

Primary Metabolites: General introduction, Detailed study with respect to Chemistry, Sources, Preparation, Evaluation, Preservation, Storage, Therapeutic used and Commercial Utility as Pharmaceutical Aids and/or Medicines for the following Primary metabolites:

Carbohydrates: Acacia, Agar, Tragacanth, Honey.

Proteins and Enzymes: Gelatin, Casein, Proteolytic Enzymes (Papain, Bromelain, Serratiopeptidase, Urokinase, Streptokinase, Pepsin).

Lipids (Waxes, Fats, Fixed Oils): Castor Oil, Chaulmoogra Oil, Wool Fat, Bees Wax.

Marine Drugs: Novel Medicinal Agents from Marine Sources.

***

Contents

1. Introduction, Classification and Quality Control of Natural Originated Drugs

1 - 56

1.1	Definition, History, Scope and Development of Pharmacognosy	1.1
	1.1.1 Definition	1.1
	1.1.2 History	1.3
	1.1.3 Scope of Pharmacognosy	1.7
	1.1.4 Applications of Pharmacognosy	1.11
1.2	Sources of Drugs – Plants, Animals, Marine and Tissue Culture	1.12
	1.2.1 Natural Products	1.12
	1.2.2 Drugs obtained from Animal Sources	1.15
	1.2.3 Drugs obtained from Marine Sources	1.15
	1.2.4 Plant Tissue Culture	1.16
1.3	Organized Drugs and Unorganized Drugs	1.17
1.4	Classification of Drugs	1.17
	1.4.1 Alphabetical Classification	1.17
	1.4.2 Morphological Classification	1.18
	1.4.3 Taxonomical Classification	1.20
	1.4.4 Pharmacological Classification	1.21
	1.4.5 Chemical Classification	1.22
	1.4.6 Chemo-taxonomical Classification	1.23
	1.4.7 Serotaxonomic Classification	1.24
1.5	Quality Control of Drugs of Natural Origin	1.25
	1.5.1 Adulteration of Drugs of Natural Origin	1.26
	1.5.2 Evaluation by Organoleptic, Microscopic, Physical, Chemical and Biological Methods and Properties	1.33
•	Exercise	1.52

2. Cultivation, Collection, Processing and Storage of Drugs of Natural Origin

2.1 - 2.42

2.1	Cultivation and Collection of Drugs of Natural Origin	2.1
2.2	Concept of Good Agricultural Practices (GAPs)	2.2
2.3	Factors Influencing Cultivation of Medicinal Plants	2.4
	2.3.1 Atmospheric Factors	2.5
	2.3.2 Soil Factors	2.10
2.4	Plant Hormones and their Applications	2.30
2.5	Polyploidy, Mutation and Hybridization with reference to Medicinal Plants	2.32
	2.5.1 Polyploidy	2.32
	2.5.2 Mutation	2.32
	2.5.3 Hybridization	2.33
2.6	Conservation of Medicinal Plants	2.34
•	Exercise	2.37

3. Plant Tissue Culture and its Applications   **3.1 - 3.28**

3.1   Plant Tissue Culture   3.1

3.2   Historical Development of Plant Tissue Culture   3.1

3.3   Types of Cultures   3.4

3.4   Nutritional Requirements, Growth and their Maintenance   3.16

3.5   Applications of Plant Tissue Culture in Pharmacognosy   3.21

3.6   Edible Vaccines   3.22

•   Exercise   3.24

4. Traditional System of Medicines and Plant Secondary Metabolites   **4.1 - 4.58**

4.1   Allopathy   4.1

    4.1.1   Role of Pharmacognosy in Allopathy   4.2

4.2   Ayurveda, Siddha, Unani and Homeopathy   4.2

    4.2.1   Ayurveda   4.2

    4.2.2   Siddha   4.5

    4.2.3   Unani   4.7

    4.2.4   Homeopathy   4.9

    4.2.5   Chinese Systems of Medicine   4.10

4.3   Alkaloids   4.14

    4.3.1   Classification   4.15

    4.3.2   General Extraction Methods   4.22

4.4   Glycosides   4.23

    4.4.1   Classification   4.25

    4.4.2   Functions of Glycoside   4.31

4.5   Flavonoids   4.32

    4.5.1   Classification   4.33

4.6   Tannins   4.38

    4.6.1   Classification   4.39

4.7   Volatile Oil   4.44

4.8   Resins   4.47

    4.8.1   Classification of Resins   4.49

•   Exercise   4.52

5. Study of Primary Metabolites, Plant and Marine Sources Natural Drugs

5.1 - 5.62

5.1 Plant Products	5.1
5.1.1 Fibres	5.1
5.1.2 Natural Allergens	5.12
5.2 Primary Metabolites	5.13
5.2.1 Carbohydrates	5.13
5.2.2 Carbohydrate Related Drugs	5.17
5.3 Proteins and Enzymes	5.27
5.3.1 Protein Related Drugs	5.30
5.4 Proteolytic Enzymes	5.33
5.5 Lipids (Waxes, Fats, Fixed Oils)	5.40
5.5.1 Lipid	5.40
5.5.2 Fatty Acids	5.41
5.6 Marine Drugs	5.52
5.6.1 Factors Affecting Distribution and Occurrence of Marine Drugs	5.53
5.6.2 Cardiovascular Active Agents from Marine Sources	5.55
• Exercise	5.57
• Bibliography	B.1 - B.3

***

INTRODUCTION, CLASSIFICATION AND QUALITY CONTROL OF NATURAL ORIGINATED DRUGS

♦ LEARNING OBJECTIVES ♦

After completing this unit, reader should be able to:

❖ Know about the detail history, modern scope and the recent development of Pharmacognosy.

❖ Know about the sources of drugs and their various forms.

❖ Know about various classification of crude drugs.

❖ Know about Quality control of natural originated drugs with respect to adulteration and its identification and various Quantitative microscopic determinations.

❖ Know drug evaluation and their classification.

1.1 DEFINITION, HISTORY, SCOPE AND DEVELOPMENT OF PHARMACOGNOSY

1.1.1 Definition

Plants from the natural sources are serves for the benefits of man kinds. The drugs that are procured from natural sources belong to the branch of Pharmacognosy. Earlier only the external morphological characters were used to identify a drug. At the beginning, Pharmacognosy had developed mainly on the botanical side, being particularly concerned with the description and identification of drugs, both in their whole state and in powder form. Modern aspects of Pharmacognosy include not only the crude drugs but also their natural constituents and derivatives. The word Pharmacognosy is derived from the Greek words "Pharmakon" (drug), and "gnosis" (knowledge). The term Pharmacognosy was used for the first time by the Austrian physician Schmidt in 1811 and 1815 by Crr. Anotheus Seydler, who first coined this term in his dissertation entitled *'Analecta pharmacognostica'*. Pharmacognosy is closely allied to medicine, developed during early 19th century as a branch of *Materia Medica* and applied biology.

Pharmacognosy is the study of drugs having their origin in plant and animal kingdom. The subject Pharmacognosy can also be expressed as an applied science that deals with biological, biochemical, therapeutic and economic features of natural drugs and their constituents. Pharmacognosy is a subject in which plant parts are identified or authenticated using macroscopical anatomical phytochemical characters. Therefore Pharmacognosy is "the science of medicines from natural sources". In other way, Pharmacognosy is knowledge of the history, distribution, cultivation, collection, selection, preparation, commerce, identification, evaluation, preservation and use of drugs and economic substances that affects the health of men and other animals. During the 19th century and the beginning of the 20th century, "Pharmacognosy" was used to define the branch of medicine or commodity sciences, which deals with drugs in their crude, or unprepared form. Crude drugs are the dried, unprepared material of plant, animal or mineral origin and they are used as such as they occur in nature without any processing except, drying and size reduction for medicines. Plant originated crude drugs consist of entire plants or their parts. For example, Ephedra and datura are entire plants, senna leaves and podes, nux-vomica seeds, cinnamon and cinchona bark, Rauwolfia roots, clove is a flower bud. Crude drugs may also be obtained by physical processes like drying (opium) or extracting with water (catechu, agar). Several other useful substances affecting the health of animals and human being are also included along with crude drugs in the study of Pharmacognosy but have no pharmacological action. These substances include allergens, flavoring agents, colors, pesticides, immunizing agents, vehicles disintegrants, stabilizers, filtering and supporting media and diagnostic aids. Animal source originated crude drugs include beeswax, gelatin, wool fat, silk, vitamins etc. Some of the mineral originated crude drugs like talc, chalk, bentonite etc. are used in various pharmaceutical preparations. In addition, antibiotics, hormones etc. may also be involved. Marine organisms (plants and animals), which have special potent pharmacological actions, are recent focus in the search for new drugs.

Study of the materials obtained from natural sources in pharmakognosie was first developed in Europe especially in German populated areas, while other language areas often used in the book named *Materia Medica* that taken from the works of Galen and Dioscorides. Drogenkunde ("science of crude drugs"), the German term is also used in the same way. As late as the beginning of the 20th century, Pharmacognosy is still in growing importance, particularly for identification and quality control purposes and resulted rapid development in all other areas in the subject.

With above discussion, finally a brief definition of Pharmacognosy is described as: *"It is a branch of science and a tool for crude drug standardization which deals with the scientific and systematic study of structural, physical, chemical and biological characters and evaluation of crude drugs along with geographical sources, history, method of cultivation, collection and preparation for the market, their proper storage and their application in the improvement of health."*

Hence, Pharmacognosy science is concerned with studying the following subjects:

1. Taxonomy of plants and the natural sources of drugs.
2. Distribution of natural products worldwide.
3. Description of plants such as Trees (Cinnamon, cinchona, Salix), shrub, (Vinca), Perennials (Peppermint).
4. The active constituents from natural sources (active groups) like (glycosides, alkaloids, volatile oils, tannins, etc.).
5. The biosynthesis and storage places of the active constituents in organisms (plants, animals etc.).
6. The part used from the natural sources in medicine and pharmacy such as leaf (Senna, Mint, Digitalis), roots (Liquorice), seeds (Nux Vomica, Coffee bean), bark (Cinnamon).
7. Collection and Storage of the part used.

To understand the basic concept of Pharmacognosy, some general functions of Pharmacognosist is:

*   Identification of the drug sources.
*   Determination of the morphological character.
*   Investigation of potency, purity, and admixture.
*   Planning and designing of the cultivation of medicinal plants.
*   Prescription of the detail processes of collection, drying and preservation.
*   Knowledge about extraction and isolation procedures.
*   Knowledge about active constituents, phytoconstituents, chemical nature and uses.
*   Knowledge about physical, chemical, biological and microbial evaluation of drugs.

1.1.2 History

The early man sought to alleviate his sufferings of illness and injuries by using plants. They acquired knowledge of medicinal properties of plants by guesswork or trial and error, while searching for food, by superficial resemblance between the plant parts and the affected organs, i.e., by examining the "Signature of Nature", by observing other animals, instinctive discrimination between toxic and palatable plants or by accidental discovery.

In course of time a group of people emerged in each community who acquired expertise in collecting, testing and using medicinal plants for treating diseases. These people later became known as `Medicine Men'. They transferred this secret knowledge only to their trusted predecessors of the successive generations, who gradually increased the volume of knowledge about drugs and their medicinal uses. Initially the transfer of the acquired knowledge from generation to generation used to be done verbally by the use of signs and symbols. As civilization progressed, transfer and recording of the knowledge were done in writing.

According to Old History:

The history of herbal medicine is from the beginning of human civilization. In that era, maximum plant based medicines were used. Before the beginning of Christian era, many ancient documents revealed that plants were used largely by the Asian namely China, India,

Egypt and Greece. In China, medicinal plants had been in use since 5000 BC. In around 3000 BC, *Shen Nung* wrote a book on herbal document *"Pentaso"*which is very old documentary book. During the same period, meticulous efforts had been progressing in India, for classification of herbs through proper examination. Finally, Charaka made 50 groups of 10 herbs, each of which was meant for specific diseases whereas Sushrutha enlisted only 760 herbs in 7 groups, based on their common properties.

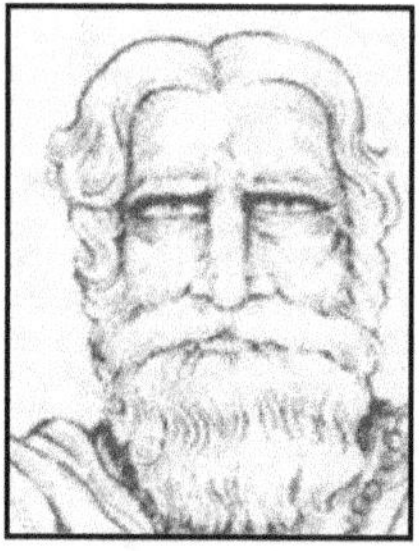

Sushrutha

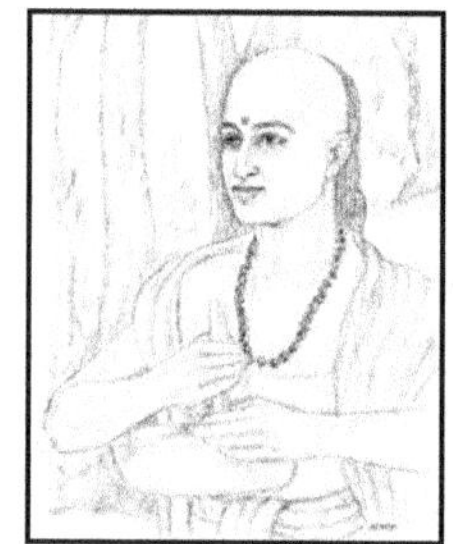

Charaka

In India, the medicinal properties of the plants are first described in two Vedas, Rigveda and in Atharvaveda (3500-1500 B.C) from which Ayurveda has developed. The earliest plant medicines used in the Ayurvedic system were described with a list of 127 plants. The binomial classification of plants, introduced by Swedish botanist Carl Linnaeus in 1700s, was further developed by Bentham and Hooker (1862-1863). Gregor Mendel's important observations on plant hybrids came in 1865. Soon microscope was introduced as an important analytical tool; techniques like clearing, staining, mounting etc. came in to focus. Thus, anatomical atlas of crude drugs was published in 1865. In the 20th century, tremendous work was been done in this field and Phytochemistry evolved as a distinct branch in science. Constituents isolated from the plants were not only used as such, but they were also used for semi-synthetic and synthetic drugs.

This section has tried to give basic information about origination of Pharmacognosy so that readers can get an idea about the history of the same.

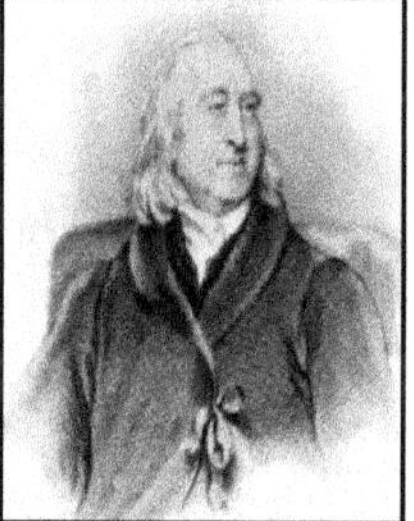

Bentham

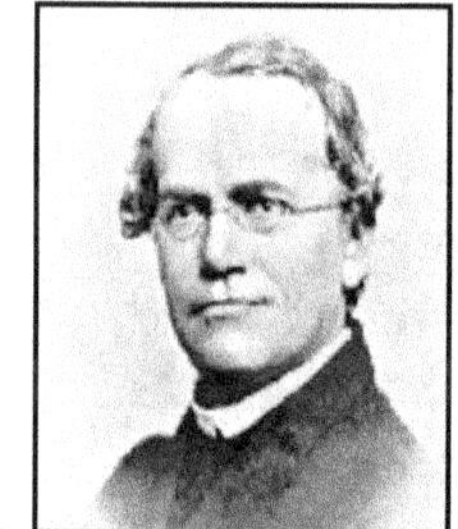

Gregor Mendel

Contribution of the Scientists in Significant Development of Pharmacognosy:

Hippocrates (460-370 B.C), a Greek scientist, is known as the father of medicine. He worked on human anatomy and Physiology, particularly circulatory system and nervous system. He prepared famous oath for physicians, which is still taken by them. Further **Aristotle** (384-322 B.C) and **Theophrastus** (370-287 B.C), well known philosopher and scientist are known for their writing animal and plant kingdom respectively. **Dioscorides** (1st

Century AD), a Greek Physician, published five volumes of a book, entitled "**De Materia Medica**" in 78 AD, in which the described more than 600 medicinal plants with their collection, storage and uses. **Pliny de Elder** (23-70 AD), a Greek botanist, collected and described a large number of medicinal plants with their uses.

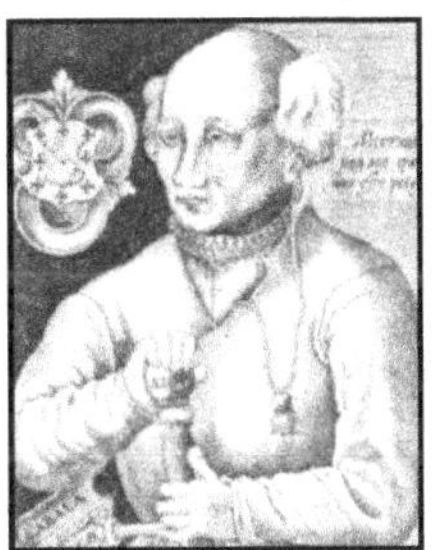

Theophrastus

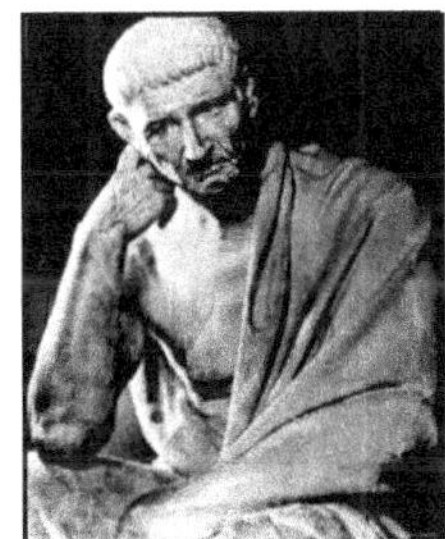

Aristotle

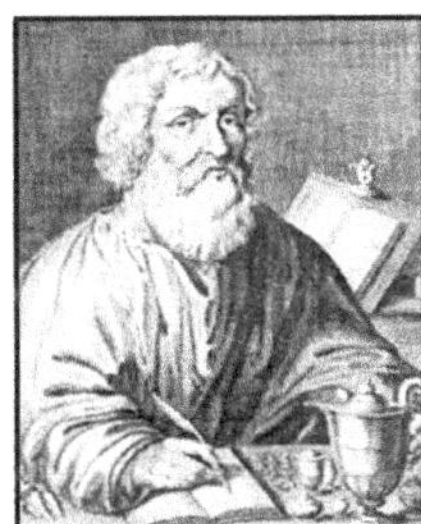

Hippocrates

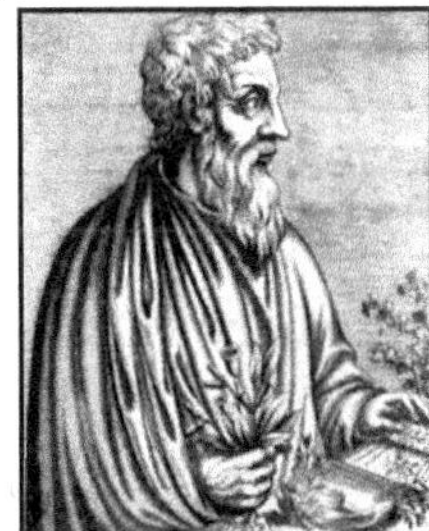

Dioscorides

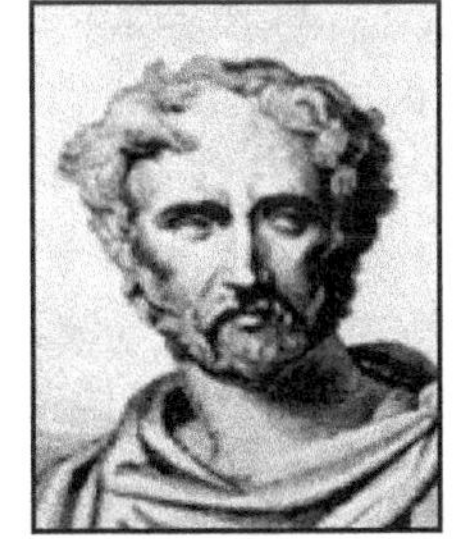

Pliny de Elder

Work of Seydler:

Seydler was a German scientist and he wrote a book *"Analecta Pharmacognostica"* in 1815. In that book he introduced the word Pharmacognosy. He coined this word first time by combining two Greek words "Pharmakon": Drug "Gignosco": To acquire knowledge of. Hence Pharmacognosy means to acquire knowledge about drugs.

Work of Galen: (131 – 200)

Galen was a Greek pharmacist. He worked on extraction of chemical constituents from the plants. He developed various methods of plant part extraction and is under the branch of Galenical Pharmacy which deals with the extraction of chemical constituents from plants and animals.

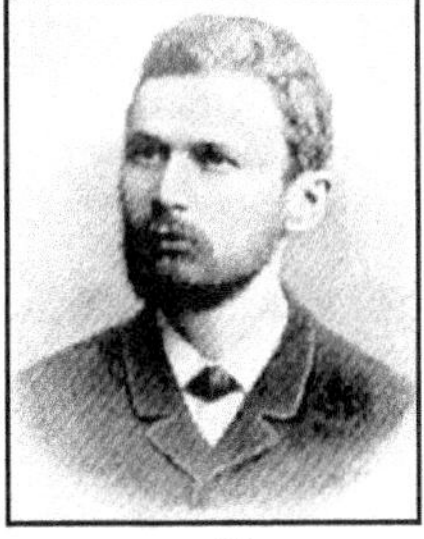

Seydler

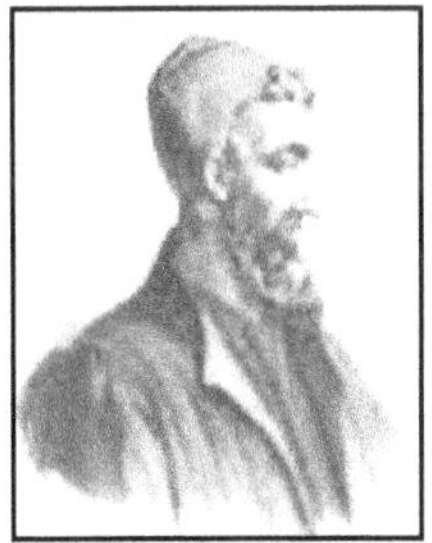

Galen

Some of the biological scientists and their important discoveries:

Table 1.1: Famous scientists with their invention

Year	Name of scientist	Work carried out
1805	Friedrich Wilhelm Adam Serturner	Meconic acid present in opium
1828	Wilhelm Heinrich Posselt and chemist Karl Ludwig Reimann	Nicotine from tobacco
1860	Albert Niemann	Cocaine from coca species
1875	Gerrard and Hardy	Pilocarpine from pilocarpus
1885	Nagayoshi Nagai	Ephedrine from ephedra
1891	Kuersten	Podophylotoxin from Podophyllum

Modern Pharmacognosy:

The development of modern Pharmacognosy began during the period of 1930-1960 by the application of a broad spectrum of biological and socio-scientific subjects, including botany, ethno botany, medical anthropology, marine biology, microbiology, herbal medicine, chemistry, biotechnology, phytochemistry, pharmacology, pharmaceutics, clinical pharmacy and pharmacy practice along with modern analytical techniques like paper and thin layer chromatography (TLC), gas chromatography (GC), High performance liquid chromatography (HPLC), Extreme and ultra-pressure liquid chromatography (XLC, UPLC), high pressure thin layer chromatography (HPTLC), Mass spectroscopy, Liquid chromatography combined with mass spectroscopy (LC/ MS), High Resolution Mass Spectroscopy (HRMS) etc. During this period isolation, structure elucidation and various pharmacological activity of different phytoconstituents were studied. Examples like isolation of penicillin in 1928 by Alexander Fleming from microorganisms and later on commercial production of the same in 1941 by Florey and Chain. Gradually, other antibiotics were isolated and their chemistry was studied and among them streptomycin, chloramphenicol, tetracycline are most important.

Some of the important isolated constituents are reserpine from Rauwolfia root (responsible for anti-hypertension action), vincristine and vinblastine from vinca plant (responsible for treatment of leukemia), digitoxin from digitalis plant (only one potent cardiac drug which is used directly as an allopathic medicine), morphine (a potent analgesic) and codeine (a potent antitussive) isolated from dried latex of Opium poppy, ergotamine from ergot (have potent oxytocic activity) etc. Several steroidal hormones were also isolated from plants. E.g., progesterone from diosgenin (from dioscorea plant). Gradually biosynthetic pathways were also identified with the help of radioisotopes for the study of accumulation and synthesis of primary and secondary metabolites. Some of the important pathways are Calvin's cycle for photosynthesis (biosynthesis of carbohydrate, a primary metabolite), shikimic acid pathway for synthesis of aromatic compounds, acetate pathway for anthracene glycoside synthesis, isoprenoid pathway for synthesis of terpenes and steroids etc. Development of structure activity relationship of the phytoconstituents helped in the identification of the structure of the constituents, as well as effects of addition or deletion of the organic or inorganic groups in the mother structure. This tracer study is also useful to make derived plant products through biotransformation which shows more therapeutic activity. For example, hypotensive and tranquillizing actions of reserpine are attributed to the trimethoxy benzoic acid moiety, which is essential; presence of lactone ring is essential for the action of cardiac glycosides; oxytocic activity of methyl ergometrine is more than that of ergometrine. 9 : 10 position hydrogenation in ergotamine suppressed oxytocic activity but increases spasmolytic activity. Similarly, etoposide, a semi synthetic derivative of podophyllotoxin (isolated from podophyllum plant), has more potent anticancer activity than podophyllotoxin. After 1960, several drugs were discovered with the help of isolated plant constituents. Plant products are also used in various pharmaceutical aids. Examples: acacia, tragacanth are used as binding and suspending agents, Guar gum is used as a thickening agent; Isphagula and linseed are used as demulcents or as soothing agents, agar is used as laxatives by osmosis and is also used as an emulsifying agent etc. During 1980-1990, huge growth occurred in pharma world market which resulted in combinatorial chemistry and nutraceutical products. Nutraceutical products are used as food supplements. Year 2000 onwards to till date, nano level research on plant based products brought revolution in the world market. Nanomedicines, nanofertilizers, gold particles etc. are the current focus towards new drug discovery especially in the field of cancer research, AIDS and other critical diseases. Hence, Pharmacognosy is a multidisciplinary science that developed over the years but adapted challenges of the future with continuous changing environment. Among that application of molecular docking techniques is most attractive and new dimension for the natural drug discovery. Further molecular pharmacognosy is also concerned with gene regulation of metabolic pathway and developed as a new borderline discipline. This system helps in herbal and animal drug populations by molecular marker assay, conserving and utilizing wild resources based on genetic diversity, investigating the mechanism of active compound accumulation and obtaining new high quality resources through genetic engineering.

1.1.3 Scope of Pharmacognosy

India also has a diverse cultural heritage due to its biodiversity. Though at present Indian health care delivery consists of both traditional and modern systems of medicines, both organized traditional systems of medicine like Ayurveda, Siddha and Unani and unorganized systems like folk medicine have been flourishing well. Ayurveda and Siddha are of Indian origin and account for about 60% health care delivery in general, and 85% of rural Indian population depends on these traditional systems. It is estimated that roughly 1500 to 1600 plant species in Ayurveda and 1200 to 1500 plant species in Siddha have been used for drug preparation. In Indian folk medicine use, about 7500 to 9,000 plant species are recorded as medicinal plants. In 1998 the latest figures available for Europe, the total OTC market for herbal medicinal products reached about $ 6 billion, with consumption for Germany of $ 2.5 billion, France $ 1.6 billion and Italy $ 600 million. In the US, the market for all herb sales reached a peak in 1998 of $ 700 billion. Medicines became a huge business with an annual growth of 6-9% and it is presently estimated that global sales of pharmaceuticals will top in 2017 with $ 1.5 trillion. Hence the demand of herbals is increased gradually in the world market especially in India. The scope of Pharmacognosy has expanded from the traditional morphological description of plants and other organisms, to encompass the most modern aspects of molecular science relating to the exploration of naturally occurring bioactive compounds, their mode of action and their applications in world market and to the social activities. Nature is a source of bioactive products from which new drugs have been developed and marketed. Hence by understanding and exploiting the biodiversity, it is essential to establish integrative programs like conservation of species, bioactivity, chemical analysis, chemical synthesis and their proper storage. This is clearly mentioned in the below Fig. 1.1.

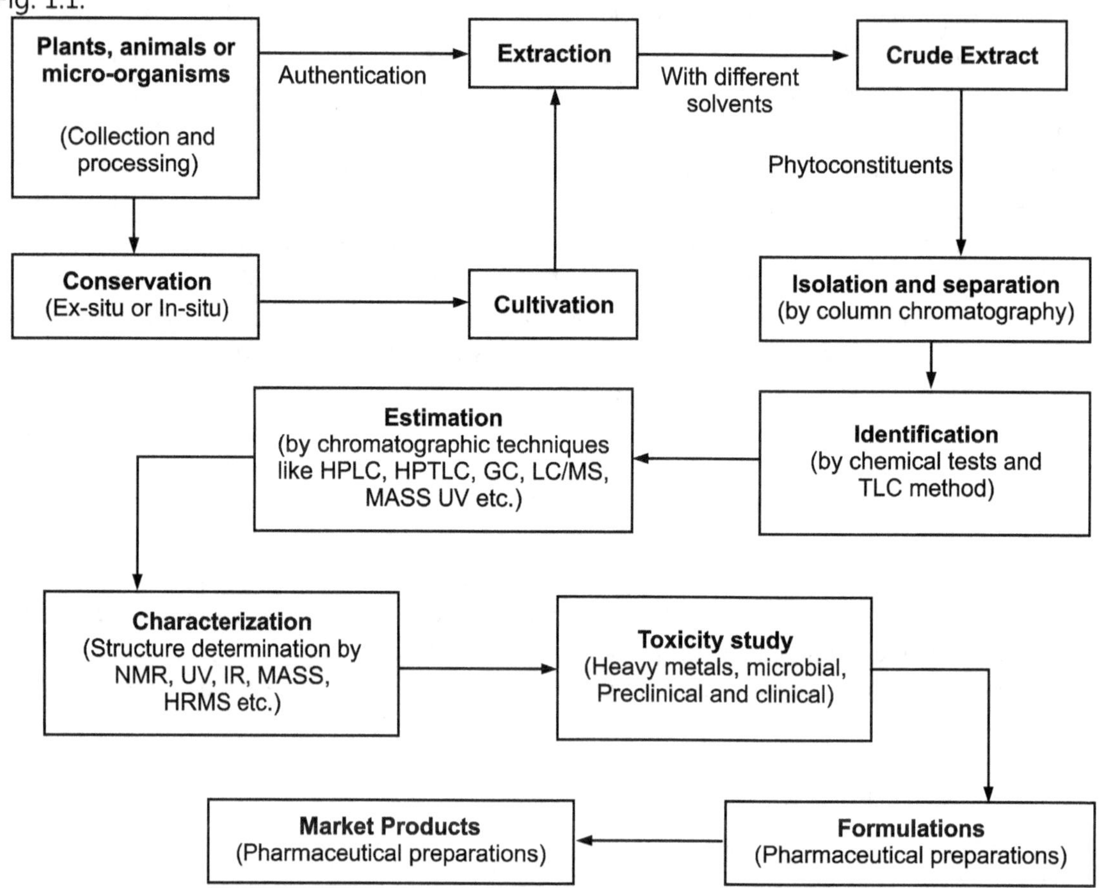

Fig. 1.1: Sequential development of herbal products

Contribution to the Advancement of Natural and Physical Science:

In a broad sense, Pharmacognosy embraces the knowledge of the history, distribution, cultivation, collection, selection, preparation, commerce, identification, evaluation, preservation, standardization, transfer, storage of drugs and economic substances for therapeutic drug discovery and use of drugs and economic substances affecting the health related matters in human. Such useful economic products extend beyond the category of crude drugs and their derivatives that included commercial products like allergens, allergenic extracts, antibiotics, biological products, flavoring agents, beverages and pesticides.

(a) The drug-drug, drug-food interactions are studied in Pharmacognosy which helps to avoid the untoward effects of severe interactions with optimal therapeutic outcomes. The most important category drugs include the following; cardiac glycoside, blood thinners etc.

(b) Bioassay Guided fractionation helps in the extraction of the crude drugs from the natural sources based on their physio-biochemical activities.

The extraction of active compounds from various plants and parts of plants and their utilization has revolutionized the health sciences.

(c) In the pharmaceutical industry, various herbal drugs are used in drug manufacture process includes:

- Aloe Vera used for healing burns and wound healing.
- Blackberry (*Rubus fruticosus*) reduces the wrinkling of skin, aging effect.
- Digitoxin (*Digitalis purpures*) used for the cardiac diseases.
- Calendula (*Calendula officinalis*) used for the treatment of constipation and cramps.
- Echinacea (*Echinacea angustifolia*) used for action against rhinovirus colds.
- Grapefruit (*Naringenin*) used for obesity treatment.
- Green tea (*Camelia sinensis*) cures the breast cancer.

(d) The revolution in herbal medicine has increased the demand for research in Pharmacognosy with concern to:

- Quality Control to assure the identity, purity and uniform consistency of drug substances.
- Efficacy to determine the therapeutic effects, indications, clinical aspects and pharmacological effects.
- Safety research to study the adverse toxic reactions, drug interactions, contraindications and precautions.

With the view of above applications of Pharmacognosy is linked with various allied sciences.

Link between Pharmacology and Medicinal Chemistry

Pharmacognosy gives a sound knowledge of the vegetable drugs under botany and animal drugs under zoology. It also includes taxonomy, breeding, pathology and genetics of plants. Pharmacognosy knowledge helps to improve the cultivation methods for both medicinal and aromatic plants. Now-a-days photochemistry (plant chemistry) has undergone significant improvement. This includes a variety of substances that are accumulated by plants and synthesized by plants. Newly detected plant drugs (purified phytochemicals) are converting into medicines. Pharmacognosy is essential for drug discovery because crude drugs are used for the preparation of galanicals or as sources of therapeutically active metabolites. Phytopharmaceuticals, i.e., synthesized drugs are finally formed in a suitable dosage forms and in which the crude drugs can act as an intermediates (Fig. 1.2).

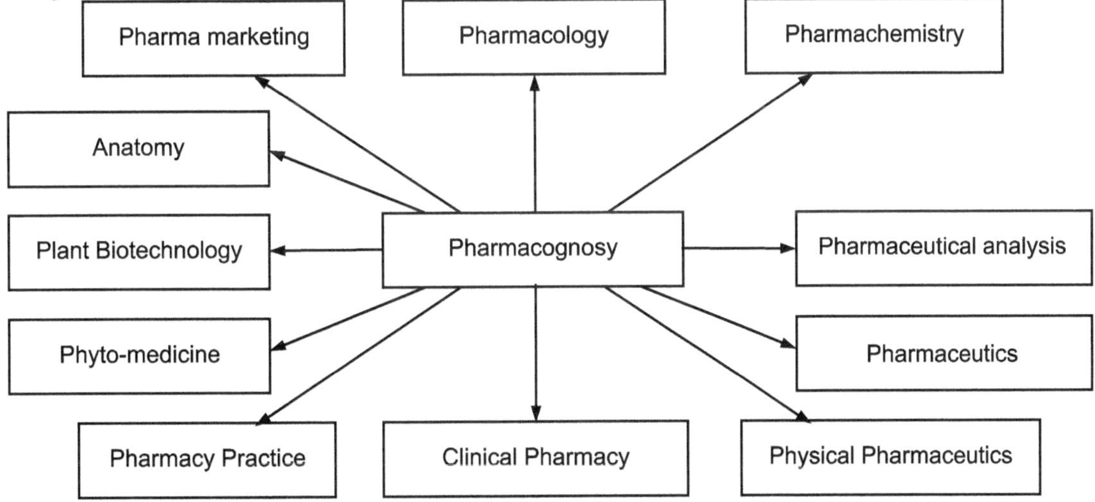

Fig. 1.2: Interrelation between Pharmacognosy with other branches

Pharmacognosy is a link between pharmaceuticals, basic sciences, traditional ayurvedic and allopathic medicines (Fig. 1.3). So Pharmacognosy is a science of active principles of crude drugs, which can help in dispensing, formulating and manufacturing of dosage forms. In other way Pharmacognosy provides help in industries, as a research tools and in new drug delivery systems, and all the departments of pharmaceuticals can improve the healthcare facilities across the world. Today molecular biological techniques especially DNA fingerprints viz. RAPD, RFLP, AFLP) are used to identify and authenticate the herbs. Some US patents were also issued for identifying the herbs using DNA fingerprints.

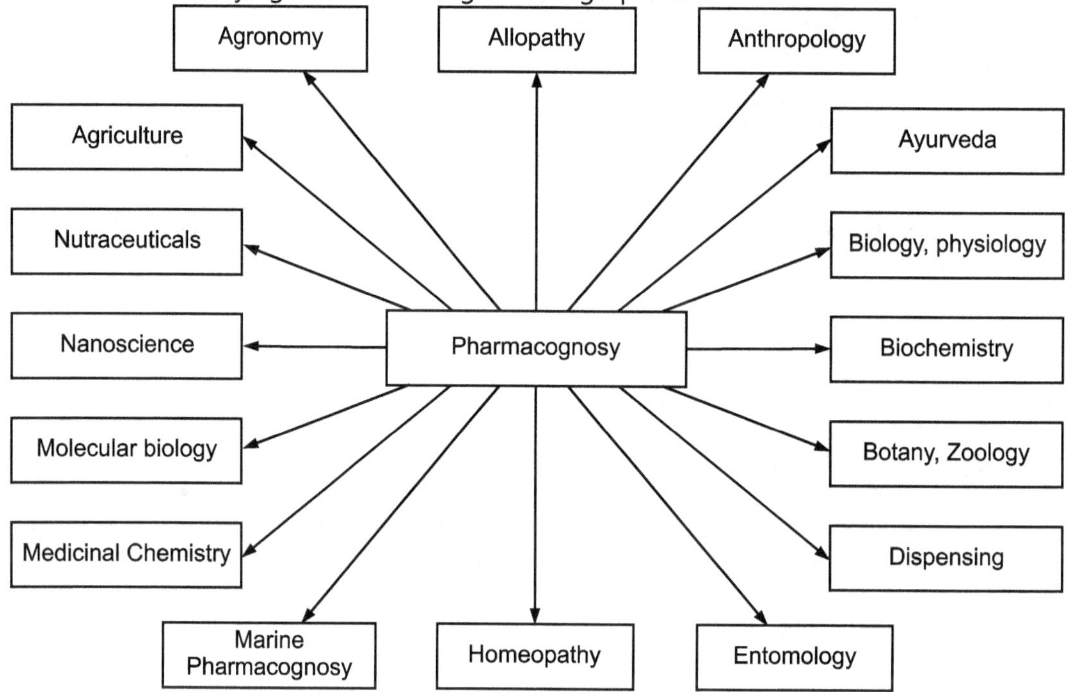

Fig. 1.3: Linkage between Pharmacognosy with other basic sciences

Agricultural science is encompasses the parts of natural, economic and social sciences, whereas agronomy is the application of a combination of sciences-biological sciences, earth science and genetics. The agronomy method is stepwise cultivation of plants where crop rotation, irrigation, drainage, plant breeding, plant physiology, soil classification, soil fertility, weeding, pesticides are important. Anthropology is the study of humans, past and present. It draws and builds upon knowledge from the biological sciences as well as physical and social sciences. Entomology is the scientific study of insects, a branch of arthropology, which in turn is a branch of biology. Molecular biology is a biological branch, deals with the molecular basis of biological activity. This field also correlates with genetics and biochemistry. The term molecular biology first described by Warren Weaver in 1938.

Marine science is a branch of Pharmacognosy concerned with pharmacologically active substances present in plants and animals from aquatic source. Marine Pharmacognosy discovers new therapeutic agents for various disease treatments. Nanotechnology is the science of developing materials at the atomic and molecular level with no change of special electrical and chemical properties. It deals with devices typically less than 100 nanometres in size, is making a significant contribution also to the fields of biotechnology, manufacturing and energy. The term "nanotechnology", originally coined by Norio Taniguchi in 1974, was unknowingly appropriated by Drexler in his book "Engines of Creation: The Coming Era of Nanotechnology. The term nutraceutical further came in world science which is derived from the words "nutrition" and "pharmaceuticals", coined by Stephen DeFelice in 1989. It is a dietary supplement, provides therapeutic efficacy, including the prevention and treatment of disease. They are available in the form of isolated nutrients, dietary supplements, genetically engineered foods, herbal marketed products and cereals, soups, beverages. They provide all the essential substances, energy and nutrient supplements that should be present in a healthy diet for the human. Nutraceuticals are widely used in the food and pharmaceutical industries.

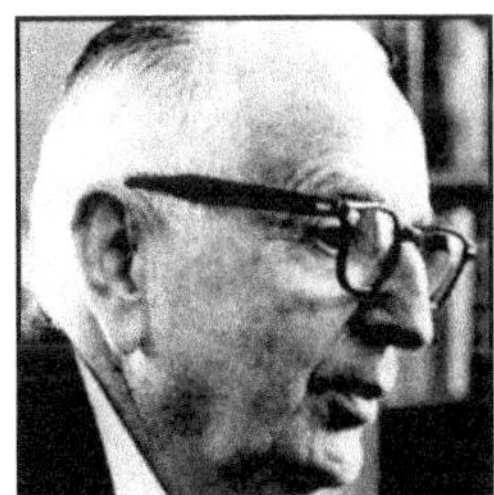

Warren Weaver

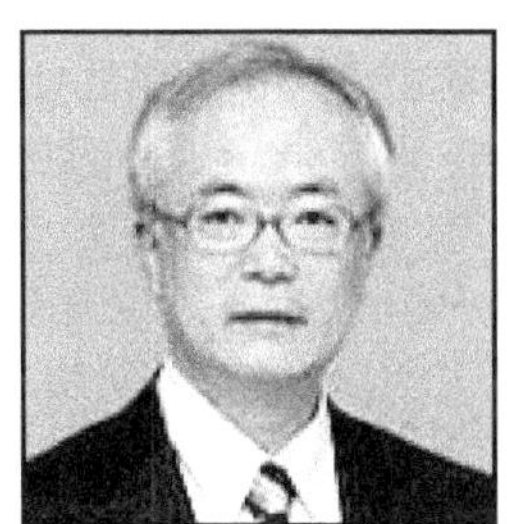

Norio Taniguchi

1.1.4 Applications of Pharmacognosy

1.   **Plant Bioactive extraction and isolation:** The extraction of plant material and isolation of plant constituents typically require tedious protocols that are essential for isolating biologically active compounds and understanding their role in disease prevention and treatment. Bioactives isolated from leaf, stem, root, bark, flower, fruit, seed or other plant materials are often identified using a Bioassay-Guided approach. This type of approach is useful for the investigation of alkaloids, antioxidants, bioflavonoids, terpenoids and other compounds as promising therapeutics from an immense pool of plant biodiversity.

2.   **Development of plant biomarkers:** DNA fingerprinting is the technique based on the use of polymerase chain reaction (PCR), to reveal the specific DNA profile of a particular organism which is as unique as a fingerprint. DNA fingerprinting can distinguish plants from different families, genera, species, cultivars and even sibling plants. Chromatographic techniques such as High Performance Thin-Layer Chromatography and High Performance Liquid Chromatography give the profiling of various secondary metabolites of a plant. Combining the use of DNA fingerprinting and chemical fingerprinting will be an effective tool in authentication and quality control of herbs. Some examples of *biomarkers* are:

(a)   Curcumin isolated from *Curcuma longa* rhizome which is recently under clinical trial for curing head and neck squamous cell carcinoma.

(b)   Withanolide-D isolated from *Withania somnifera* roots, the recent clinical trial projected that it induces apoptosis in leukemia.

(c)   Kutkoside isolated from *Picrorhiza kurroa*, the recent clinical trial established as a serum *biomarkers* for liver cirrhosis.

3. Development of nano fertilizers and nano medicines: Nanotechnology in drug delivery is exemplified by nanocrystals, liposomes, nanoparticle-protein conjugates, magnetic nanoparticles, nanogels and biodegradable nanoparticles. Fertilizer particles can be coated with nano membranes that facilitate slow and steady release of nutrients thereby reducing loss of nutrients and enhancing its use efficiency of medicinal plants. Recent study revealed the use of nanotechnology in *in vitro* and *in vivo* drug and gene delivery. With the incorporation of this innovative technology, the safety, quality, and freshness of food can be assured, which will lead the nanotechnology being the key technology for developing health food. In herbals, there are already preliminary results obtained from trials with turmeric, black pepper, berberine, trifla using nano formulations and more that give strong evidence to prove the concept of improved efficacy in reduction in these herbal preparations. Recently, Stevioside nano-bioconjugated on PEG-PLA nanoparticles of size 150-170 nm showed the initial burst phase followed by the slow controlled release of 2 hours and 21 days respectively which helped in the development of antidiabetic nanomedicine. The coating induces the plants to swallow the particles, effectively inserted genes inside the plant cell walls. The biologists have succeeded in using this technology to introduce DNA into tobacco and corn plant, among others. Cassia twigs, liquorice root, sealwort are used in nanotechnology to reduce their active ingredients to smaller sizes, thus enabling them to enter cancerous cells without damaging healthy cells.

4.   Nutraceuticals towards biochemical mechanisms of healthy aging: In fact, the global herbal supplement and remedies market is expected to reach $ 93 billion by 2015, according to a new report by San Jose, CA-based Global Industry Analysts, Inc. Nutraceutical are a group of natural substances that include certain herbs and products such as cholesterol-lowering margarines, psyllium-fortified products as dietary supplements. Some herbs like ginseng, ginkgo, nuts, grains, tomato, soy phytoestrogens, curcumin, melatonin, vitamins, carnitine, carnosine, ubiquinone, etc. can prevent diseases. Phytosterols, green tea, herbal antioxidant and natural sweeteners are the botanicals that successfully crossed the threshold of functional foods. Stevia leaves (from *Stevia rebaudiana*), brazzein, pentadin (from *Pentadiplandra brazzeana* Plant), curculin (Fruit of *Curculigo latifolia*), monk fruit or luo han guo (from *Siraitia grosvenorii* fruit) etc. are the recent focus for sugar supplement and use as natural non caloric sweeteners.

1.2 SOURCES OF DRUGS – PLANTS, ANIMALS, MARINE AND TISSUE CULTURE

1.2.1 Natural Products

A natural product a chemical compound or substance produced by a living organism - found in nature is that usually has a pharmacological or biological activity for use in pharmaceutical drug discovery and drug design. A *natural* product can be considered as such even if it can be prepared by total synthesis. Natural products may be extracted from tissues of terrestrial plants, marine organisms or microorganism fermentation broths. A crude (untreated) extract from any one of these sources typically contains novel, structurally diverse chemical compounds, which the natural environment is a rich source of. The basic difference between active constituents and phytoconstituents is also important to identify the therapeutic active principles in the plants. Phytoconstituents are the whole chemical constituents that are present in the plants and active constituents are the specific chemical constituents that are therapeutically active or are responsible for medicinal activity that are isolated from other extracted chemical constituents.

The most important things are to identify the natural origin plant sources like shrub, tree, creeper and herbs that are the most basic criteria for authentication of the plant. Further traditional plants, complementary/alternative medicine, endangered plants, medicinal plants, aromatic plants and natural products are also important terminologies that are quite similar, but exact knowledge of these will provide good skill to the Pharmacognosists for research and to develop new drug molecules.

Shrub: A shrub is distinguished from a tree by its multiple stems and shorter height, usually under 6 m (20 ft) tall.

Tree: A tree is a perennial woody plant. It typically has many secondary branches supported clear of the ground by a single, self-supporting main stem or trunk.

Creeper: It is a prostate or trailing plant that spreads by means of stems that creep. These plants creep along the soil surface, though unlike climbers, they have strong stems and firm grip on the soil.

Herb: As per the botanists, an herb is a plant with no woody stem above ground distinguished from tree or a shrub. In general terms, any part of the vegetable species that can be used for medicine, cosmetic, culinary or such purposes is known as herb. The roots, leaves, bark, fruits, flowers, stem or any part of the plant can be used for these purposes.

Traditional plant medicine: It is a system of plant based on cultural beliefs from generation to generation and practices handed down to formulate the medicines for curing the diseases. Traditional medicine is the total of the knowledge, skills, and practices based on the theories, beliefs, and experiences indigenous to different cultures, whether explicable or not, used in the maintenance of health as well as in the prevention, diagnosis, improvement or treatment of physical and mental illness.

Complementary/alternative medicine (CAM): The terms "complementary medicine" or "alternative medicine" are used interchangeably with traditional medicine in some countries. They refer to a broad set of health care practices that are not part of that country's own tradition and are not integrated into the dominant health care system.

Endangered plant species: An endangered plant species is a population of plants which is facing a high risk of becoming extinct because it is either few in numbers, or threatened by changing environmental or predation parameters such as habitat destruction, climate change, or pressure from invasive species.

Medicinal plants: Medicinal herbs are plants or parts of plants used for therapeutic or medical benefit.

Aromatic plants: Plants that produce and exude aromatic substances (largely ether oils), which are used in making perfumes, in cooking and in the food, pharmaceutical and liquor industries.

Plant source is the old source of the drugs. Whole parts of the plants are used like leaves, stem, bark, fruits, roots etc. Some important natural drugs that are procured from, plant sources are listed in table 1.2.

Table 1.2: Various sources of plant drugs

Name	Biological source and family	Chemical constituents	Uses
Source: Leaves			
Senna	B.S: *Cassia angustifolia* F: Leguminosae	Sennoside A, B, C and D	Laxative
Digitalis	B.S: *Digitalis purpurea* F: Scrophulariaceae	Digitoxin, Digoxin	Cardio tonic
Eucalyptus	B.S: *Eucalyptus globulus* F: Myrtaceae	Eucalyptol	Cough syrup
Belladona	B.S: *Atropa belladonna* F: Solanaceae	Atropine	Pain reliever, muscle relaxer
Source: Flower			
Clove	B.S: *Eugenia caryophyllus* F: Myrtaceae	Eugenol	Dental Analgesic Myrtaceae
Vinca	B.S: *Catharanthus roseus* F: Apocynaceae	Vincristine, Vinblastine	Anticancer
Hibiscus	B.S: *Hibiscus rosa sinensis* F: Malvaceae	Cyanidin-3,5-diglucoside, Quercetin-3-diglucoside	Antiulcer
Source: Fruits			
Amla	B.S: *Emblica officinalis* F: Euphorbeaceae	Vitamin-C	Antioxidant
Bael	B.S: *Aegle marmelos* F: Rutaceae	Marmesinin, Aegelin	Antidiarrhoeal Antidysenteric
Mango	B.S: *Mangifera indica* F: Anacardiaceae	Mangiferin	Antioxidant
Source: Seeds			
Nux vomica	B.S: *Strychnos nuxvomica* F: Loganaceae	Strychnine, Brucine	CNS stimulant
Castor	B.S: *Ricinus communis* F: Euphorbiaceae	Ricinoleic acid, Oleic acid	Laxative
Mustard	B.S: *Brassica nigra* F: Cruciferae	Oleic acid	Antiarthritis
Source: Bark			
Cinchona	B.S: *Cinchona officinalis* F:Rubiaceae	Quinine	Antimalarial
Quassia	B.S: *Picrasma excelsa* F: Simaroubaceae	Quassin	Antitumor

Cinnamon	B.S: *Cinnamomum zeylanicum* F: Lauraceae	Cinnamaldehyde, Cinnamic acid	Antimicrobial
Source: Roots			
Ipecac	B.S: *Cephaelis ipecacuanha* F: Rubiaceae	Emetine	For amoebic dysentery
Rauwolfia	B.S: *Rauwolfia serpentine* F: Apocynaceae	Reserpine	Antihypertensive
Ashwagandha	B.S: *Withania somnifera* F: Solanaceae	Withanolides	Adaptogen
Source: Stems			
Kalmegh	B.S:*Andrographis paniculata* F: Acanthaceae	Andrographolide, Kalmeghin	Hepatoprotective
Tree turmeric	B.S: *Coscinium fenestratum* F: Menispermaceae	Berberine	Bitter tonic
Ephedra	B.S: Ephedra gerardiana F: Ephedraceae	Ephedrine	Increase heart rate

1.2.2 Drugs obtained from Animal Sources

The drugs that are procured from the animal sources are depicted in table 1.3.

Table 1.3: Various sources of animal based drugs

Name of product	Source	Uses
Insulin	Pancreas of Human (B.S: *Homo sapiens*)	Antidiabetic
Thyroxin	Sheep thyroid (B.S: *Ovis aries*)	Anti-hypertension
Cod liver oil	Cod fish (B.S: *Gadus morhua*); Family: Gadidae	Source of vitamin D and A
Honey	Bees (B.S: *Apis mellifera, A. Dorsata*) Family: Apidae	Wound healing, burns
Cochineal	Female insect (B.S: *Dactylopius coccus*); Family: Dactylopiidae	Coloring agents for foods, drugs
Blood	Animal	Vaccine preparation
Shark liver oil	Shark fish (B.S: *Rhincodon typus*); Family: Rhincodontidae	Anticancer
Spermaceti	Sperm Whale (B.S: *Physeter macrocephalus*); Family: Physeteridae	Ointments, cosmetic creams

1.2.3 Drugs obtained from Marine Sources

There are more than 5 lakhs species of marine organisms available in seas and ocean. They are used for many important therapeutic activities. The enormous ecological resources of the sea and ocean have been exploited since ancient times and the use of marine animals like fish and preparations from algae are included as the sources of medicine. Oceans contain more than 80% of diverse plant and animal species. Such organisms like sponges, tunicates, fishes, soft corals, nudibranchs, sea hares, opisthobranch Molluscs, echinoderms, bryozoans, prawns, shells, sea slugs and marine microorganisms are sources of bioactive compounds. The drugs that are procured from the marine sources are depicted in tables 1.4 and 1.5.

Table 1.4: Marine anticancer natural products

Organism	Compound	Chemistry
Ascidian	Aplidine	Depsipeptide
(*Cion intestinalis*)	Fucoxanthinol	Carotenoid
Bryozoan (Moss animal)	Bryostatin-I	Macrolide
Mollusk (*Tonicella lineata*)	Kahalalide F	Depsipeptide
Sea Hare (*Aplysia californica*)	Aplyronine	Macrolide
Yellow Sponge (*Aplysina fistularis*)	Aaptamine	Alkaloid
	Agosterol A	Steroid
Tube worm (*Riftia pachyptila*)	Cephalostatin	Steroid

Table 1.5: FDA approved drugs from marine sources

Name of drug	Source	Chemistry	Uses
Cytarabine (Ara-C)	Caribbean sponge species *Tethya crypta*	Synthetic pyrimidine nucleoside	Leukemia
Vidarabine (Ara-A)	Caribbean sponge *T. Crypta*	Synthetic purine nucleoside	Antiviral
Trabectedin	Tunicate species *Ecteinascidia turbinate*	Alkaloid	Soft-tissue sarcoma and in relapsed cases of platinum-sensitive ovarian cancer
Ziconotide	Venom of marine snail *Conus magus*	Peptide	Analgesic

Many of the drugs from marine sources are in clinical phase.

1.2.4 Plant Tissue Culture

It is an *in-vitro* cultivation of plant cells, tissues and organs in liquid or semi-solid nutrient media under aseptic and controlled environment. In this method primary and secondary plant metabolites are regenerates. The basic criteria for plant tissue culture are totipotency and plasticity. Totipotency is defined as regeneration capacity of the selected plant parts whereas plasticity is the withstand capacity of plants in any stressful condition. The plant tissue culture technique is important because isolation of bioactive compounds from the medium is very easy, rare and endangered plant species are micropropagated and cultivated in mass scale, production of immobilized plant cell for future use and even biochemical conversion is easy etc.

Applications:

- Mass scale production of plants.
- Conservation of endangered plant species.
- Cultivation of disease resistance plants.
- Production of micropropagated plants.

Advantages:

- Some plants, which do not multiply by seeds, can be propagated through plant tissue culture technique.
- More amounts of secondary metabolites are produced.
- Large number of plants can be produced in a short time.
- Chemicals which are used in the tissue culture increase the capacity of produced plants to resist with biocidal chemicals, environment stress and competitive to survive over weed.
- Isolation of constituents from plant is easy.
- Mass propagation of plants is easy.

1.3 ORGANIZED DRUGS AND UNORGANIZED DRUGS

All crude drugs are mainly two types based on their sources. If the drugs are procured from cellular parts of plants in raw form is known as organized crude drugs whereas the drugs that are procured from non-cellular parts of plants are known as unorganized crude drugs. The details of these two categories of drugs are discussed in below morphological classification.

1.4 CLASSIFICATION OF DRUGS

Alphabetical, morphological, taxonomical, chemical, pharmacological, chemo and sero taxonomical classification of drugs.

In India there are more than 17500 flowering plants, out of which 2000 plants are used in various classical systems of medicine like Ayurveda, Siddha and Unani. Traditionally, about 8000 species of wild plants are used as medicine. The drugs used in Indian System of Medicine are 90% based on plant material and are considered to be safe, cost effective and with minimal or no side effects when genuine ingredients are used. To follow the study of the individual drugs, one must adopt some particular sequence of arrangement, and this is referred to a system of classification of drugs. A method of classification should be simple, easy to use; and free from confusion and ambiguities. Due to diversity, drugs are classified as:

1. Alphabetical classification.
2. Morphological classification.
3. Taxonomic classification.
4. Pharmacological classification.
5. Chemical classification.
6. Chemo-taxonomical classification.
7. Sero-taxonomical classification

1.4.1 Alphabetical Classification

This classification provides arrangement of crude drugs in alphabetical order of their Latin and English names or sometimes local names. This method is adopted in many books like Indian Pharmacopoeia, British Pharmacopoeia, United States Pharmacopoeia and National Formulary, British Herbal Pharmacopoeia, British Pharmaceutical Codex, European

Pharmacopoeia (Latin Titles), Encyclopedia of common Natural ingredients used in Drugs and cosmetics. In Indian Pharmacopoeia 1966 names changed to English, like Amylum changed to starch, Acacia gum changed to Indian gum etc.

Example: Acacia, Benzoin, Cinchona, Dill, Ergot, Fennel, Gentian, Hyoscyamus, Ipecacuanha, Jalap, Kurchi, Liquorice, Myrrh, Nux-Vomica, Opium, Podophyllum, Quassia, Rauwolfia, Senna, Uncaria Gambier, Vasaka, Wool Fat, Yellow Bees Wax, Zedoary.

Advantages:

- This method provides quick reference search of the crude drugs.
- Study of drugs by this method is easy once the name of the drug is known.
- In this system location, tracing and addition of drug entries is easy.

Disadvantage:

- There is no relationship between the previous and successive drug entries

1.4.2 Morphological Classification

All crude drugs are arranged according to the external characters of the plant or animal parts i.e., leaves, roots, stems, flowers from plants etc. This class of drug is further classified as organized and unorganized drug. The organized drugs are obtained from the cellular tissues and dried parts of the plants like, Rhizomes, barks, leaves, fruits, entire plants, hairs, fibres etc. The plant drugs are prepared by some intermediate physical processes like incision, drying or extraction with a solvent and some are do not contain any cellular plant tissues which are called unorganized drugs, e.g., aloe juice, opium latex, agar, gelatin, tragacanth, benzoin, honey, beeswax, lemon grass oil etc. The differences are given in table 1.6.

Table 1.6: Differences between Organized and Unorganized Crude Drugs

Organized drugs	Unorganized drugs
They are the sources from plants and animals.	They are the sources of plants, animals, and minerals.
They procured directly from the above sources.	They are products of plants and animals and obtained by extraction, distillation, incision methods.
They have proper cellular structures like, leaves, flowers, fruits, barks, roots, woods etc.	They do not have well defined cellular structure like gum, mucilage, resin etc.
They are identified by morphological characters.	They are identified by organoleptic properties.
They are solid in nature.	They are solid, semi-solid and liquid in nature.
To study their characters, transverse section is used for drugs under microscope.	To study their characters, physical parameters like density, optical rotation, viscosity, refractive index, chemical tests are important.
Examples: **Woods:** Quassia, sandal wood. **Leaves:** Digitalis, Eucalyptus, Mint, Senna,	**Examples:** **Dried Latex:** Opium, Papain. **Dried Juice:** Aloe, Kino.

Organized drugs	Unorganized drugs
Spearmint, Squill, Hyoscyamus, Belladonna. **Barks:** Cascara, Cassia, Cinchona, Wild cherry. **Flowering Parts:** Clove, Pyrethrum, Saffron, and Chamomile. **Fruits:** Anise, Capsicum, Caraway, Cardamom, Colocynth, Coriander, Cumin, Dill, Fennel. **Seeds:** Bitter almond, Black Mustard, Cardamom, Colchicum, Linseed, Nux vomica. **Roots and Rhizomes:** Aconite, Colchicum, Garlic, Ginger, Ginsing, Glycyrrhiza, Podophyllum, Rauwolfia, Rhubarb, Turmeric, Squill. **Plants and Herbs:** Ergot, Ephedra, Yeast, Vinca, Datura. **Hair and Fibers:** Cotton, Hemp, Jute, Silk, Flax.	**Dried Extracts:** Agar, Black catechu, Pale catechu, Pectin. **Waxes:** Beeswax, Spermaceti, Carnauba wax. **Gums:** Acacia, Guar gum, Indian gum, Resins: Asafoetida, Benzoic, Colophony, Tolo balsam, Storax. **Volatile Oil:** Coriander, Peppermint, Rosemary, Sandalwood, Cinnamon, Caraway, Clove, Eucalyptus. Fixed Oils and Fats: Arachis, Castor, Cotton seed, Linseed, Olive, Cod liver. **Animal Products:** Bees wax, Cod liver oil, Gelatin, Halibot liver oil, Honey, Shark liver oil, Shellac, Spermaceti wax, Wool fat. **Fossil Organism and Minerals:** Bentonite, Kaolin, Kiesslguhr, Talc.

Gum and Mucilage:

Gums containing crude drugs are amorphous substances, pathological products produced by the plants under injured or unfavourable conditions.

Mucilages are thick, gluey substances produced from plants and some microorganisms. The differences between gums and mucilages are given in table 1.7.

Table 1.7: Differences between Gums and Mucilages

Gums	Mucilages
They are produced by plant when it is injured or unfavourable conditions like diseased by a process Gummosis.	Mucilages are the normal products of plant growth.
It is produced outside the plant cell.	It is produced inside the cell.
They are soluble in water and form adhesive solution.	It is insoluble in water and forms slimy solution with water.
They are made up of sugar, salt of uronic acid. Example: gum acacia, Tragacanth gum.	They are made up of ester and sulphuric acid. Example: Senna, Agar, Isphagol.

Advantages:

- Easy method to study of plant drugs.
- Even if the chemical content or action of drug is not known the drug can be studied properly.
- It gives idea about the source of drugs.
- It gives idea whether it is organized or unorganized.
- Easy to identify and detect the adulteration.

Disadvantages:

- During collection, drying and packing, morphology of drug changes; they are difficult to study.
- No correlation between chemical constituents with therapeutic actions.
- Repetition of drugs or plants occurs.

1.4.3 Taxonomical Classification

This is the systematic naming of organisms into similar groups. Plant taxonomy uses the gross morphology like flower form, leaf shape, fruit form, etc. of plants to separate them into similar groups. Quite often the characteristics that distinguish the plants become a part of their name. For example, a white oak (*Quercus alba*) is named because of the white leaf. Taxonomical classification is purely a botanical classification; it is based on principles of natural relationship and evolutionary developments. They are grouped in Kingdom, Phyllum, Order, Family, Genus and Species. The entire plant is not used as drug; only a part of plant is used as a drug. E.g. cinnamon bark. It is classified scientifically as follows:

Kingdom: Plantae

      Division: Magnoliophyta

        Order: Proteales

          Family : Proteaceae

            Subfamily: Grevilleoideae

              Genus: *Telopea*

                Species: *Speciosissima*

Taxonomists classify two species together in the same genus (the plural is *genera*). For example, the horse *Equus caballus* and the donkey *Equus assinus* are both placed in the genus *Equus*. Similar genera are brought together to form a *family*. Similar families are classified within an *order*. Orders with similar characteristics are grouped in a *class*. Related classes are grouped together as *divisions* or *phyla* (the singular is *phylum*). For plants and fungi divisions are used while phyla are used for animals and animal-like organisms. The largest and broadest category is the *kingdom*.

Examples:

  Phylum: Spermatophyta

    Division: Angiospermae

      Class: Dicotyledons

        Order: Rosales

          Family: Leguminosae

           Sub-family: Papilionaceae

             Genus: Glycyrrhiza, Astragalus, Myroxylon

              Species: *Glycyrrhiza glabra, Astragalus gummifer, Myroxylon balsamum*

Phylum: Spermatophyta
    Division: Angiospermae
        Class: Dicotyledons
           Sub-class: Sympetalae
               Order: Tubiflorae
                  Family: Solanaceae
                     Genus: Atropa, Hyoscyamus, Datura
                        Species: *Atropa belladona, Hyoscyamus niger, Datura stramonium*

Advantages:
- Knowledge about taxonomical details will give proper idea about species and varieties of the organisms.
- It is helpful for studying evolutionary developments of crude drugs.

Disadvantages:
- No idea about organized/unorganized.
- No idea about chemical nature.
- No correlation between the chemical constituents and biological activity of drugs.

1.4.4 Pharmacological Classification

System in which the drugs are grouped according to their pharmacological action or most important constituent or their therapeutic use is termed as pharmacological or therapeutic classification of drug. This classification is more relevant and mostly followed method. Drugs like digitalis, squill and strophanthus having cardiotonic action are grouped together irrespective of their parts used or phylogenetic relationship or the nature of phytoconstituents they contain. Hence as per pharmacological actions various drugs are classified in to same action (Table 1.8).

Table 1.8: Classification of various drugs as per pharmacological action

Pharmacological action	Drugs
Antianthelmintic	Artemisia, Male- fern, Quassia
Carminatives	Fennel, Dill, Coriander, Clove
Cardiotonics	Digitalis, Squill, Strophanthus
Purgatives	Cascara, Aloe, Senna
Anticancer	Podophyllum, Vinca
CNS Stimulant	Nux vomica
Expectorant	Vasaka, Liquoric

Advantages:
- It is easy to study the drug based on pharmacological activity.
- If the drugs are not available at a particular place or point of time, based on activity substitutes of drugs may possible.

Disadvantages:
- Some crude drugs have two different pharmacological actions, therefore it is difficult to classify them. For example, Nux-vomica is CNS stimulant as well as bitter tonic, cinchona is bitter tonic as well as antimalarial and antipyretic.

- Drugs that have different mechanism of action have to be grouped together. e.g. castor oil is irritant purgative and isapgol is bulk purgative, but they are placed in one group.
- No idea whether drugs are organized or unorganized.
- This method does not give any idea of source of drugs.

1.4.5 Chemical Classification

The crude drugs are divided into different groups according to the chemical nature of their most important constituent. The pharmacological activity and therapeutic significance of crude chemical classification of drugs is dependent upon the grouping of drugs with identical constituents. The classification is as follows:

(a) Carbohydrates: Carbohydrates are polyhydroxy aldehydes or ketones containing an unbroken chain of carbon atoms.

Examples: Gums – Acacia, Tragacanth.

Mucilages – Plantago seed, others – Starch, Honey, Agar, Pectin, Cotton.

(b) Glycosides: Glycosides are compounds which upon hydrolysis give rise to one or more sugars (glycone) and non–sugar (aglycone).

Anthraquinone Glycosides: Senna, Aloe, Cascara, Rhubarb etc.

Saponins Glycosides: Quillaia, Glycyrrhiza;

Cyanophore Glycosides: Wild cherry bark,

Isothiocyanate Glycosides: Mustard,

Cardiac Glycosides: Digitalis, Strophantus,

Bitter Glycosides: Gentian, Calumba, Quassia

(c) Tannins: Tannins are complex organic, non–nitrogenous derivatives of polyhydroxy benzoic acids.

Examples: Pale catechu, Black catechu, Ashoka bark, Amla

(d) Volatile Oils: Monoterpines and Sesquiterpenes obtained from plants.

Examples: Cinnamon, Fennel, Dill, Caraway, Coriander, Cardamom, Orange peel, Mint, Clove, Valerian.

(e) Lipids: Fixed oils – Castor, Olive, Almond, Shark liver oil. Fats: Theobroma, Lanolin. Waxes: Beeswax.

(f) Resins: Complex mixture of compounds like resinols, resin acids, resinotannols, resenes.

Examples: Colophony, Podophyllum, Cannabis, Capsicum, Turmeric, Balsam of Tolu and Peru, Myrrh, Ginger.

(g) Alkaloids: Nitrogenous substance of plant origin;

Pyridine and Piperidine: Lobelia, Nicotiana;

Tropane – Coca, Belladonna, Datura, Stramonium, Hyoscyamus, Henbane.

Quinoline – Cinchona;

Isoquinoline – Opium, Ipecac, Calumba,

Indole – Ergot, Rauwolfia.

Amines – Ephedra,

Purine – Tea, Coffee,

Protein – Gelatin, Ficin, Papain.

Advantages:

- If the chemical constituent is known then it is easy to study the drug.
- It is a popular approach for phytochemical studies.
- Medical uses are known.

Disadvantages:

- This method does not give any idea about the source of drug.
- Some drugs contain two important chemicals so it is difficult to classify them. For example, nutmeg contains volatile oil as well as fat; Cinchona contains glycoside as well as alkaloid.
- No idea whether drug is organized or unorganized.

1.4.6 Chemo-taxonomical Classification

This system of classification relies on the chemical similarity of taxon i.e., it is based on the existence of relationship between constituents in various plants. This gives birth to completely new concept of chemotaxonomy that utilizes chemical facts/characters for understanding the taxonomical status, relationships and the evolution of the plants. Generally, tropane alkaloids are belongs to the members of Solanaceae, thereby serving as a Chemotaxonomic marker. Similarly plant metabolites can serve as the basis of classification of crude drugs. The berberine alkaloid in Berberis and Argemone; Rutin in Rutaceae members, ranunculaceous alkaloids among its members etc. are examples. It is the latest system of classification and gives more scope for understanding the relationship between chemical constituents, their biosynthesis and their possible action.

Basic Principle: It consists of investigation of distribution of chemical compounds or group of biosynthetically related compounds in a series of related plants.

Classifications:

(a) Bentham and Hooker's (1817-1911) classification: They adopted a comprehensive natural system of classification in their published work "General Plantarum" which dominated the botanical science. According to this system, the plant kingdom comprises about 97205 species of seed plants which are distributed in 202 orders that are further divided into families. Dicots have been divided in three divisions on the basis of floral characters viz., polypetalae, gamopetalae and monochlamydeae.

(b) Engler's (1844-1930) classification: This is a natural system of classification which is based on the relationship and is compatible with evolutionary principles. He has published his system of classification in "Die Naturlichen Pflanzenfamilien" in 23 volumes, covering the whole plant kingdom. The increasing complexity of the flowers is considered for classification.

(c) Hutchinson's system of classification: He has published his work "The families of flowering plants" in 1926 on dicots and in 1934 on monocots. He has further revised this system in 1959 and as per that he placed the Gymnosperm first, then the Dicots and lastly Monocots. This system indicates the concept of phylogenetic classification and is an advanced system over Bentham and Hooker's system.

(d) Modern system of classification: It is based on ultrastructure chromosomal information using higher microscope like electron microscope, scanning electron microscope etc. In this system, genetic and phylogenetic relationship was reflected and divided in broadly two groups viz. micromolecules and macromolecules. Micromolecules are compounds with a molecular weight less than 1000 e.g., alkaloids, terpenoids, fatty acids, amino acids, simple carbohydrate etc. Macromolecules are compounds with a molecular weight 1000 or more, e.g., complex polysaccharides, proteins, DNA, RNA etc. In this system serotaxonomy is gaining importance.

Advantages:

- It gives more scope for understanding the relationship between chemical constituents, their biosynthesis and their possible action.
- The characters most often studied are secondary metabolites of pharmaceutical significance such as alkaloids, glycosides, flavonoids, DNA hybridization, amino acid sequencing in proteins etc.
- It provides degree of hybridization and breeding analysis

Disadvantages:

- This system is fails to identify the organized and unorganized crude drugs in their morphological studies.
- This system fails to understand the therapeutic nature of the crude drugs.

1.4.7 Serotaxonomic Classification

Serotaxonomy is the application of serology, serology is the study of antigen and antibody reactions. Therefore, serotaxonomy is the experimentation of antigen and antibodies. These experiments are mostly done with plants. In the immune system, a specific protein molecule produced by plasma cell is known as antibody. These antibodies combine chemically with specific antigen and in combination elevate an immune response. The application of serology in solving taxonomic problems is known as serotaxonomy.

The main importance of serological data is used to classify angiosperms. Examples:

- Fairbrothers (1983) used serological data in classification of orders and families in Apiales, Fagales, Rubiales, Magnoliales, Ranunculales etc.
- Fairbrothers and Jhonson separated six species of Bromus based on the serological data in 1959.
- The relationship between Nymphaeaceae and nelumbonaceae based on serological data was established by Simon (1971).
- Klos applied serotaxonomic data in the classification of Leguminosae.

Advantages:

- The size of the data used in molecular taxonomy studies is enormous.
- The analysis of the cladograms is done using statistical methods.
- If the molecule is unchanged (Like genes coding for ribosomal RNA), the relationships are traced far back in time.
- Non-heritable variations are avoided in molecular taxonomy studies.

Disadvantages:

- There is no record of past changes in characters.
- There is no familiar intermediate condition between characters and no primitive condition for a given DNA site is recognized.

- The tracing of functional correlates of characters is very rare.
- It is very difficult indeed to root a tree derived from molecules. Moreover the likelihood of convergence is usually impossible.

1.5 QUALITY CONTROL OF DRUGS OF NATURAL ORIGIN

Quality of herbal drugs are defined as the status of a drug that is determined by its evaluation in terms of identity, purity, content and other physical, chemical and biological properties and manufacturing processes for formulated drugs. Whereas, quality control involves in processes, involve in maintaining the quality and validity of manufactured products especially for herbal products. As per Pharmacopoeial definition, the quality control of herbal drugs are based on three terms likely Identity, Purity and Assay.

Identity: Authentication of the plant is very important to know their particular species. It is achieved by correct morphology and microscopic examinations. Identity helps us to recognize the required plant species for the particular experimentation. Herbal plants are classified according to sensory, macroscopic and microscopic characteristics. An examination to determine these characteristics is the first step towards establishing the identity and the degree of purity of such plant materials. Macroscopic identity of plant materials is based on shape, size, colour, surface characteristics, texture, fracture characteristics and appearance. For instance, pollen morphology is used in the case of flowers to identify the species and the presence of certain microscopic structures such as leaf stomata is used to identify the plant part used. These characteristics are judged subjectively for external characters of the plant drugs but the substitutes or adulterants if closely resemble to the genuine material, it is often necessary to find differentiation by microscopy analysis. Microscopic inspection of herbal materials is indispensable for the identification of broken or powdered materials by treated with chemical reagents.

Purity: It is mainly safety use of drugs. The experiments that are required to know the purity is ash values, foreign matters, heavy metals, microbial contamination, aflatoxins, radioactivity, pesticide residue etc. To determine all these generally chromatographic methods such as Thin Layer Chromatography (TLC), High Performance Liquid Chromatography (HPLC), Gas Chromatography (GC) are used as analytical methods.

Assay: The content or assay is the most important and difficult part of quality control to perform because the active constituents of most of the herbal drugs are unknown. Sometimes to determine assay the biomarkers are used as standard drugs but where chemical nature of plants are unknown as well standards are not available then percentage extractable matters with a solvent is used as a form of an assay. Pesticide determination is also required for the safety of the herbal drugs. Herbal drugs are liable to contain pesticide residues that accumulate by spraying, treatment of soils during cultivation and administering of fumigants during storage. Chlorine containing pesticides are measured by analysis of total organic chlorine. Thereafter insecticides containing phosphate are detected by measuring total organic phosphorus. Various impurities are removed by partition and/or adsorption and individual pesticides are measured by GC, MS or GC/MS.

Various parameters for determination of quality control of herbal drugs:

- Macro and microscopic examination.
- Determination of ash value.
- Determination of foreign matters by Lycopodium spore method.
- Determination of heavy metals by atomic absorption spectrophotometer.
- Determination of pesticide residue.
- Determination of microbial contamination.
- Determination of aflatoxin.

1.5.1 Adulteration of Drugs of Natural Origin

The adulteration and substitution are major problem in growing herbal industries. It causes major threat in the research on commercial natural products. The deforestation and extinction of many species and incorrect identification of many plants has resulted in adulteration and substitution of raw herbal drugs. In ancient times most of the drugs used for cure of health problems were of plant origin but lack of proper description and proper authentication has made difficult to provide correct identity of the herbal drugs. Not only that, due to lack of standardization method, the herbal drugs are still in confusion and controversies for choice of the allied species, which results in adulteration of the herbal drugs. The term is derived from the Latin adultero, which in its various inflections signifies to defile, to debase, to corrupt, to sophisticate, to falsify, to counterfeit. Ultimately it is defined as a practice of substituting original crude drug, partially or wholly, with other similar looking substances, but the latter is either free from or inferior in chemical or therapeutic properties or adulteration is defined as mixing or substituting the original drug material with other spurious, inferior, defective, spoiled, useless other parts of same or different harmful substances or drug that do not comply with the official standards. The constituents that are added to the original substances are known as *adulterants* and the practice or process is known as *adulteration*. The whole admixed products are known as *adulterated products*. The plant based drugs are adulterated by substitution with sub-standard commercial varieties, inferior drugs or artificially manufactured commodities.

Objectives:

- To increase the bulk or weight of the article.
- To improve its appearance.
- To give it a false strength.
- To rob it of its most valuable constituents.
- To make product cost benefit.
- Scarcity of drugs.

Conditions of Adulteration:

- **Deterioration:** It is the impairment in the quality of a drug. This condition is due to destruction or abstraction of valuable constituents by bad treatment or aging or to the deliberate extraction of the constituents and the sale of the residue as the original drugs. Apart from this condition, the crude drugs are also prone to deterioration on storage. The shelf-life of crude drugs is influenced by many factors which include not only the quality of storage conditions but also the stability of the secondary metabolites present. Several factors are to be considered for the detrimental effects on the stored products.
- **Admixture:** It is the addition of one article to another due to ignorance or carelessness or accidentally. Example: inclusion of soil on an underground organ or the co-collection of two similar species.

- **Sophistication:** It is the intentional or deliberate type of adulteration by adding spurious or inferior material with intent to defraud. Such materials are carefully produced and may appear at first sight to be genuine. E.g., powder ginger may be diluted with starch with addition of little coloring material to give the correct shade of yellow colour.
- **Substitution:** It occurs when some totally different substance is added in place of original drug. e.g., supply of cheap cottonseed oil in place of olive oil.
- **Inferiority:** It refers to any sub-standard drug. This condition is like a crop is taken whose natural constituent is below the minimum standard for that particular drug. It can be avoided by more careful selection of the plant material.
- **Spoilage:** The deterioration due to the attack of microorganisms. This condition makes the product unfit for consumption, which can be avoided by careful attention to the drying and storage conditions.

Adulteration generally takes place either directly (intentionally) or indirectly (unintentionally).

Direct adulteration: This type of practice is mainly encouraged by traders who are reluctant to pay premium prices for herbs of superior quality and hence are inclined to purchase only the cheaper products. Therefore producers and traders sell the herbs of inferior quality. In this type of adulteration, a herbal drug is substituted partially or fully with other inferior products which have morphological resemblance to the authentic herb and many other inferior commercial varieties.

They may or may not have any chemical or therapeutic potential. This practice is most common in the case of volatile oil containing materials. Foreign matters like any other parts of the same plant with no active ingredients, fine sand and stones, dust, dried clay, manufactured artefacts and synthetic inferior principles are used as substitutes (Fig. 1.4).

Indirect adulteration: This type of adulteration is also known as unintentional or undeliberate adulteration that accidentally occurs without any intention of the manufacturer or supplier. Sometimes due to improper evaluation, an authentic drug partially or fully replaced with the active ingredient which enters in the market. Generally, this practice happens at geographical sources, growing conditions, processing and storage conditions that influence the quality of the drug.

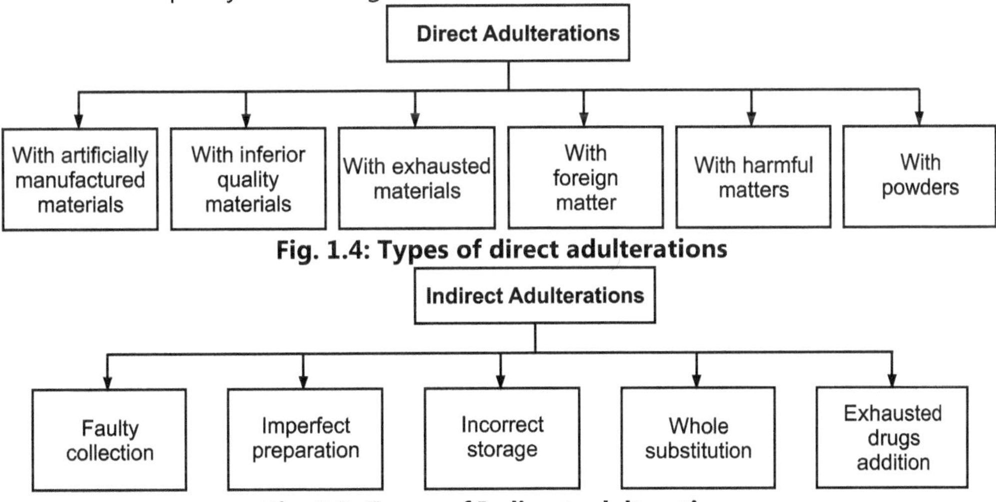

Fig. 1.4: Types of direct adulterations

Fig. 1.5: Types of Indirect adulterations

Types of Adulteration:

1. **With artificially manufactured substances:** This type of adulteration is done for costlier drugs. Artificially prepared substances resemble the original drug and are not separated or identified by naked eyes and these products are used as substitutes. Generally they are colored substances. Examples: Compressed Chicory in place of coffee, yellow coloured praffin wax for bees wax, properly cut and shaved baswood for nutmeg, artificial invert sugar for honey, Musk is adulterated with dust and dried blood; *Tinospora cordifolia* extract adulterated with arrow root powder.

2. **Superficially similar inferior drugs:** These drugs are with or without chemical or therapeutic values as that of original drug. Due to their morphological resemblance to the authentic drug, they are marketed as adulterants. Ailanthus leaves are used to substitute belladonna leaves, *Carthamus tinctorious* flowers are mixed with costly saffron flowers and bees wax is substituted with Japan wax and mother clove with original clove, *Strychnous nux-blanda* or *S.potatorum* in place of *S. nux-vomica*, *Capsicum annuum* in place of *C.minimum*, Indian senna is substituted with Arabian senna (*Cassia angustifolia*) or dog senna (*Cassia obovata*), medicinal ginger (*Zingiber officinale*) is substituted with *Zingiber mioga*, or Cochin ginger.

3. **Exhausted materials:** The exhausted material may be used entirely or in part as a substituent for the genuine drug. e.g., umbelliferous fruits and cloves (without volatile oils) are adulterated with exhausted (without volatile oils) drugs, exhausted jalap and Indian hemp (without resins) are used as adulterant.

4. **Use of synthetic chemicals:** They are sometimes used to enhance the natural character as in case of addition of benzyl benzoate to balsam of peru, citral to citrus oils like oil of lemon and orange oil, etc.

5. **Substitution with exhausted drug:** The same drug is admixed but is devoid of any medicinally active constituents as they are already extracted out. This practice is common with volatile oil containing drugs like fennel, clove, coriander, caraway etc. Colour and odour of exhausted drugs are manipulated by adding other additives and then it is substituted. e.g., exhausted gentian made bitter with aloes, artificial colouring of exhausted saffron, almond oil adulterated with ground nut oil and cotton seed oil etc.

6. **Harmful adulterants:** In this type of adulteration, the waste from the market are collected and admixed with the authentic drug. This practice is noticed in case of liquids or unorganized drugs. Examples include pieces of amber coloured glass in colophony, limestones in asafoetida, lead shot in opium, white oil in coconut oil, cocoa butter mixed with stearin or paraffin. The addition of rodent feacal matter to cardamom seed is a very harmful adulteration.

7. **Adulteration of powders:** The powdered forms are frequently found to be adulterated with original drugs. Examples: dextrin in ipecacuanha, powered liquorice or gentian admixed with powdered olive stones, exhausted ginger powder in powdered colocynth or ginger, red-sanders wood in capsicum, *Mallotus phillippinesis* is mixed with fine brick powder etc.

8. **Faulty collection:** Herbal adulteration sometimes occurs due to the carelessness of herbal collectors and suppliers. The correct part of genuine plant should be collected. Moreover collection should be carried out at a proper season and time when the active constituents reach maximum. Examples: *Datura strumarium* leaves should be collected during flowering stage and wild cherry bark in autumn etc. Collection from other plant by ignorance, due to similarity in the appearance, color, lack of knowledge may lead to adulteration. Examples: In place of Aconitum napellus, the other *Aconitum deinorhizum* may be collected or in place of *Rhamnus purshiana* (cascara bark) *Rhamnus colifornica* is generally collected. Often in different states the same plant is known by different vernacular names, while quite different drugs are known by same name. This creates confusion which is best illustrated by Punarnava and Brahmi. The Indian pharmacopoeia drugs *Trianthema portulacastrum* L. and *Boerhavia diffusa* L. are both known by the same vernacular name "Punarnava". Sometimes lack of authentic source may lead to adulteration. Example: Nagakesar is one of the important drugs in Ayurveda. Original drug, *Mesua ferrea* is adulterated with flowers of *Calophyllum inophyllum* and is sold as Nagakesar in market. Authentic flowers can be easily identified by the presence of two-celled ovary, whereas in case of spurious flowers they are single-celled.

9. **Imperfect preparation:** Collection of the plant parts should be clear by the collectors. Sometimes stems are collected with leaves, flowers, fruits which are not necessary. Sometimes undesirable parts should not be collected, like cork should be removed from ginger rhizome. Sometimes neglected drying process may lead to unintentional adulteration. e.g. if digitalis leaves are dried above 65°C, decomposition of glycosides by enzymatic hydrolysis occurs. Use of excessive heat in separating the cod liver oil from livers but the proportion of vitamins, odor and color etc. are adversely affected.

10. **Incorrect storage:** Deterioration, especially during storage, leads to the loss of active ingredients and production of non-active toxic metabolites. Physical factors such as oxygen, humidity, light, and temperature can bring about deterioration directly or indirectly. These factors also help in development of the growth of organisms such as molds, mites and bacteria. Oxidation of essential oils can lead to rancid. Moisture or humidity and elevated temperatures can accelerate enzymatic activities, leading to changes in the physical appearance and decomposition of the herb. For example, volatile oils should be protected from light and stored in well closed containers in cool place. Belladonna leaf should be stored in moisture free containers, which may cause enzymatic action leading to decomposition of medicinally active constituents.

11. **Presence of vegetative matter in the same plant:** In the same field, sometimes other miniature plants are grown along with medicinal plants that are admixed accidentally with the authentic drug due to their morphological resembling i.e. colour, odour etc. The lower plants like moss, liverworts and epiphytes are grown on bark portion and are mixed with cascara or cinchona. The stem portions are

mixed along with leaf drugs like stramonium, lobelia and senna. *Mucuna pruriens* is adulterated with other similar Papilionaceae seeds having similarity in morphology. *M. utilis* and *M. deeringiana* are popular adulterants. Apart from this, *M. cochinchinensis, Canavalia virosa* and *C. ensiformis* are also sold in Indian markets.

Substitution:

Pharmacognostically, it is defined as "whole replacement of an entirely different article that is used or sold in place of the original article". Examples: Cottonseed oil substituted in place of olive oil, American saffron substituted in place of Spanish saffron etc.

Reasons for Substitution:

1. **Non-availability of the drug:** If the part of the plant is not available, then similar looking part of other plant is used as replacement. Example: In case of nonavailability of leaf of the *Abies webbiana* (Talisa patra), leaf of the *Abies baccata* is used.

2. **Uncertain identity of the drug:** Sometimes due to the confusion of the authenticity of the plant, drug identity becomes uncertain. Like Chichona bark it has different species like *Cinchona calisaya, C. officinalis, C. ledgeriana* etc. are considered.

3. **Cost of the drug:** Some costly drugs are not always available in market and hence similar type of drugs are sold in market in lesser price that of original drugs. Examples: Kumkuma (*Crocus sativas*) being costly herb is substituted by Kusumbha (*Carthamus tinctorius*).

4. **Geographical distribution of the drug:** Depending on the geographical location and plant distribution, the different plants are sold in same name in the market. For example, in North India *Premna integrifolia* is used as Agnimantha, whereas in South India, Arani (*Clerodendrum phlomidis*) is used as Agnimantha.

5. **The adverse reaction of the drug:** Vasa is a well-known drug that cures bleeding disorder, but due to its abortificiant activity, its utility in pregnant women is limited, instead drugs such as Laksha, Ashoka etc. are substituted for similar therapeutic effect.

6. **Seasonal availability of drugs:** Some drugs are available in a specific season so other drugs can be introduced in their absence which has same action. For example, *Trianthema portulacastrum* can be used in seasonal absence of *Boerhavia diffusa*.

Types of Substitutions:

Substitution with totally different drugs: This practice is generally done in case of oil. Like cotton seed oil in place of olive oil. Sometimes barks also substitute original bark.

Substitution of species in the same family: This practice is done in case of dried leaves, roots or stems. Example: Dog senna in place of Indian seena, but both have same family (Leguminosae), Leaves of *Datural metal* with *D. stramonium* (family: Solanaceae), Cinchona bark can be easily substituted with other species of same family (Rubiaceae) i.e., *Cinchona ledgeriana, C. succirubra*.

Substitution of different species: Dried fruits, flowers and leaves are easily substituted with different species with different family but the genus are same. For example, Brahmi, which has two species like Centella asiatica and Baccopa monerii and both belong to different families of Umbelliferae and Scrophulariaceae, respectively. Two types of Gokhru viz. *Tribulus terrestris* (Zygophylaceae) and *Pedalium murex* (Pedaliaceae) of which, *T. terrestris* has the chemical constituents like chlorogenin, diosgenin, rutin, rhamnose and alkaloids. While *P. murex* has sitosterol, ursolic acid, vanilin, flavonoids and alkaloids. Both the species have proved lithotriptic, diuretic and hepatoprotective activities.

Substitution of different parts of same plant: Depending on the pharmacological activities and therapeutic active principles present, the substitution of the plant parts are practiced. Example: The root of *Sida cordifolia* and the whole plant of *Sida cordifolia*. Root has the chemical constituents such as sitoindoside, acylsteryglycoside, while the whole plant has alkaloid, hydrocarbons, fatty acids and ephedrine. Various extracts of the whole plant showed antibacterial, antioxidant, hypoglycemic, hepatoprotective and cardio tonic activities.

Substitution of the plant parts due to same action: Based on the pharmacological activities, this practice is carried out for the substitution of the plants. Different plant sources have same action but have the same part of the plant. Like leaves of Datura, Belladona, Hyoscyamus etc. They belong to tropane alkaloids but have different biological sources. They possess anticholinergic activities with the same useful plant part of leaves and flowers.

Some of the examples of original drugs that are adulterated and substituted in the market, depicted in table 1.9.

Table 1.9: Adulteration and substitution of natural crude drugs

Drug Name	Botanical name	Part used	Substitute	Adulterant
Aconite	*Aconitum nephallus*	Roots	*Aconitum chasmanthum*	*Gloriosa superba*
Belladona	*Atropa belladonna*	Leaves	*Atropa acuminate*	*Althaea officinalis*
Wormseed	*Chenopodium hybridum*	Leaves	*Chenopodium ambrosioides*	*Datura stramonium*
Digitalis	*Digitalis purpurea*	Leaves	*Verbascum Thapsus*	*Inula racemosa*
Sicklewort	*Prunus comuta*	Karnel oil	*Prunus amygdalus*	*Telfairia pedata*
Rauwolfia	*Rauwolfia serpentine*	Root	*Rauwolfia tetraphylla*	*Rauwolfia densiflora*
Chirata	*Swertia chirayita*	Dried plant	*Swertia decussate*	*Andrographis paniculata*
Quinine	*Cinchona officinalis*	Bark	*Cinchona lencifolia*	*Swietenia mahagoni*
Kurchi	*Holarrhena antidysenterica*	Stem bark	*Wrightia tomentosa*	*Wrightia tinctoria*

Method of Detection of Adulteration and Substitution

Generally adulterants and substituents are detected in the original drug morphologically, microscopically, chemical tests, physical evaluation method, microbiological techniques and instrumental methods. These all are have been explained in detail in evaluation method in earlier chapter. Oils are detected by odor, viscosity, color, clarity, followed by specific gravity, optical rotation, refractive index and finally by gas chromatography (GC) analysis.

Some of the detection tests for the original crude drugs with adulterants are given in table 1.10.

Table 1.10: Test for detection of original natural drugs with their adulterants

Original drugs	Adulterant	Detection test
Honey	Water	A cotton wick dipped in pure honey burns when ignited with a match stick. If adulterated presence of water will not allow the honey to burn, if it does will produce a cracking sound.
Coffee	Chicory	Gently sprinkle the coffee powder on surface of water in a glass. The coffee floats over the water but chicory begins to sink down within few seconds and powder particles leave behind them a trail of colour, due to presence of large amount of caramel.
Tea	Colored tea	Rub leaves on white paper, artificial colour comes out on paper.
Turmeric, chilly, curry powder etc.	Colors	Extract the sample with Petroleum ether and add 13N H_2SO_4 to the extract. Appearance of red colour indicates the presence of added colours. However, if the colour disappears upon adding distilled water the sample is not adulterated.
Coriander powder	Dung powder	Soak in water. Dung will float and can be easily detected by its foul smell.
Cardamom big	Cardamom small	Separate out the seeds by physical examination. The seeds of Big cardamom have nearly plain surface without wrinkles or streaks while seeds of small cardamom have pitted or wrinkled ends.
Red chilli powder	Brick powder grit, sand, dirt, filth etc.	Brick powder settles fast chilli powder settles slowly when put in water.
Cumin seeds (Black jeera)	Grass seeds coloured with charcoal dust	Rub the cumin seeds on palms. If palms turn black adulteration in indicated.
Mustard seeds	Argemone seeds	Argemone seeds have rough surface and mustard seeds on pressing is yellow inside while Argemone seed is white.

Original drugs	Adulterant	Detection test
Turmeric powder	Lead chromate	Ash the sample. Dissolve it in 1:7 H_2SO_4 and filter. Add 1 or 2 drops of 0.1% dipenylcarbazide. A pink colour indicates presence of Lead Chromate.
Black pepper	Papaya seeds/ light berries	Float the sample in alcohol or Carbon tetrachloride. The mature black pepper berries sink while papaya seeds and light black pepper float.
Asafoetida	Soap stone or earthy matter	Shake a little portion of sample with water and allow to settle. Soap stone or earthy matter will settle down at the bottom.
Saffron	Colored dried tendrils of maize cob	Pure saffron will not break easily like artificial. Pure saffron when allowed to dissolve in water will continue to give its colour so long as it lasts.
Vegetable oil	Castor oil	Take 1 mL. of oil in a clean dry test tube. Add 10 mL. of acidified petroleum ether. Shake vigorously for 2 minutes. Add 1 drop of Ammonium Molybdate reagent. The formation of turbidity indicates presence of Castor oil in the sample.

1.5.2 Evaluation by Organoleptic, Microscopic, Physical, Chemical and Biological Methods and Properties

Therapeutic efficacy of medicinal plants depends upon the quality and quantity of chemical constituents. It has been established that chemical constituents of a plant species vary with respect to climatic and seasonal changes. Plant species grown in different geographical localities also show quantitative variation in their chemical constituents. Variation in biological compounds exists not only at species level but at variety and cultivar levels too. Many varieties within a species show variations in anatomical and phytochemical aspects and these differences exist among varieties of commonly occurring medicinal plants. These variations might be climatic, altitudinal, geographical or genetical in nature. Hence drug evaluation is required because of three reasons:

(a)   Biochemical variation of the crude drugs.

(b)   Deterioration due to treatment and storage.

(c)   Substitution and adulteration present, as a result of carelessness, in the crude drugs.

To fulfil these requirements, comparative analysis of the variations in morphological, phytochemical and pharmacological aspects of varieties of medicinal plants should be performed that give results of similarities and dissimilarities in morphological, anatomical, microscopical, physicochemical and phytochemical characters of the varieties of plants.

Hence **drug evaluation** is completely defined as the confirmation and complying of drug (identity), determination of its quality, purity and detection of nature of adulteration. In another way drug evaluation can be expressed as method of estimation of active principles present in the crude drug, its morphology and microscopic analysis, its physical evaluation, the biological behaviour and determination of pharmacological evaluation.

Types of Evaluation:

- Organoleptic evaluation
- Microscopic evaluation
- Physical evaluation
- Chemical evaluation
- Biological evaluation
- Analytical evaluation
- **Organoleptic and Morphologic Evaluations:** Basically, organoleptic character (also known as *sensory evaluation*) and morphological character (also known as *macroscopic method*) are the preliminary identification methods. These two methods (*organoleptic and morphologic methods*) are together known as *diagnostic characters* of the crude drugs. These refer to evaluation of drugs by systemic morphological characters such as leaves, barks, fruits, flowers, roots and rhizomes etc. (by size, shape and special features) and further identification by sensory characters like color, odor, taste and consistency (touch and texture). The general appearance of the crude drug indicates it is likely to comply with standard. For example fractured surface in cinchona and cascara are important characteristics. Seeds of different species of caraway, dill, leaves of senna species, disc- shaped structure of nuxvomica, conical shape of aconite etc., can be distinguished. Leaves of different species of menthe can be differentiated by smell. Smell can also identify the adulterated crude drugs like clove and exhausted clove. By taste, bitter drugs like quassia, chirata, kalmegh, neem, sweet tasted drugs like glycyrrhiza, Stevia, pungent tasted drugs like ginger, capsicum, spice drugs like black pepper, nut meg, caraway etc. can be identified. Texture and nature of fracture also provide important information like liquorice is hard and its fracture is fibrous. Fracture of ipecac is brittle, aconite and nuxvomica are horny etc.
- **Microscopic Evaluation:** This evaluation is also known as anatomical evaluation or histological evaluation of crude drugs. This method can be used to identify the organized drug in powdered form by their histological characters or anatomical cell or tissue arrangements. Various reagents (like chloral hydrate, conc. HCl, glycerin) and stains (phuloroglucinol for identification of lignified cells and tissues like xylem, phloem etc., Iodine for detection of starch grains etc.) can be used to differentiate cellular structure. This evaluation also covers study of the constituents by application of chemical method to small quantities of powdered drug. This is known as chemomicroscopy. The elements such as stomata, trichomes, vessels, fibres, stone cells, starch grains, medullary rays, oil cells, calcium oxalate crystals are present in powdered condition and are used in microscopic identification of crude drugs. For example, leaves contain epidermis cells included trichome, stomata, calcium oxalate crystals (if present); bark contains phloem elements (cinchona), stone cells (Kurchi) or sometimes both (cascara); trichome (nuxvomica); fruits contain oil cells, endosperm, pericarp, epicarp, mesocarp etc. This evaluation method is also useful in identification of closely related drugs or species. Hence microscopy is two types viz. Qualitative and Quantitative. Qualitative microscopy is only detection and identification of cellular structures of drugs whereas Quantitative

microscopy is to determine particular cellular substances like linear measurement as diameter of starch grains, length of fibres, vessels, quantitative microscopic constant as stomatal index, vein islet number, palisade ratio, Lycopodium spore method etc. using camera lucida method using two types of micrometers viz. Stage and eye piece micrometers (Figs. 1.6, 1.7 and 1.8).

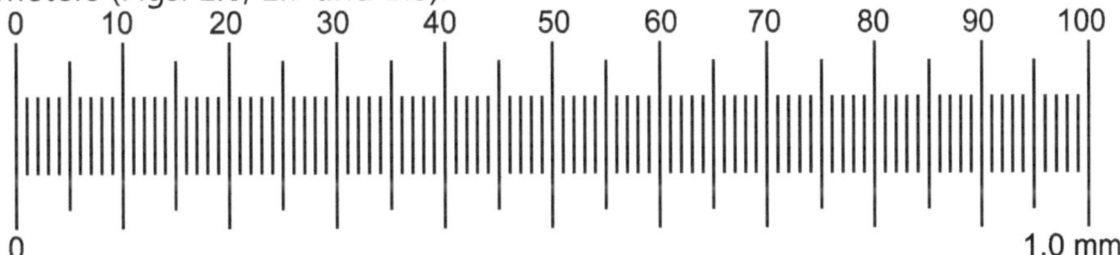
Fig. 1.6: Scale of Stage micrometer

Each big division of stage micrometer is total 1.0 mm in length. It has 100 divisions. Each division is 1/100 = 0.01 mm.

Fig. 1.7: Scale of Eye Piece micrometer

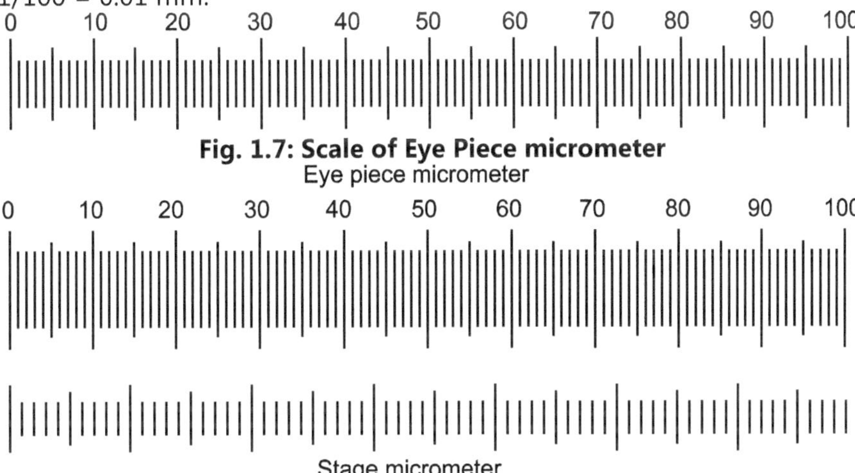

Fig. 1.8: Eyepiece and stage micrometers together

Eyepiece micrometer: It is a circle of glass with a scale etched on the surface. It is a scale of 1 mm length with 100 divisions.

Calibration:

Both the eyepiece and stage micrometers are kept in their respective position and coincided with any line of eyepiece and any line of stage micrometer. Thereafter the number of lines counted which are coincide further (Fig. 1.8). Then the divisions of eyepiece and those of stage micrometer present between the two coincided lines are counted.

Calculation:

Now, if 7 division of eyepiece coincided with 4 division of stage micrometer,

Then the value of one division of eyepiece micrometer is calculated as:

1 division of stage micrometer = 0.01 mm = 10 μ

Therefore, 4 division of stage = 10 × 4 = 40 μ

Now, 7 division of eyepiece = 4 division of stage = 40 μ

Hence, 1 division of eyepiece = 40/7 = 5.71 μ

This is known as calibration factor.

With the help of this calibration factor (5.71 μ) further quantitative microscopy like starch grain diameter, fibre length determination etc. are carried out. For these two experiments there is not required any camera lucida. Directly by observed sample slide calculated the length or diameter of sample with the help of eyepiece micrometer and readings are recorded. Finally all the readings are multiplied by calibration factor.

Example: Starch grain diameter of one starch is measured by eyepiece micrometer are 8 divisions. Then 8 × 5.71 μ = 45.68 μ is the actual dimension of one starch grain.

Camera Lucida:

It is an optical device or instrument in which rays of light are reflected by a prism to produce an image on a sheet of paper, from which a drawing is made. It works on simple optical principle reflecting beam of light through a prism and a plane mirror.

There are two types of camera lucida namely Swift Ives and Abbe model camera lucida. The Abbe camera lucida consists of a prism fitted over the eyepiece of the microscope. A side arm is carrying a mirror that supported vertical over the tracing paper (Fig. 1.9 b and c).

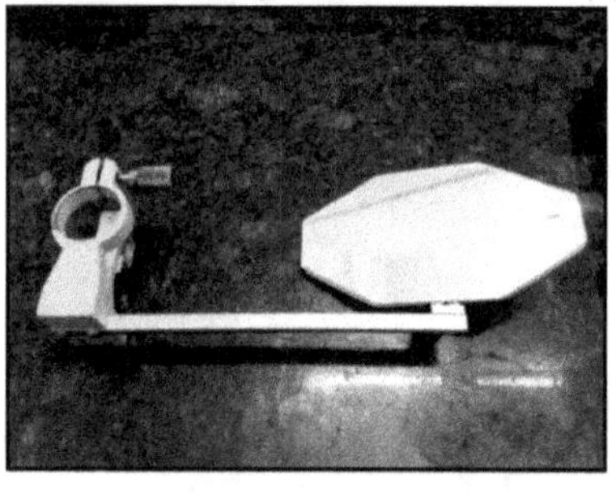 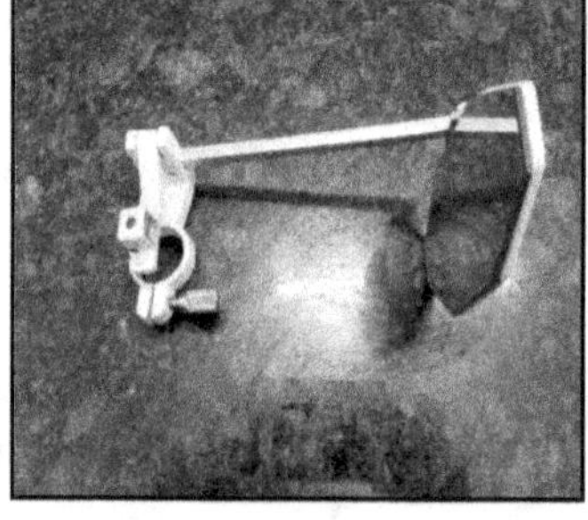 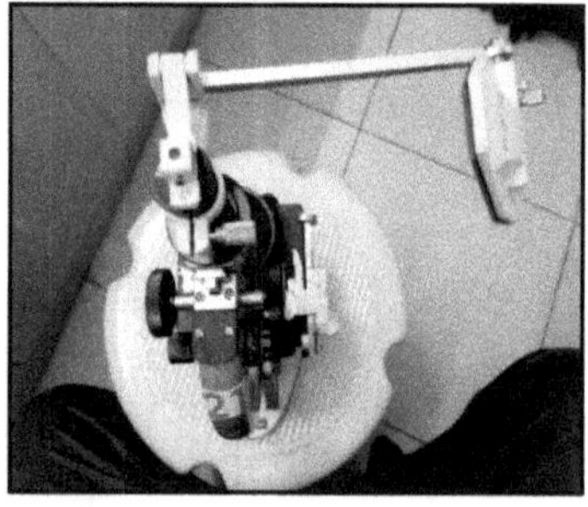

(a)   (b)   (c)

Fig. 1.9: Set up of Abbe camera lucida with microscope

In Swift Ives Camera lucida the plane mirror is replaced by a small right angled prism. It is a small size and fitted over the eyepiece of the microscope with a screw.

Principle:

During use, the light from the drawing board is reflected by the plane mirror into the prism and further reflected into the observer's eye that is seeing the drawing paper and the pencil in the direction of the stage of the microscope. The prism has a small opening through which the observer is seeing the image of the object. As a result, the superimposed image then conveniently traces the microscopic object (Fig. 1.10).

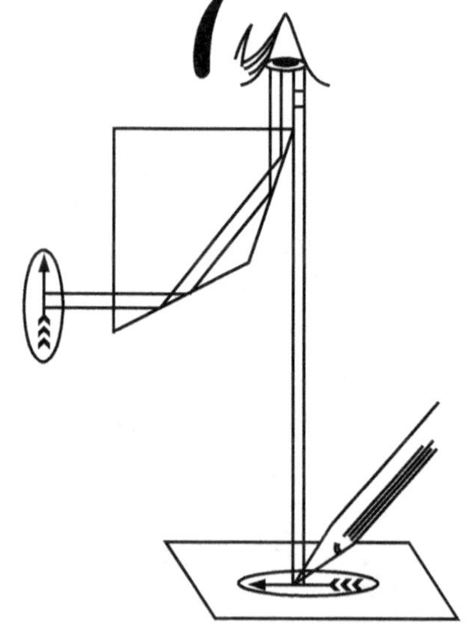

Fig. 1.10: Principle of Camera lucida

Stomata:

Stomata are the minute epidermal opening present in the aerial part of the leaves. Mainly it helps in gaseous exchange. It consists of two kidney shaped cells with middle tiny pore. Broadly four types of stomata viz. Moss type, Gymnospermous type, Gramineous type and Dicotyledonous type. As per arrangement of stomata in dicot plants they are classified into paracytic (stomata two guard cells covered by two subsidiary cells, e.g.: Senna), Diacytic (Guard cell is covered by two subsidiary cells on right angle, e.g.: Peppermint), Anisocytic (Stomata number of guard cells are two but covered by three subsidiary cells, e.g.: Datura), Anomocytic (Stomata is surrounded by varying number of subsidiary cells, e.g.: Digitalis) and Actinocytic (Two guard cells are surrounded by radiating subsidiary cells, e.g.: *Banksia conferta*), Cyclocytic (stomata is surrounded by four or more subsidiary cells, e.g.: *Baccharis articulata*) (Fig. 1.11).

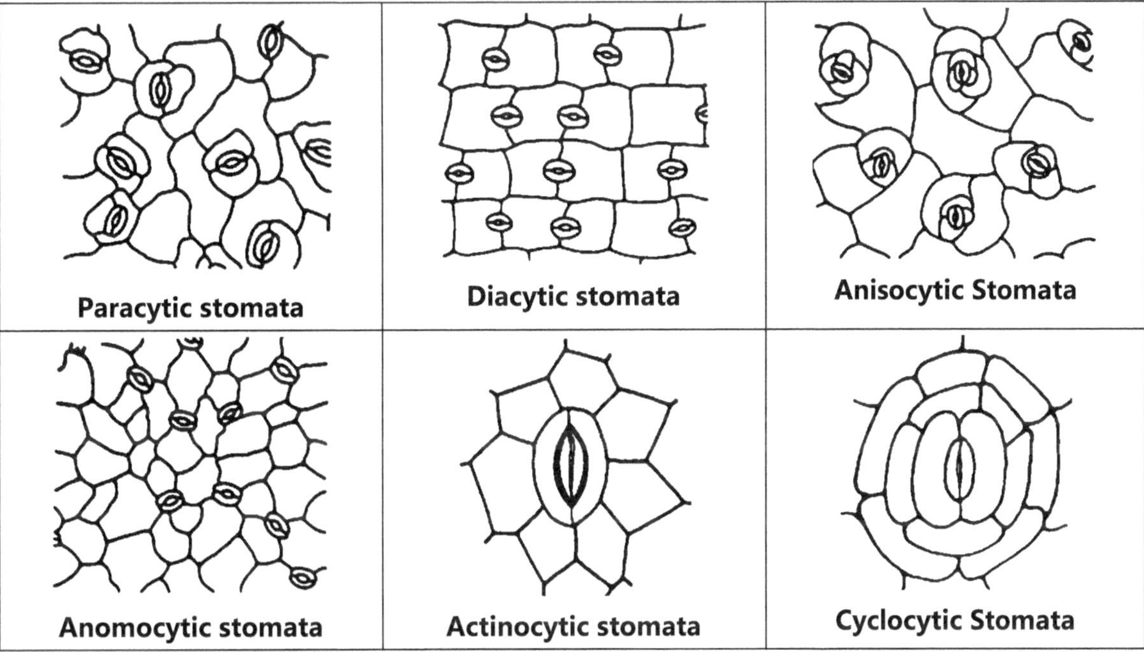

Fig. 1.11: Types of stomata

Trichome:

Trichomes are hair-like components, found on the epidermis of several types of plant stems and leaves. Sometimes in seeds also observed (*Nux vomica*). Generally they are colorless under microscope but lignified in case of *Nux vomica*. They are various types viz. Covering trichomes (Unicellular and multicellular), glandular and hydathodes. Multicellular covering trichomes are two types namely branched and unbranched (Fig. 1.12).

Examples:

Unicellular covering trichomes: Senna, Nuxvomica, Cannabis, Tea, Lobelia.

Multicellular unbranched trichomes: Datura, Digitalis, Belladona.

Multicellular Branched trichomes: Artemisia, Pyrethrum.

Glandular trichomes: They are two types namely Unicellular and multicellular.

Unicellular glandular trichomes: Betel, Vasaka, Piper.

Multicellular glandular trichomes: Digitalis.

Hydathodes: Present in Piper betal.

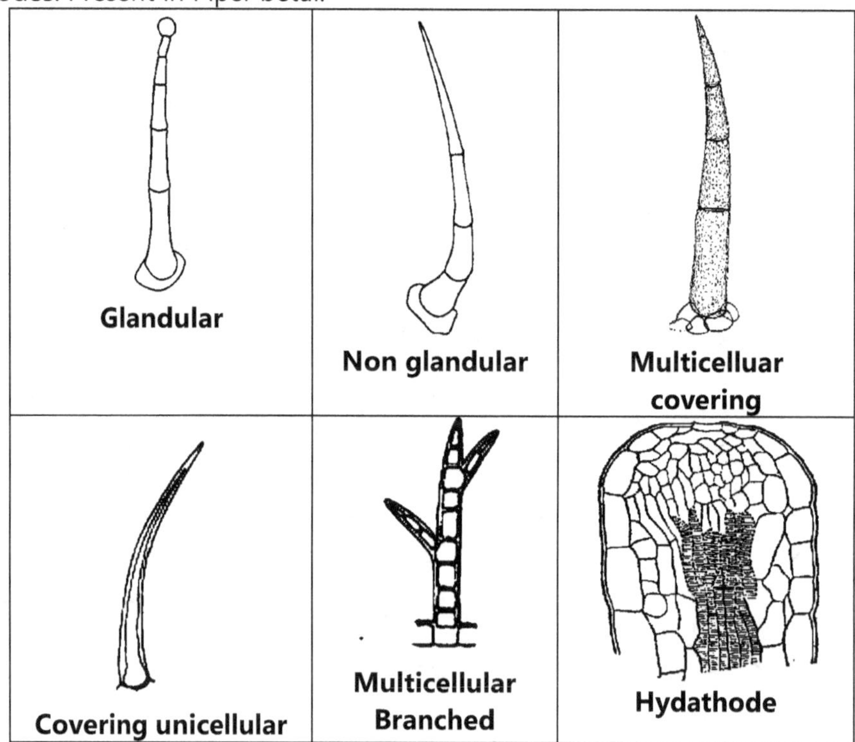

Fig. 1.12: Various types of Trichomes

Functions:

- They control the rate of transpiration.
- They reduce the heating effect of sunlight.
- They aid in the protection of plant body from environmental injuries.

Calcium Oxalate Crystal:

Calcium oxalate crystals are present in almost all parts of the plant. The Ca oxalate crystals are either the monohydrate whewellite form or the dihydrate weddellite form. They are identified by X-ray diffraction, Raman microprobe analysis and infrared spectroscopy are the most accurate. Under microscope they are visible as colourless when treated with chloral hydrate solution.

Types: Morphologically they are different types viz. Prisms (Large, single and well defined; Example: Liquorice, clove), Cluster crystals (Group of prisms; Example: Senna, Rhubarb), Rosette (Large mass form in spherical mass; Example: Arjuna, Rhubarb), Acicular (Needle like slender, long pointed at the end. Example: Cinnamon, Ipecac), Microcrystals or crystal sand (Amorphous mass in a cell, present in large number; Example: Cinchona, Belladona) (Fig. 1.13).

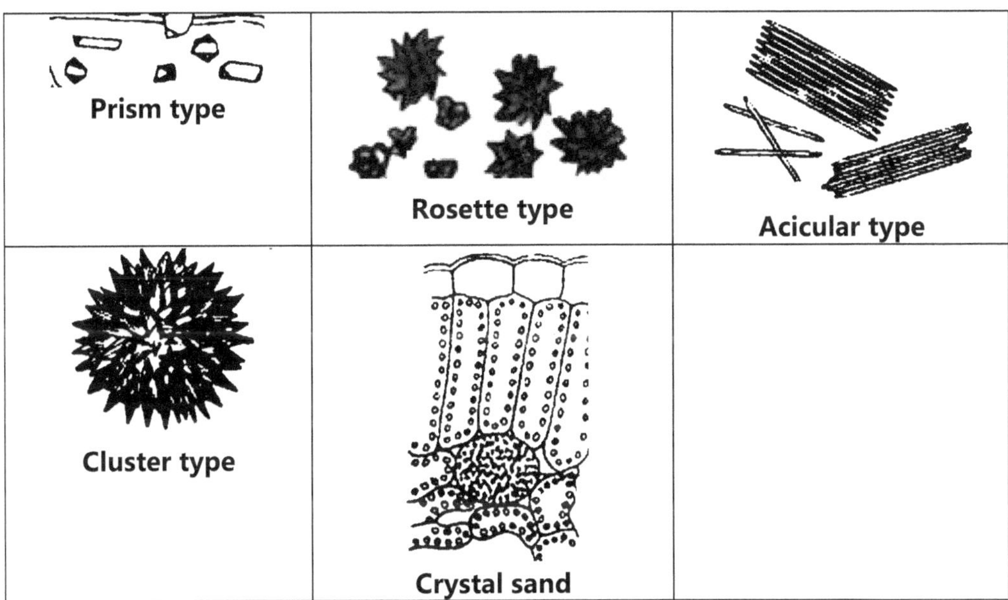

Fig. 1.13: Types of various calcium oxalate crystals

Functions:

- They give protection to the plant against environmental stress.
- They help in identification of crude drugs.
- They help in detection of adulterants.
- They help in identification of plants in same family.

Leaf constants:

1. Stomal Index: The stomatal index is the percentage of the number of stomata formed by the total number of epidermal cells, including the stomata, each stoma being counted as one cell. Place leaf fragments of about 5 × 5 mm in size in a test tube containing about 5 mL of chloral hydrate solution and heat in a boiling water-bath for about 15 minutes or until the fragments become transparent. Transfer a fragment to a microscopic slide and prepare the mount, the lower epidermis uppermost, in chloral hydrate solution and put a small drop of glycerol-ethanol solution on one side of the cover-glass to prevent the preparation from drying.

$$\text{Calculation: Stomatal Index} = \frac{S \times 100}{S + E}$$

Where S = the number of stomata in a given area of leaf; and E = the number of epidermal cells (including trichomes) in the same area of leaf.

2. Stomatal number: It can be defined as the average number of stomata per square millimeter area of epidermis cell. Stomatal number can be determined by treating the lamina of the leaves with chloral hydrate and then the part of the epidermal surface is removed carefully and observed under microscope.

Place leaf fragments of about 5 × 5 mm in size in a test tube containing about 5 mL of chloral hydrate solution and heat in a boiling water-bath for about 15 minutes or until the fragments become transparent. Transfer fragments to a microscopic slide and prepare the mount the lower epidermis uppermost, in chloral hydrate solution and put a small drop of glycerol-ethanol solution on one side of the cover glass to prevent the preparation from drying. Examine with a 40*x* objective and a 6*x* eye piece, to which a microscopical drawing apparatus is attached. Mark on the drawing paper a cross (*x*) for each stomata, and calculate the average number of stomata per square millimeter for each surface of the leaf.

3. Palisade ratio: Palisade ratio is the average number of palisade cells under one epidermal cell. Place leaf fragments of about 5 × 5 mm in size in a test tube containing about 5 mL of chloral hydrate solution and heat in a boiling water-bath for about 15 minutes or until the fragments become transparent. Transfer a fragment to a microscopic slide and prepare the mount of the upper epidermis in chloral hydrate solution and put a small drop of glycerol solution on one side of the cover-glass to prevent the preparation from drying. Examine with a 40x objective and a 6x eye piece, to which a microscopical drawing apparatus is attached. Trace four adjacent epidermal cells on paper; focus gently downward to bring the palisade into view and trace sufficient palisade cells to cover the area of the outlines of the four epidermal cells. Count the palisade cells under the four epidermal cells. Where a cell is intersected, include it in the count only when more than half of it is within the area of the epidermal cells. Calculate the average number of palisade cells beneath one epidermal cell, dividing the count by 4; this is the "Palisade ratio". For each sample of leaf make no fewer than ten determinations and calculate the average number.

Examples: *Atropa belladonna*: 6 - 10; *Datura stramonium*: 4 - 6; *Mentha piperita*: 5.1 - 8.1.

4. Vein Islet Number: The mesophyll of a leaf is divided into small portions of photosynthetic tissue by a stomosis of the veins and veinlets; such small portions or areas are termed "Vein-Islets". Vein-islets present in per square millimeter is known as "Vein-Islet number". This value has been shown to be constant for any given species and, for full-grown leaves, to be unaffected by the age of the plant or the size of the leaves. The vein-islet number has proved useful for the critical distinction of certain nearly related species.

Take pieces of leaf lamina with an area of not less than 4 square millimeters from the central portion of the lamina, excluding the midrib and the margin of the leaf. Clear the pieces of lamina by heating in a test tube containing chloral hydrate solution on a boiling water-bath for 30 to 60 minutes or until clear and prepare a mount in glycerol-solution or, if desired, stain with safranin solution and prepare the mount in *Canada balsam*. Place the stage micrometer on the microscope stage and examine with 4*x* objective and a 6*x* eye piece. Draw a line representing 2 mm on a sheet of paper by means of a microscopical drawing apparatus and construct a square on the line representing an area of 4 square millimeters. Move the paper so that the square is seen in the centre of the field of the eyepiece. Place the slide with the cleared leaf piece on the microscope stage and draw in the veins and veinlets included within the square, completing the outlines of those vein-islets which overlap two adjacent sides of the square. Count the number of vein-islets within the square including those overlapping on two adjacent sides and excluding those intersected by the other two sides. The result obtained is the number of vein-islets in 4 square millimeters. For each sample of leaf, make no fewer than three determinations and calculate the average number of vein-islets per square millimeter.

Examples: *Cassia angustifolia*: 19 - 23; *Digitalis purpurea*: 2 - 5.5; *Cassia acutifolia*: 25-30.

5. Lycopodium spore method: This method is use to identify the crude drugs when the chemical and physical methods are inapplicable. This method is also useful to detect the adulteration present in the crude drugs containing starch grains.

Examples: Adulterated drug containing starch can be determined by counting the number of starch grains per mg and calculating the amount from the known number of starch grains per mg of the pure starch. The percentage purity of an authentic powdered ginger is calculated using the following equation:

$$\% \text{ purity} = \frac{N \times W \times 94000 \times 100}{S \times M \times P}$$

Where,

N = Number of characteristic structures (starch grain) in 25 fields.

W = Weight in mg of lycopodium taken.

S = Number of lycopodium spores in the same 25 fields.

M = Weight in mg of the sample, calculated on the basis of sample dried at 105°C.

P = 2,86,000 in case of ginger starch grains powder.

Significance:

- Determination of foreign organic matter.
- Determination of percentage purity of drugs.
- Detection of adulterant

Physical Evaluation:

Physical standards are to be determined for drugs which is constant for crude drugs and helps in drug evaluation. Physical constant such as specific gravity, refractive index, swelling factor, optical rotation, viscosity etc., are useful in determining the identity, purity and quality of the drugs (Figs. 1.14 and 1.15).

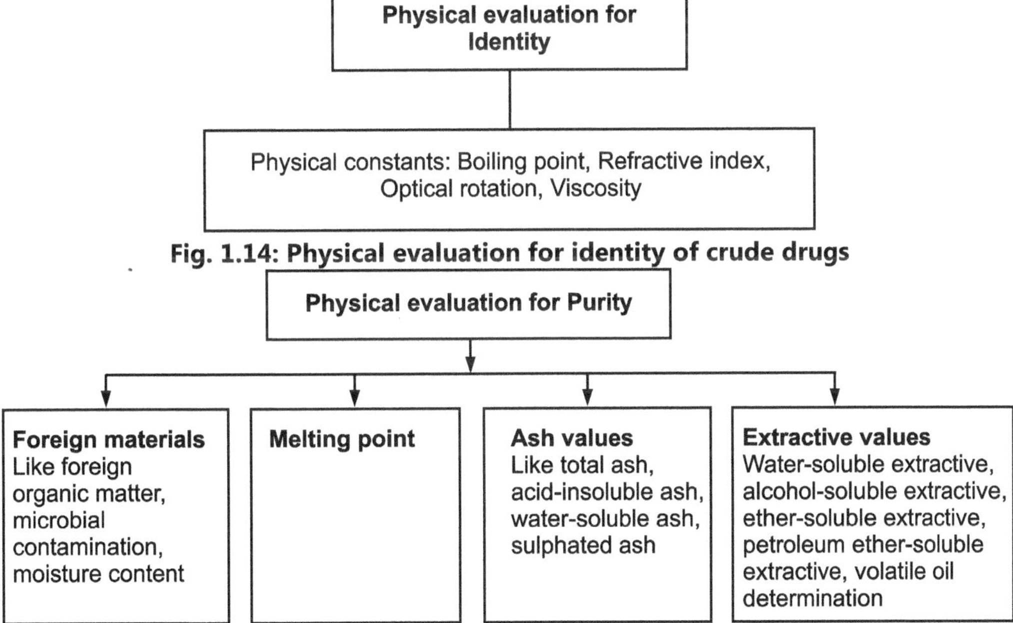

Fig. 1.14: Physical evaluation for identity of crude drugs

Fig. 1.15: Physical evaluation for purity of crude drugs

Boiling point: The boiling point of a substance is the temperature at which the vapour pressure of the liquid equals the pressure surrounding the liquid and the liquid changes into a vapour. A liquid in a vacuum has a lower boiling point than when that liquid is at atmospheric pressure. Boiling points are approximately related to their molecular weight. The higher the molecular weight, the higher is the boiling point.

Refractive index (R_i): This method is used for determination of refractive index to essential and fixed oils and also for detection of adulteration present in the oils. It is defined as the ratio between the velocity of light in the air and in the oil. It can be determined with refractometer. It is denoted as, n = sin i/sin r. Where, n = refractive index, sin i = sine of angle of incidence and sin r = sin e of angle of refraction. It is measured at 20°C ± 5°C temperature. Sometimes Abbe refractometer is used for accurate measurements of R_i .

Examples: Clove oil: 1.530 – 1.531 at 20°C., Castor oil: 1.475 – 1.479 at 20°C.

Optical rotation: Basically volatile oils show the ability to rotate in the plain of polarized light to left or right side, and likewise they are called laevorotatory or dextrorotatory respectively. It is measured by using polarimeter at 20°C.

$$\frac{\text{Angular rotation per dm of solution}}{\text{Gram of substance per ml of solution}} = \frac{100\,\alpha}{Ldp}$$

where, α = Observed rotation, L = Length of observed layer in drug, d = Density and p = gm of substance in 100 g of solution.

Viscosity: Viscosity is a measure of the resistance of a fluid which is being deformed by either shear or tensile stress. The most common method of determining kinematic viscosity in the lab utilizes the capillary tube viscometer.

Examples: Clove oil: 0° to – 1.5°, Cinnamon oil: 0° to – 2°.

Melting Point: The melting point of a solid is the temperature at which it changes state from solid to liquid. At the melting point the solid and liquid phase exist in equilibrium. The melting point of a substance depends (usually slightly) on pressure and is usually specified at standard pressure. Freezing point or crystallization point is the temperature of the reverse change from liquid to solid. It can be determined by capillary method. In this method, a thin glass capillary tube containing a compact column of the substance to be determined is introduced into a heated stand (liquid bath or metal block) in close proximity to a high accuracy thermometer. The temperature should continue at fixed rate until the sample in the tube transitions into the liquid state. While determining melting point, several observations and the temperatures are recorded.

Examples: Cocoa butter: 30 – 35°C; Wool fat: 34 – 44°C

Foreign Organic Matters: Anything extra present in the drug which is not complying with the authentic drug may be considered as a foreign matter. The foreign matter can be present in the drug due to improper harvesting. The source of foreign organic matter can be animal excreta, insect or mould and is determined by sedimentation or floatation method.

Examples: Curcumin – not more than 2.0%; Neem – not more than 1.5%

Ash Value: After the incineration of the crude drugs, the remnants are known as ash. Ash contains mostly inorganic salts. It gives the idea about the quality and purity of the crude drugs. It can be determined by (a) Total ash: Carbon and organic matters of the crude drugs are converted to ash at temperature about 900°C. It mostly contains carbohydrate, phosphates, silicates and silica. This total ash is further used with water soluble ash and acid insoluble ash. Water soluble ash is produced by separating the water-soluble materials, which is dried to yield water-soluble ash. Further, total ash, when treated with dilute hydrochloric acid, removes many inorganic salts to yield mainly silica in the residue. This is known as acid-insoluble ash. When the crude drug is incinerated with dilute sulphuric acid at temperature above 600°C, the ash obtained by this method is known as sulphated ash. This method converts all oxides and carbonates to sulphate salt.

Total Ash Value: 2 g of the ground air-dried sample is to weigh into previously ignited, dried and tarred silica crucible. Spread the material in an even thin layer. It is then kept on a gas burner under a low flame and is ignited slowly to obtain a carbonized residue. It is then placed in the muffle furnace and the temperature of the muffle is adjusted to 450-500°C and ignition is then allowed   in the muffle furnace. After 3 hours, switch off the muffle furnace and allow it to cool and remove the silica crucible. Further cool in a desiccator and weigh. If carbon free ash cannot be obtained in this manner, moist residue with 2 mL of water or saturated solution of ammonium nitrate. (This is to expose bits of unashed carbon). Then it is dried on water bath and then on hot plate, and after that ignite in muffle furnace to constant weight. Remove from muffle furnace and allow cooling for 30 minutes in a desiccator and weight. Finally percentage of ash is calculated.

Acid Insoluble Ash: To the silica crucible containing the total ash obtained, 25 mL of hydrochloric acid (~70 g/*l*) is added. Cover with a watch glass and boil gently for 5 minutes on a hot plate or burner. Rinse the watch glass with 5 mL of hot water and add these washings to the crucible. The insoluble matter will collect on an ash less filter paper by filtration and rinse the filter paper repeatedly with hot water until the filtrate becomes neutral/free from acid. Transfer the filter paper containing the insoluble matter to the original crucible, dry on a hot plate, and ignite to a constant weight in the muffle furnace at 450-500°C. Remove the silica crucible from the muffle furnace and allow cooling the matter in a desiccator for 30 minutes, and then weighing without delay. The content of acid insoluble ash will be calculated as percentage.

Water-Soluble Ash: The ash is boiled for few minutes with required amount of water, collect the insoluble matter in a silica crucible and then wash with hot water and ignite for 15 minutes at a temperature not exceeding 450°C. The weight of the insoluble matter will be subtracted from the weight of the ash. The difference in weight represents the water-soluble ash. The percentage of water-soluble ash is calculated with reference to the air dried drug.

Calculation:

Total ash/Acid insoluble ash/Water soluble ash % = (B – C) × 100/A

Where, **A** - Sample weight in g; **B** - Weight of dish + contents after drying (g) **C** - Weight of empty dish (g).

Determination of Sulphated Ash:

Heat a silica or platinum crucible to redness for 10 minutes, allow to cool in a desiccators and weigh. Put 1 to 2 g of the substance, accurately weighed, into the crucible; ignite gently at first, until the substance is thoroughly charred. Cool, moisten the residue with few mL of sulphuric acid and then ignite at 800° ± 25°C until all black particles have disappeared. Conduct the ignition in a place protected from air currents. Allow the crucible to cool, add a few drops of sulphuric acid and heat. Ignite as before, allow cooling and weighing. Repeat the operation until two successive weighing do not differ by more than 0.5 mg.

Examples: Ashwagandha: Total ash: <7% w/w; acid insoluble ash: <1.2% w/w.

Rauwolfia: Total ash: <8% w/w; Acid insoluble ash: <1.2% w/w.

Significances of Ash Values:

- Determine authenticity and purity of crude drug sample
- Determine the presence of inorganic salts like carbonates, phosphates, silicates etc. in crude drugs.
- Useful to detect adulterated products.
- Useful to detect exhausted products.
- Useful to detect earthy matter in the products.

Moisture Content: Moisture content in the drug provides enzymatic activity or facilitates the growth of microbes, which results in deterioration. The crude drugs heated at 105°C to constant weight and calculate the total loss of weight. The methods used for the determination of moisture contents are (a) Loss on drying (b) Azeotropic distillation method (c) Karl Fischer method (d) Directly with the moisture pan balance. Toluene distillation method is used for the determination of moisture content in the volatile oil containing drugs.

2 gm of powdered drug is transferred into a shallow weighing bottle and the contents will be distribute evenly to a depth not exceeding 10 mm. The full bottle is then heated at 105°C in hot air oven and weighed until a constant weight is obtained. The difference is calculated from the weight after drying and initial weight is the moisture content. The amount of calculated moisture content is confirmed with moisture pan balance.

Ultrasound wave for moisture content: Air-coupled ultrasonic spectroscopy is enabled ultrasonic waves to be applied to the on-line and real-time assessment of the water content of different fresh plant materials.

Examples: Senna leaf: Not more than 10% w/w; Digitalis: not more than 5% w/w; Aloes: not more than 10% w/w.

Significances of Moisture Content:

- Excess of moisture present in drugs is leads to degradation of quality.
- Excess moisture content is leads to microbial attack to the drugs
- Moisture content determination is also helpful in quality of drug.

Extractive Values: All the chemical constituents are soluble either in polar, semi polar or organic solvents. Total soluble constituents of the drug in any particular solvent or mixture of solvents may be called its extractive value or percent extractive.

Alcohol Soluble Extractive Value:

Prepare coarse powder of air dried drug. Take 100 mL of ethanol (specified strength) in a conical flask. Macerate 5 g of powdered drug in conical flask, close the flask for 24 hours. Shake the flask frequently during first 6 hours; allow it to stand for 18 hours. Filter rapidly taking precaution against loss of ethanol. Evaporate 25 mL of the filtrate to dryness in a tarred flat bottomed shallow dish. Dry at 105°C and weight it. Calculate the % of alcohol soluble extractive with reference to the air dried drug.

Water Soluble Extractive Value:

Prepare coarse powder of air dried drug. Take 100 mL of chloroform water in conical flask. Macerate 5 g of powdered drug in a conical flask, and close the flask for 24 hours. In between the flask is shake for first 6 hours and then stand for 18 hours. Filter rapidly by decanting the water extract and then evaporate 25 mL of the filtrate to dryness in a tarred flat bottomed shallow dish. Dry at 105°C and weight it. Calculate the % of water soluble extractive with reference to the air dried drug.

Calculation:

The percentage of water soluble extractive value/alcohol soluble extractive value

$$= (B - A) \times 4 \times 100/W$$

where,

A: Empty weight of the dish (g); B: Weight of dish + residue (g);

W: Weight of plant material taken (g)

Significances of Extractive Values:

- This method is important when the constituents of drugs can't be readily estimated by any other means.
- It indicates the nature of chemical constituents present in drugs.
- It helps in identification of adulterants.

Examples:

Alcohol soluble extractive value of Ashwagandha is not less than 60% w/w, water soluble extractive value of senna is not less than 30% w/w.

Volatile Oil Determination: Generally volatile oil can be determined with the Clevenger's apparatus by hydro-distillation method. Recently microwave assistance Clevenger apparatus has been used for more yields with less time consumption. Volatile oil content present in the drug gets separated at the temperature of boiling water or steam and deposited as a layer on top of the water layer. During hydro-distillation, 5 to 10% glycerin is to be added, which gives better yields with elevation in boiling point of water. Volatile oil can be collected and measured with the graduated receiver. Further the volatile oil is separated from the water, and the excess of water is removed by adding anhydrous sodium salt and keeping it overnight. The oil should be stored in a dry and cool place.

Examples: Clove: Not less than 15% w/w; Fennel: Not less than 1.4% w/w; Dill: Not less than 2.5% w/w; Caraway: Not less than 2.5% w/w.

Physical Evaluation for Quality:

Quality is the most important factor that greatly affects the economy of the crude drugs. Various factors like collection, storage and geographical location are most important to get the pure quality of the products.

Bitterness Value: This experiment is performed only for those drugs which have a strong bitter taste and are used for their bitterness property as appetizing agent. The bitter property of the drug is determined by comparing the threshold bitter concentration of an extract of the material with that of dilute solution of quinine hydrochloride. Bitter value is expressed in units' equivalent to bitterness of solution containing 1 gm of quinine HCl in 2000 ml concentration of quinine HCl (0.04-0.058 mg/ mL in 9 different test tubes).

Bitterness value is calculated in units/gm using following formula:

$$\frac{2000 \times C}{a \times b}$$

where,

        a = Concentration of stock solution,

        b = Volume of sample in test tube with threshold bitter conc.,

        c = Concenration of quinine HCl in test tube with the threshold bitter conc.

Haemolytic Activity: This test is done for drugs belonging to the family Caryophyllaceae, Araliaceae, Sapindaceae and Dioscoraceae. The drugs belonging to these families contain saponins, which have the ability to cause haemolysis. When added to blood, saponins produce changes in erythrocytes membranes causing haemolysis. The activity is compared with reference material saponin.

$$\text{Haemolytic Index} = \frac{1000 \times a}{b}$$

where,

        a = Quantity of saponin that produces total haemolysis,

        b = Quantity of plant material that produces total haemolysis

     1000 = Haemolytic activity of saponins in relation to Ox blood

Swelling Index: Some specific plant materials are of specific therapeutic utility because of their swelling properties, specially gums, hemicellulose, pectin and mucilage. The swelling index is the volume in mL taken up by swelling of 1 gm of plant material under specific condition.

Take 50 mL glass stoppered measuring flask. To this add 25 mL water and 1 g drug. Then shake the sample at every 10 minutes for 1 hour. Let it stand for 3 hours and then measured the volume in mL occupied by the plant material.

Example: Isphagula: swelling index minimum 9.

Foaming Index: Plant materials containing saponins cause persistent foam when the decoction is shaken. Foaming ability of plant material and their extracts is measured by foaming index.

Take 1 gm drug and add to 100 mL boiled water. Heat for 30 minutes. Cool and filter into a 100 mL vol. flask. Make-up the volume with water. Then pour this solution into 10 different stopper test tubes in different vol. (1- 10 mL) and adjust the volume up to 10 mL with water. Shake well for 15 seconds and then allow to stand for 15 minutes. Measure the height of foam.

If height of the foam in every test tube < 1 cm, it indicates that the foaming index will be < 100.

If height of the foam is 1 cm in any test tube, then foaming index will be 1000/a
where a = Volume of decoction in that test tube.

If this is the 1st and 2nd test tube of the series then intermediate dilution is prepared in similar manner. If the height of the foam in every test tube > 1 cm, then foaming index will be over 1000.

Chemical evaluation:

With this method active constituents in the drugs are determined. There are various methods for chemical evaluation (Fig. 1.16).

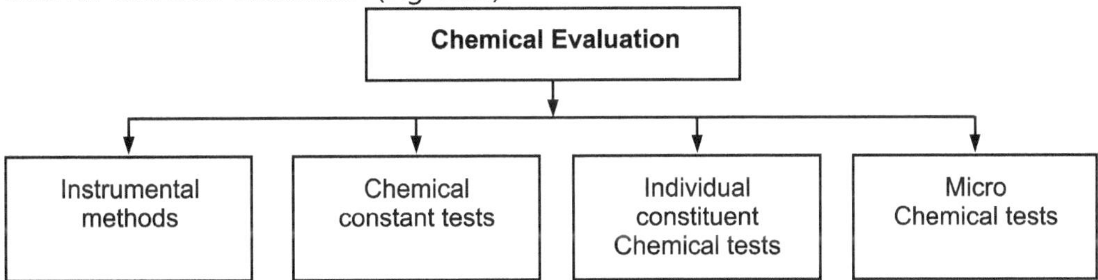

Fig. 1.16: Types of chemical evaluation

(a) Instrumental methods: Various instrumental methods like colorimetry, fluorimetry, spectrophotometry etc. are used for the evaluation.

Colorimetric Method: It is a method of determining the concentration of a chemical element or chemical compound in a solution with the aid of a color reagent. It is applicable to both organic and inorganic compounds and may be used with or without an enzymatic stage. The method is widely used in medical laboratories and for industrial purposes, e.g., the analysis of water samples in connection with industrial water treatment.

Photometric Method: It is the set of methods of quantitative chemical analysis based on the relationship between the concentration of a substance in a solution or gas and the absorption of radiation. In this method the intensities of the monochromatic components of transmitted radiation are scanned.

Fluorimetric Method: It is an analytical technique for identifying and characterizing minute amounts of a substance by excitation of the substance with a beam of ultraviolet light and detection and measurement of the characteristic wavelength of fluorescent light emitted.

Gravimetric Method: It is the quantitative determination of a substance by the precipitation method of gravimetric analysis involving isolation of an ion in solution by precipitation reaction, filtering, washing the precipitate, conversion of precipitate to a product of known composition, and finally weighing the precipitate and determining its mass by difference. There are four fundamental types of gravimetric analysis: physical gravimetry, thermogravimetry, precipitative gravimetric analysis, and electrodeposition.

Volumetric Method: It is a quantitative analysis of liquids or solutions by comparing the volumes that react with known volumes of standard reagents, usually by titration. A reagent is prepared as a standard solution, acts as titrator. A known concentration and volume of titrant reacts with a solution of analyte or titrand to determine concentration.

(b) Chemical Constant Tests: Various tests like acid value, iodine value, Saponification value etc. are used for the evaluation of fixed oils and fats.

Saponification value: It is the number of milligrams of potassium hydroxide required to saponify 1g of fat under the specific conditions. It is a measure of the average molecular weight of all the fatty acids present.

Calculation:

$$\text{Saponification value} = 28.05 \, (y - x)/w$$

where,   w = Weight of substance in g.

Examples: Castor oil: 176–187; Yellow bees wax: 90–103

Acid value: It is the number of milligrams of potassium hydroxide (KOH) necessary to neutralize the fatty acids in 1 gram of sample.

Calculation:

Acid value: 5.61 n/w

where,   n = mL of 0.1 m Potassium hydroxide solution required.

w = Weight of sample in g.

Example: Acid value of crude castor oil = 1.114

Significance:

(a) to know the freshness of oil.

(b) to know the degree of rancidity of oil.

Iodine value: It is the mass of iodine in grams that is consumed by 100 grams of a chemical substance. Iodine numbers are often used to determine the amount of unsaturation in fatty acids. The higher the iodine number, the more C=C bonds are present in the fat.

Iodine value = 1.269 (y – x)/w where, w is weight of sample in g.

Examples: Castor oil: 82–90; Cocoa butter: 35–40; Lard: 52–56.

Significance:

(a) To determine the quality of any unsaturated oils.

(b) It measures the degree of unsaturation in a fat or oil.

(c) It provides degree of rancidity.

(c) Individual Constituent Chemical Tests: Various chemical tests are carried out for identification of individual components. For each plant drugs there are some common test for identification of group of plant secondary metabolites as well as specific tests for identification of individual constituents.

Molish test for detection of sugars, Lieberman Burchard test for detection of steroids, Borntrager test for detection of anthraquinones, ferric chloride test for tannins, Keller- Kiliani test for deoxy sugars, ninhydrine test for the detection of amino acids and proteins etc.

(d) Microchemical Tests: These tests are carried out on slide. Example: Eugenol in clove oil is precipitated as potassium euginate when potassium hydroxide is added on slide containing clove oil. Under microscope clove oil shows needle shaped crystal of potassium euginate.

Biological evaluation: This method is carried out when the drugs are not evaluated by any other methods, or chemical nature of the drug is unknown or chemical methods are not available or drugs which have different chemical composition but same biological activity. Generally in this method, the response produced by the test drug on a living system is compared with that of the standard preparation.

This method is used for:

1. Measurement of the pharmacological activity of new or chemically undefined substances.

2. Investigation of the function of endogenous mediators.
3. Determination of the side effect profile, including the degree of drug toxicity.
4. Measurement of the concentration of known substances.
5. Assessing the amount of pollutants being released by a particular source such as waste water.

Example: Cardiac glycosides are evaluated by this method using frogs, cats, pigeons etc.

Significance:

- This method is used when the standardization is not done by physical or chemical method.
- When the quantity of drug is very less or drug itself not available
- This method is performed on living animals.

Microbiological Assay:

The method of measuring compounds such as vitamins and amino acids using microorganisms. The principle is based on a comparison of the inhibition of growth of microorganisms by measured concentration of the antibiotics to be examined with that produced by known concentrations of a standard preparation of the antibiotic having a known activity.

As per IP, two methods are used for assay viz. the cylinder plate method or cup plate method and the turbidity method. The cup plate method is depends upon diffusion of the antibiotic from a vertical cylinder through a solidified agar layer in a petri dish or plate to an extent such that growth of the added microorganism is prevented entirely in a zone around the cylinder containing a solution of the antibiotic. The method depends on the microbial growth inhibition in the culture of uniform antibiotic. This is favorable to the rapid growth in the absence of the antibiotic.

- **Analytical Evaluation:** In this method various chromatographic as well as spectroscopic methods are used for the sample.

Thin Layer Chromatography (TLC): It is a chromatographic technique used to separate mixtures with the principle of adsorption. Thin layer chromatography is performed on a sheet of glass, plastic or aluminum foil which is coated with a thin layer of adsorbent material, usually silica gel, aluminium oxide or cellulose known as stationary phase. The sample has been applied on the plate and the mobile phase is drawn up the plate via capillary action and based on their affinity towards stationary phase the separation is achieved.

Advantages:

(a) This method is easy and simple.
(b) Always available to be used.
(c) Any type of samples can be used.
(d) Neutral, basic, acidic or purely aqueous eluents can be employed.

Calculation:

$$\textbf{Retention factor } (R_f): = \frac{\textbf{Distance travelled by the solute}}{\textbf{Distance travelled by the solvent}}$$

High Performance Thin Layer Chromatography (HPTLC): HPTLC system is a versatile modern analytical technique with reference to its excellent automation, optimization, multidimensional applications. The process is based on fundamental principle, theory of separation, experimental details, handling understanding and implementation. Phytochemical analysis, fingerprint analysis, authentication, biomedical analysis, drug quantification, analytical analysis, quantitative analysis and validation are carried out by this method. Application of HPTLC in combinatorial approach provided new dimension to its high potential. HPTLC-MS coupling, laser desorption-HPTLC chromatography coupled with chemical ionization mass spectrometry etc. that is used in identity, purity, quality, and stability of raw materials, extracts and finished herbal products.

Advantages:

(a)   Simultaneous processing of sample and standard, better analytical precision and accuracy, less need of analytical standard.

(b)   Several analysts work simultaneously.

(c)   Lower analysis time and less cost per analysis.

(d)   Simple sample preparation.

(e)   No prior treatment for solvents like filtration and degassing.

(f)   Low mobile phase consumption per sample.

(g)   Fresh stationary and mobile phases for each analysis but no contamination.

(h)   Visual detection possible-open system.

High Performance Liquid Chromatography (HPLC): It is a highly improved form of column chromatography. By this method solvent allowed passing through the stationary column with high forced under high pressure of up to 400 atmospheres. The column is made up of silica particle tightly packed material which gives a much greater surface area for interactions between the stationary phase and the molecules flowing passed it. It is a chromatographic technique used to separate a mixture of compounds in analytical chemistry and biochemistry with the purpose of identifying, quantifying and purifying the individual components of the mixture. Depends on the relative polarity of the solvent, HPLC variants are two types (a) Normal phase HPLC and (b) Reversed phase HPLC

Gas Chromatography (GC): It is used for separation and analysis of vaporized compounds which are non decomposable. The purity of a substance and separating the different components of a mixture (the relative amounts of such components can also be determined) is carried out by GC. It helps in identifying a compound. Preparative GC is used to prepare pure compounds from a mixture. The *mobile phase* (or "moving phase") is a carrier gas, usually an inlet gas such as helium or an inert gas such as nitrogen. The *stationary phase* is a liquid or polymer on an inert solid support, called as column. It is also known as vapor-phase chromatography or gas–liquid partition chromatography (GLPC).

Spectroscopic Methods:

UV-visible Spectrophotometer: This method refers to absorption spectroscopy or reflectance spectroscopy in the UV-visible spectral region. This means it uses light in the visible and adjacent (near-UV and near infrared (NIR)) ranges. 190 nm to 380 nm is UV region and 380 nm to 900 nm is known as visible region. The absorption in the visible range directly affects the color of the chemicals. In this region molecules undergo electronic transitions. It is applicable for determination of transition metal ions, highly conjugated organic compounds and biological macromolecules. Examples: Morphine is determined at 286 nm, Anthraquinones are determined at 505 nm,

Infra-Red Spectroscopy (IR): It is the spectroscopy that deals with the infrared region of the electromagnetic spectrum i.e., light with a longer wavelength and lower frequency than visible light. It is used to identify and study chemicals. Fourier transform infrared (FTIR) spectrometer is used in this method. The three regions of IR are: the near, mid and far region, named for their relation to the visible spectrum. The near IR (14000–4000 cm^{-1}) range molecules excite harmonic vibrations whereas mid-infrared (4000–400 cm^{-1}) is used for the fundamental vibrations associated with rotational vibrational structure. Thereafter far-infrared (400–10 cm^{-1}) is considered as the microwave region, used for rotational spectroscopy. It is used for identification of functional group and structure elucidation, identification of substances, detection of impurities etc.

Nuclear Magnetic Resonance Spectroscopy (NMR): This technique deals with the magnetic properties of certain atomic nuclei to determine physical and chemical properties of atoms or the molecules in which they are contained. It provides information about the structure, dynamics, reaction and chemical nature of molecules. Most frequently, NMR spectroscopy is used by chemists and biochemists to investigate the properties of organic molecules, though it is applicable to any kind of sample that contains nuclei possessing spin. Proton and carbon NMR nuclei (1H or 13C) absorb electromagnetic radiation at a frequency characteristic of the isotope. The frequency and resonant energy of absorption and the intensity of the signal are proportional to the strength of magnetic field.

Mass Spectroscopy: It is an analytical technique that measures the mass to charge ratio of charged particles. It is used for determination of particle masses, elemental composition of molecule and the chemical structures elucidation of molecules like peptides and other chemical compounds. MS works by ionizing chemical compounds to generate charged molecules or molecule fragments and measuring their mass to charge ratios. The technique has both qualitative and quantitative uses for identification of unknown compounds, the isotopic composition of elements in a molecule determination and determination of the structure of a compound by their fragmentations.

X-ray Crystallography: It is a method of determining the arrangement of atoms within a crystal, in which a beam of X-rays strikes a crystal and causes the beam of light to spread into many specific directions. From the angles and intensities of these diffracted beams, a crystallographer can produce a three-dimensional picture of the density of electrons within the crystal. The mean positions of the atoms in the crystal, as well as their chemical bonds and disorder is determined. This method is useful for protein structure analysis.

LC-MS: It is a chemistry technique that combines the physical separation capabilities of liquid chromatography (or HPLC) with the mass analysis capabilities of mass spectrometry. LC-MS is used for determination of high sensitivity and selectivity of molecule. Generally its application is oriented towards the general detection and potential identification of chemicals in the presence of other chemicals (in a complex mixture). For fast and mass purification of natural products extracts, new molecular entities important to food and pharmaceutical industries, preparative LC-MS system is used. LC-MS is very commonly used in pharmacokinetic studies of pharmaceuticals, Proteomics and is thus the most frequently used technique in the field of bioanalysis.

EXERCISE

Long Essays:
1. Explain history, scope and development of Pharmacognosy.
2. Define Crude drugs. Classify them and discuss them in brief with examples.
3. Define Adulteration. Classify them. Explain the various methods of detection of adulteration.
4. Explain Morphological and chemical classification of crude drugs.
5. Define drug evaluation. Classify them. Explain microscopic evaluation.
6. Explain in details about physical method of drug evaluation.
7. Explain various leaves constant.
8. Explain various analytical methods of drug evaluation.

Short Essays:
1. Explain modern Pharmacognosy.
2. Explain the scope of Pharmacognosy.
3. Explain the application of Pharmacognosy.
4. Explain various sources of drugs.
5. Note on marine sources of drugs.
6. Explain taxonomic classification of crude drugs.
7. Note on Serotaxonomy.
8. Explain various types of Adulteration.
9. Explain substitution and their reason.
10. Explain various method of detection of adulteration with examples.
11. Explain chemical method of drug evaluation.
12. Explain biological method of drug evaluation.
13. Explain Camera Lucida with it scales.
14. Explain Stomata and Trichomes.
15. Note on spectroscopic method of drug evaluation.

Multiple Choice Questions (MCQs):
1. The meaning of "Pharmakon" is ......
   - (a) Knowledge
   - (b) Science
   - (c) Drug
   - (d) Application
2. The meaning of "Gnosis" is ......
   - (a) Knowledge
   - (b) Science
   - (c) Drug
   - (d) Herbal
3. The father of Pharmacognosy is ......
   - (a) Schmidt
   - (b) Crr. A. Seydler
   - (c) Charaka
   - (d) Shen Nung

4. The name Pharmacognosy coined in the year ......
   - (a) 1811
   - (b) 1851
   - (c) 1815
   - (d) 1814
5. The term Pharmacognosy is explained in book ......
   - (a) Medicine
   - (b) Pentaso
   - (c) Analecta Pharmacognostica
   - (d) Materia Medica
6. Mineral originated crude drug is ......
   - (a) Gelatin
   - (b) Talc
   - (c) Silk
   - (d) Coal
7. The name of the book that written by Scientist Shen Nung is ......
   - (a) Pentaso
   - (b) Materia Medica
   - (c) Pharmakognosie
   - (d) Medicine
8. Extraction of chemical constituent from plant was first carried out by ......
   - (a) Pikaso
   - (b) Charaka
   - (c) Galen
   - (d) Sushrutha
9. Anatomical Atlas of crude drugs was published in the year ......
   - (a) 1856
   - (b) 1815
   - (c) 1862
   - (d) 1865
10. First binomial classification of plants given by ......
    - (a) Bentham
    - (b) Hooker
    - (c) Bentham and Hooker
    - (c) Carl Linnaeus
11. The creator of science of genetics of plant is ......
    - (a) Gregor Mendel
    - (b) Galen
    - (c) Hooker
    - (d) Bentham
12. The father of medicine is ......
    - (a) Theophrastus
    - (b) Aristotle
    - (c) Hippocrates
    - (d) Charaka
13. Animal Kingdom was first written by ......
    - (a) Theophrastus
    - (b) Aristotle
    - (c) Hippocrates
    - (d) Charaka
14. "De Materia Medica" was written by ......
    - (a) Aristotle
    - (b) Elder
    - (c) Dioscorides
    - (d) Hippocrates
15. Penicillin was discovered by ......
    - (a) Alexander Fleming
    - (b) Willium Fleming
    - (c) Flory
    - (d) Calvin
16. Warren Weaver is famous for the discovery of ......
    - (a) Biology
    - (b) Genetics
    - (c) Molecular biology
    - (d) Biochemistry
17. The term Nanotechnology was first given in 1974 by ......
    - (a) Norio Taniguchi
    - (b) Drexler
    - (c) Elder
    - (d) Sakaguchi

18. Nutraceutical was first coined by ......
    (a) Stephen DeFelice
    (b) Drexler
    (c) Elder
    (d) Norio Taniguchi
19. Biomarker of *Withania ssomnifera* is ......
    (a) Withanin
    (b) Withanolide
    (c) Withanolide-D
    (d) Withaferin
20. The plant is having multiple stems and shorter height is known as ......
    (a) Herb
    (b) Shrub
    (c) Creeper
    (d) Tree
21. Leaf based crude drug is ......
    (a) Belladona
    (b) Clove
    (c) Vinca
    (d) Cinchona
22. Eugenol is the plant constituent of ......
    (a) Amla
    (b) Hibiscus
    (c) Senna
    (d) Clove
23. Bark containing plant drug is ......
    (a) Castor
    (b) Cinchona
    (c) Mango
    (d) Mustard
24. Stem containing crude drug is ......
    (a) Honey
    (b) Ashwagandha
    (c) Ephedra
    (c) Ipecac
25. Cochineal product is procured from ......
    (a) Human
    (b) Female insect
    (c) Cod Fish
    (d) Shark
26. Cephalostatin is the drug obtained from ......
    (a) Sea Hare
    (b) Tube worm
    (c) Mollusk
    (d) Bryozoan
27. Ara-A drug is used for the treatment of ......
    (a) Anticancer
    (b) Analgesic
    (c) Antiviral
    (d) Soft tissue sarcome
28. Resin containing crude drug is ......
    (a) Rosemary
    (b) Linseed
    (c) Storax
    (d) Yeast
29. Cocoa butter is adulterated with ......
    (a) Paraffin
    (b) Lime stone
    (c) Lard
    (d) Kokum butter
30. Almond oil is adulterated with ......
    (a) Coconut oil
    (b) Cotton seed oil
    (c) Linseed oil
    (d) Palm oil
31. *Mucuna Pruriens* is adulterated with ......
    (a) *Canavalia virosa*
    (b) *Mucuna utilis*
    (c) *Mucuna Virosa*
    (d) *Mucuna alata*

32. Prism is present in ......
    (a) Abbe camera lucida   (b) Swift Ives camera lucida
    (c) Both   (d) None
33. Diacytic stomata present in ......
    (a) Datura   (b) Digitalis
    (c) Senna   (d) Peppermint
34. Anomocytic stomata present in ......
    (a) Datura   (b) Digitalis
    (c) Senna   (d) Peppermint
35. Paracytic stomata is ......
    (a) Guard cell is covered by two subsidiary cells on right angle
    (b) Stomata two guard cells covered by two subsidiary cells
    (c) Two guard cells are surrounded by radiating subsidiary cells
    (d) Four guard cells are surrounded by radiating subsidiary cells
36. Stomata of senna is ......
    (a) Diacytic   (b) Paracytic
    (c) Anisocytic   (d) Actinocytic
37. Type of stomata present in Datura ......
    (a) Paracytic   (b) Actinocytic
    (c) Anisocytic   (d) Diacytic
38. Lignified trichome is present in ......
    (a) Belladona   (b) Digitalis
    (c) Nux vomica   (d) Tea
39. Multicellular branched trichome is present in ......
    (a) Belladona   (b) Lobelia
    (c) Pyrethrum   (d) Datura
40. Multicellular glandular trichome is present in ......
    (a) Datura   (b) Piper
    (c) Artimisia   (d) Digitalis
41. Hydathodes are present in ......
    (a) Vasaka   (b) Piper betel
    (c) Cannabis   (d) Coffee
42. Prism type calcium oxalate crystal is present in ......
    (a) Senna   (b) Digitalis
    (c) Clove   (d) Belladona
43. Rosette type calcium oxalate crystal is present in ......
    (a) Cinnamon   (b) Ipecac
    (c) Arjuna   (d) Cinchona
44. Haemolytic activity is carried out for ......
    (a) Cardiac glycoside   (b) Saponin glycoside
    (c) Cyanogenetic glycoside   (d) Flavonoids

45. Swelling index is carried out for ......
    - (a) Isphagula
    - (b) Digitalis
    - (c) Clove
    - (d) Aloes

ANSWERS

1. (c)	2. (a)	3. (b)	4. (c)	5. (c)	6. (b)	7. (a)	8. (c)	9. (d)
10. (d)	11. (a)	12. (c)	13. (b)	14. (c)	15. (a)	16. (c)	17. (a)	18. (a)
19. (c)	20. (b)	21. (a)	22. (d)	23. (b)	24. (c)	25. (b)	26. (b)	27. (c)
28. (c)	29. (a)	30. (b)	31. (b)	32. (b)	33. (d)	34. (b)	35. (b)	36. (b)
37. (c)	38. (c)	39. (c)	40. (d)	41. (b)	42. (c)	43. (c)	44. (b)	45. (a)

✸✸✸

$Unit ... 2$

CULTIVATION, COLLECTION, PROCESSING AND STORAGE OF DRUGS OF NATURAL ORIGIN

♦ LEARNING OBJECTIVES ♦

After completing this unit, reader should be able to:

❖ Know about the detail study of cultivation of medicinal and aromatic plants.

❖ Know about various factors influencing cultivation.

❖ Know about plant hormones and their application.

❖ Know about the collection procedure of crude drugs.

❖ Know about processing of crude drugs.

❖ Know about various storage conditions of crude drugs.

❖ Know about gene manipulation for crop improvement.

❖ Know about various methods for conservation of medicinal plants.

2.1 CULTIVATION AND COLLECTION OF DRUGS OF NATURAL ORIGIN

Medicinal plants have curative properties due to the presence of various complex chemical substances of different composition, which are found as secondary plant metabolites in one or more parts of these plants. These plant metabolites, according to their composition, are grouped as alkaloids, glycosides, corticosteroids, essential oils, etc. World Health Organization (WHO) has estimated that at least 85% of the world population relies on traditional systems of medicine for their primary health needs. These systems are largely plant-based. According to WHO, over 21000 plant species are useful in the preparation of medicines. Due to the growing awareness about side effects and complications of chemical and synthetic medicines, cosmetics and health supplements, usage of herbal products has gained importance both in the Eastern and Western Worlds. It is estimated that more than 70,000 plant species, from lichens to towering trees, have been used at one time or another for medicinal purposes. The herbs provide the starting material for the isolation or synthesis of conventional drugs. India is endowed with a rich wealth of medicinal plants, which ranked our country in the list of top producers of herbal medicines. The varied agro-climate conditions in India make this suitable for growing a wide range and variety of valuable medicinal plants. This production of medicinal plants generates increased employment opportunities for the farmers and enhances their incomes. But due to over population and other conditions, the total forest area is reducing, which has reduced the total cultivation/ collection of medicinal plants in India. We may lose the wealth of medicinal plants if this deforestation continues, which will affect the growth of our economy. Therefore, it is essential to cultivate at large scale and to conserve heritage of medicinal plants. Recently Indian Government has set up a national level body, the NMPB (National Medicinal Plant Board) for the growth and development of medicinal plant sectors in the country. General guidelines on good agricultural practices (GAP) for medicinal plants are required to distribute to all the growing sectors, which describes general principles and provides technical details for the cultivation of medicinal plants, their quality control measures, where applicable. We are still at the developing stage with regard to cultivation of medicinal plants because there is no standard operation procedure for the cultivation in India. Indian farmers are facing various problems in cultivation of medicinal plants because of lack of proper agro-technology, high fees for packages developed by various organizations, lack of reliable and standardized technology package, lack of planting material, market potential and system, cultivated wild plants, organic farming techniques, etc. Knowledge of post-harvest processing technology of plants for the extraction of chemicals and preparations of active formulation is still needed. Various aspects of medicinal plant cultivation include old philosophies, modern impact of traditional medicines and methods of assessing the spontaneous flora for industrial utilization, climatic variations, biological assessment, formulation, process technologies, phytochemical research and information sources. Indian herbal Industry is at blooming stage, but supply of raw materials through cultivation of medicinal plants is very difficult in all the seasons. In India, various medicinal plants are cultivated and domesticated, therefore, International trade is looking to procure medicinal plant materials from India for the production of pharmaceutical, nutraceutical and cosmeticeutical preparations.

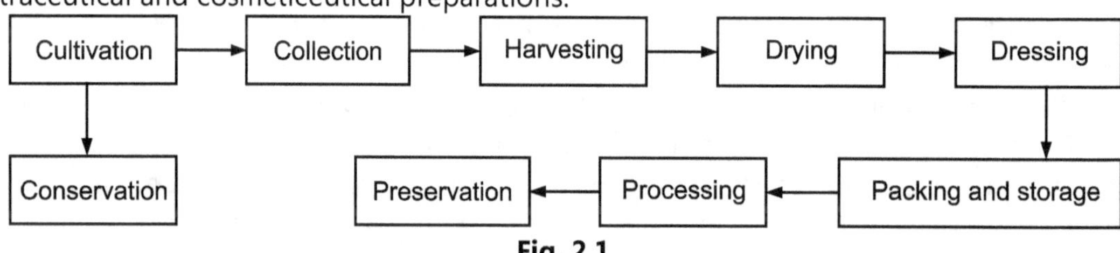

Fig. 2.1

2.2 CONCEPT OF GOOD AGRICULTURAL PRACTICES (GAPs)

These are specific methods which, when applied to agriculture, produce results that are in harmony with the values of the proponents of those practices.

Objectives:
1. Ensuring safety and quality of produce in the food chain.
2. Capturing new market advantages by modifying supply chain governance.
3. Improving natural resources use, workers health and working conditions.
4. Creating new market opportunities for farmers and exporters in developing countries.

Cultivation:

It is a scientific approach to healthy growth of medicinal plant in large scale. The growth is defined as progressive development of the organs with respect to various factors.

Some of the advantages of cultivations are:

(1) Cultivation ensures quality and purity of medicinal plants.
(2) It gives better healthy yield and therapeutic effects.
(3) It minimizes biodiversity.
(4) It supplies the raw materials to the industries throughout the year.
(5) It provides disease free plants.
(6) It increases industrialization and helps in unemployment problem.

General Steps for Cultivation of Plants:

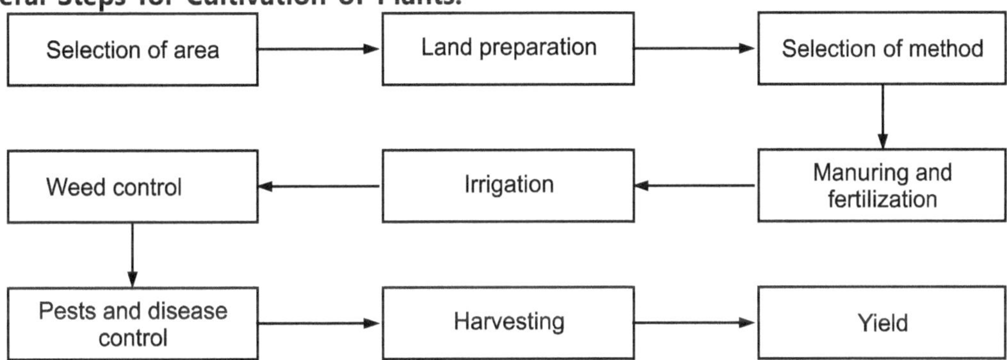

Fig. 2.2: General steps for cultivation of medicinal plants

Methods of cultivation: Generally two types of cultivation are possible.

(a) Sexual method: In this method plants are cultivated from the seeds and such plants are called seedlings. This method is also known as seed propagation. Generally good quality seeds of high germination rate should be used for cultivation. Seeds should be free from other seeds and impurities. Examples: Mango, Lichi, Methi, Coriander, papaya, tomato.

Advantages:
- It is an easy method to cultivate plants.
- It gives high yields.
- It gives more number of varieties.
- It is applicable for both monocot and dicot plants.

Disadvantages:
- Sometimes it takes more time to grow.
- Hybrid plant may not get.
- Healthy plants may not get from the same field.
- Asymmetric growth of the plants may occur.

(b) Asexual method: Vegetative part of plant, such as steam or root, is placed in such an environment that develops new plant. Examples: Jasmine, sugarcane, potato, banana, rose.

Advantages:
- It gives high yield.
- It develops hybrid plants.
- It gives fruits and flowers throughout the year.
- Quality of cultivated plant can improve.
- This method is more useful for monocot plants.

Disadvantages:
- It requires a skilled person.
- Initially temperature and soil nature have to be controlled.
- This method is time consuming.

2.3 FACTORS INFLUENCING CULTIVATION OF MEDICINAL PLANTS

The most important parameter is factors on which the growth, variation of plant species depends. It also affects the quantity of the medicinally active compounds present in the plants and this greatly depends on the plant size. The variation depends on various factors (Fig. 2.3).

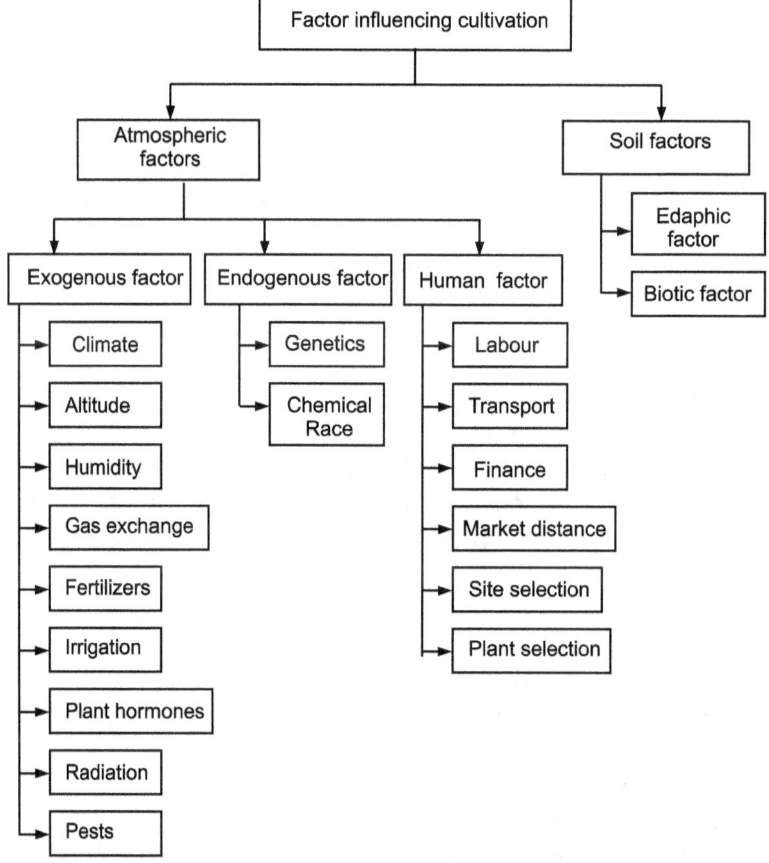

Fig. 2.3: Factors affecting cultivation of medicinal plants

An auxanometer is an apparatus for measuring increase or rate of growth in plants.

2.3.1 Atmospheric Factors

2.3.1.1 Exogenous Factors

• **Climate and Light:** Plant should be cultivated in conditions which are similar to the plant's natural habitat. Hence climate that is temperature, rainfall and length of day, plays an important role in the growth of plants. Different crops require different climatic patterns. Most of the plants can grow well in sunny, dry conditions.

Examples: In cloudy weather the amount of carbohydrates in leaves is decreased, since photosynthesis is light-dependent. As carbohydrates serve as the initial starting material for biosynthesis, their abundance affects the amount of secondary metabolites. Changes in temperature may also influence plant growth by affecting the rate of chemical reactions. Excessive temperature as well as frost also affects the growth, quality and metabolism of the medicinal plants. High temperature leads to death of the plants and low temperature infects the plants by microorganisms. Alkaloids content become lower in *Datura stramonium* during cloudy/rainy weather, volatile oils are produced more readily in warmer weather, yet very hot days lead to a physical loss of oil; growing peppermint in shade rather than the sun. The contents of alkaloids in Stramonium leaves lower in rainy and cloudy weather. For seed germination temperature should be 15–20°C. Optimum temperature for propagation is 18–28°C in which day temperature should be 21–27°C and night temperature 15°C.

• **Latitude and Altitude:** The effect of latitude is important in fat producing plants. Tropical plants (palm oil, cocao butter) contain mainly saturated fatty acids, while the subtropical plants give a larger amount of unsaturated acids. The olive, almond and sesame oils are predominant in oleic acid. The plants of temperate zones (Cottonseed, sunflower) also contain more unsaturated acids. Peanut and olive trees grown in the subtropics have a higher unsaturated fat content.

Examples: *Cinchona succirubra* grows well at low levels but alkaloids are not produced. The bitter constituents of *Gentiana lutea* are increased with altitude. The alkaloids of *Aconitum napellus* and *Lobellia inflata and* the oil content of Thyme and Peppermint decrease with altitude. Pyrethrum gives the best yields of flower-heads and pyrethrins at high altitudes on Equator (East Africa).

• **Humidity:** Humidity refers to the amount of vapour that the air holds at a given time. It is usually expressed as a percentage in relation to the maximum amount of water vapour that the air will hold at current temperatures. There are three main measurements of humidity: absolute, relative and specific. Absolute humidity is the water content of air. Relative humidity is the ratio of actual water vapour content to the saturated water vapour content at a given temperature and pressure expressed in percentage (%). Specific humidity is a ratio of the water vapour content of the mixture to the total air content on a mass basis. Humidity has a major impact upon the overall performance and final yield of the plants grown indoors.

Examples: Optimum Humidity for plant growth is 50-80%; high humidity encourages the spread of fungal diseases, whereas low humidity increases transpiration. The mean maximum relative humidity occurs in the early morning, whereas mean minimum, relative humidity occurs in the early afternoon. There are various devices used to measure and regulate humidity. A device used to measure humidity is called a psychrometer or hygrometer. Relative humidity (RH) directly influences the water relations of plant and indirectly affects leaf growth, photosynthesis, pollination, occurrence of diseases and finally economic yield. The dryness of the atmosphere as represented by saturation deficit (100-RH) reduces dry matter production through stomatal control and leaf water potential.

• **Gas exchange:** In order to carry on photosynthesis, green plants need a supply of carbon dioxide and a means of disposing of oxygen. In order to carry on cellular respiration, plant cells need oxygen and a means of disposing of carbon dioxide. Roots, stems and leaves respire at rates much lower than are characteristic of animals. Only during photosynthesis are large volumes of gases exchanged and each leaf is well- adapted to take care of its own needs. Oxygen and carbon dioxide also pass through the cell wall and plasma membrane of the cell by diffusion. High respiration rate occurs with seed germination and during advantageous root formation at the base of cuttings, so it requires more oxygen and removal of CO_2. The exchange of oxygen and carbon dioxide in the leaf occurs through pores known as stomata. Gas exchange will occur through the moist epidermal layers of the young roots. Oxygen from the soil will diffuse into the cells while carbon dioxide diffuses out of the cells into the soil. In lower plants (and also protozoans) exchange of gases takes place through the general body surface as they are not highly modified or specialized. Also, the body surface allows the diffusion of gases.

• **Fertilization:** Fertilizer dosage has to be dependent on growing media. Soilless mixes have lower nutrient holding capacity and therefore require more frequent fertilizer application. Essential elements are at their maximum availability in the pH range of 5.5 to 6.5. In general microelements are more readily available at lower pH ranges, while macroelements are more readily available at pH 6 and higher. Recently nano-fertilizers are demanded for improvement of the crop yield. Nano-fertilizers may be defined as the nanoparticles, which can directly/augment supply of essential nutrients for plant growth, have higher nutrient use efficiency and can be delivered in timely manner to a rhizosphere target or by foliar spray.

Examples: *Slow release nano nitrogen fertilizer:* Nano zeolite impregnated with urea causes slow and steady release of N. NH^+ ions occupying the internal channels of zeoloite slowly set free N allowing progressive absorption by the medicinal plants.

Slow release nano phosphate fertilizer: Surface modified zeolite (SMZ) has been found to be a well sorbent for PO^{-3} and slow release of P is achievable.

Uptake of nano micronutrients: Application of Zn nanoparticles (< 100 nm) at relatively lower level (0.28 ppm) enhanced the growth of maize plant as compared to normal zinc sulphate (0.5 ppm). The plant height, root growth and volume, dry matter weight can also improve with application of zinc oxide nanoparticles.

• **Irrigation and drainage:** Irrigation and drainage should be controlled and carried out in accordance with the needs of the individual medicinal plant species during its various stages of growth. Water used for irrigation purposes should comply with local, regional and/or national quality standards in order to ensure that the plants under cultivation are neither over- nor under-watered. First light irrigation is required during land preparation and initial sowing of the seeds. It gives fast germination rate to get plantlets.

- **Plant hormones:** Plant hormones are signal molecules produced within the plant cells. They occur in extremely low concentrations but exert strong control over plant development. They act either locally or in more distant part of the plant. There are several types of plant hormones available viz. auxin, gibberellin, cytokinin, ethylene and abscisic acid. These hormones work together or independently to influence plant growth.

- **Radiation:** Solar radiation plays an important role as regulator and controller of growth and development. Solar energy provides light required for seed germination, leaf expansion, growth of stem and shoot, flowering, fruiting and thermal conditions necessary for the physiological functions of the plant. Solar radiation also influences assimilation of nutrient and dry matter distribution. Plants require solar radiation for photosynthesis and their growth rate is proportional to the amount received, assuming that other environmental parameters are not limiting. Visible light is a composite of wavelengths between 400 and 700 nanometers (nm) and this specific waveband is defined as PAR (Photosynthetically Active Radiation). PAR consists of wavelengths that are utilized by the plant biochemical processes in photosynthesis to convert light energy into biomass. Light energy can also be defined in radiometric units, which is measured with a pyranometer. Solar radiation may be measured in radiometric units (Wm^{-2}) to determine its total energy value, or it may be measured in quantum terms (mmol s^{-1} m^{-2}) for calculation of the amount of the sunlight specifically available for plant growth during a specific growth period (mol m^{-2}). Radiation energy has three components (a) quality (b) intensity and (c) duration of light. They influence the physiological process of the plants for the healthy growth. The quality (wavelength and colour), quantity (the intensity and duration of exposure to light) greatly influence the plant growth. Quality refers to the wavelength and colour. Of the total range of electromagnetic wavelengths in the solar spectrum, light or the luminous energy includes wavelengths between 400- 750 mm (milli microns) or nm (nanometers). Quantity of light is measured in g cal/ m^2/year. Lux: It is luminous flux per unit area which is equal to one lumen per square metre. The intensity of light has much effect on the uptake of phosphorus and potassium. Oxygen intake increases with the increase of light intensity. Some species of plant produce more active constituents at night like *Nicotiana tobacum*; *Ocimum basilicum* grown in glasshouses have less phenol and terpenoids in the leaves. On the basis of reaction to the photoperiod, the plants are classified as short day, long day and intermediate day plants. Short day plant: Tobacco, menthofuran; long day: grains, menthone, menthol; intermediate day: cotton.

- **Pests:** Reduction in the quantity of the crude drugs also depends on the pests and their attack. The huge losses due to pest infestation tune to lakhs of rupees every year due to less medicinal values. Pests are detrimental for the plants and thus controlling them during cultivation of medicinal plants is essential. These pests include fungi, viruses, weeds, insects and rodents (non insect pests). Example of fungal pests are *Pythium spinosum* (rhizome rot), *Currularia prasadii* (leaf blight), *Septoria digitalis* (leaf spot), *Cercospora rauwolfiae* (leaf spot) etc. Fungus on henbane lowers the alkaloid content. Some of the viruses like tobacco mosaic virus, cucumber mosaic virus and tobacco ring spot virus attack the digitalis plant. Several insects can also cause problem in the growth of the plants, e.g., *Diaphania nilgirica* attack Rauwolfia plant, *Phytomyza atricornis* attack Menthe plants etc. Weeds are also considered as dreadful pests that are undesired plants. They can resist the growth of the original plants. Some weeds also causes allergies e.g., hey fever caused by ragweed, asthma cause by parthenium etc. Non-insect pests like rats, monkeys, birds, snails, mites, crabs also spoil the stored crude drugs.

There are some methods available to control the pests:

1.   **Mechanical method:** During preliminary stages they can be controlled by hand picking, pruning, burning and trapping.

2.   **Agricultural method:** Advanced breeding techniques are capable of gene manipulation in different stages of the plant growth to get disease free healthy plants. These methods include hybridization, polyploidy, mutation and chemical races. To control weeds, ploughing should be deep as possible so that up-rootation of the weeds is possible. Crop rotation also helps to minimize the attack of the pests.

3.   **Biological control:** This is very useful method by combating the pests with other living organisms. Example, the chemical substances produced (7,8-epoxy-2-methyloctadecane) and released by gypsy moth are capable to elicit sexual response from the opposite sex and that can control the pests. Mexican brittle can control the parthenium by sucking the root sap of parthenium weeds; Australian lady bug feeds on damaging insect called cottony cushion scale insect on citrus crop etc.

4.   **Chemical control:** The use of chemical pesticides also helps to control the pests like insecticides, fungicides, herbicides and rodenticides. When necessary, only approved pesticides and herbicides should be applied at the minimum effective level, in accordance with the labelling and/or package insert instructions of the individual product and the regulatory requirements that apply for the grower and the end-user countries.

Some examples are Rodenticides: Warfarin, strychnine red squill etc. Insecticides: DDT, parathion, gammaxine etc. Fungicides: Bordeaux mixture, chlorophenols etc; Herbicides: 2,4-dichlorophenoxy acetic acid, calcium arsenate etc.

2.3.1.2 Endogenous Factors

•   **Genetic factors:** Genetic differences are responsible for morphological variety and biochemical diversity. Information on genetic divergence is essential for sustained genetic improvement of a crop. Genetic markers are used for the improvement of the crop production. They represent genetic differences between individual organisms or species. Molecular markers are being increasingly used for divergence studies and are known as genotypic markers. They do not affect the phenotype of the trait of interest because they are located only near or linked to genes controlling the trait. All genetic markers occupy specific genomic positions within chromosomes called loci. They are of three types.

(1)   Morphological markers, which themselves are phenotypic traits or characters.

(2)   Biochemical markers, which include allelic variants of enzymes called isozymes.

(3)   DNA markers, which reveal sites of variation in DNA. They are of three types: RFLP (Restriction Fragment Length Polymorphism), polymerease chain reaction based on

RAPD (Random Amplified Polymorphic DNA) and DNA sequence based on SNP (Single Nucleotide Polymorphism).

Application: This method is (1) used for characterization and identification of cultivars, varieties and natural populations; (2) used to understand the genetic variability of population; (3) provides protection of variety by fingerprinting; (4) determines the phylogenetic relationships between species and (5) assesses varietal uniformity.

- **Chemical races:** It is also known as chemodemes. They are regarded as a group of plants of a species which have identical morphological characters, but differ in their chemical nature. Hence chemodemes are considered as chemically separate groups within species. The chemical characters of chemodemes are hereditary. Genotype and phenotype are together responsible for chemical races. Genotype refers to the genetic traits in an organism. Current methods of genotyping include restriction fragment length polymorphism identification (RFLP) of genomic DNA, random amplified polymorphic detection (RAPD) of genomic DNA, amplified fragment length polymorphism detection (AFLPD), polymerase chain reaction (PCR), DNA sequencing, allele specific oligonucleotide (ASO) probes and hybridization to DNA microarrays or beads. Phenotype refers to observable, physical manifestations of an organism.

  Examples: *Withania somnifera* has three chemical races, Chemotype I and II contains same compounds withaferin and chemotype III contain withanolides, where both these active constituents have different medicinal action. Chemical races have also been reported in *Claviceps purpurea, Digitalis purpurea, Digitalis lanata, Cinnamomum zeylanicum, Ocimum sanctum* etc.

2.3.1.3 Human Factors

- **Labours:** All farms need either human labour or machinery to do the work. Some farm types use very little labour, e.g. sheep farming. Others require a large labour force, e.g., rice farming in India.

- **Market:** This is the customer who buys farm produce. Farmers need to sell their crops and animals to make a profit. Perishable crops such as soft fruits fetch a high price, but need to be grown with a short travelling distance of the market.

- **Finance:** Profits are used to pay the wages and to re-invest in the farm e.g., buying seeds, fertilizer, machinery and animals. This is known as feedback within the farming system.

- **Transport:** Transportation is an economic factor of production of goods and services, implying that relatively small changes can have substantial impacts in on costs, locations and performance. It provides market accessibility by linking producers and consumers. Improvements in transportation and communication favor a process of geographical specialization that increases productivity and spatial interactions.

- **Site selection:** Medicinal plant materials derived from the same species can show significant differences in quality when cultivated at different sites, owing to the influence of soil, climate and other factors. These differences may relate to physical appearance or to variations in their constituents, the biosynthesis of which may be affected by extrinsic environmental conditions, including ecological and geographical variables and should be taken into consideration.

- **Selection of plants:** The species or botanical variety selected for cultivation should be the same as that specified in the national pharmacopoeia or recommended by other authoritative national documents. In the absence of such national documents, the selection of species or botanical varieties specified in the pharmacopoeia or other authoritative documents of other countries should be considered. In the case of newly introduced medicinal plants, the species or botanical variety selected for cultivation should be identified and documented as the source material used or described in traditional medicine of the original country.

2.3.2 Soil Factors

Soil plays an important role in plant growth. It is classified into two types viz. edaphic and biotic factors (Fig. 2.4).

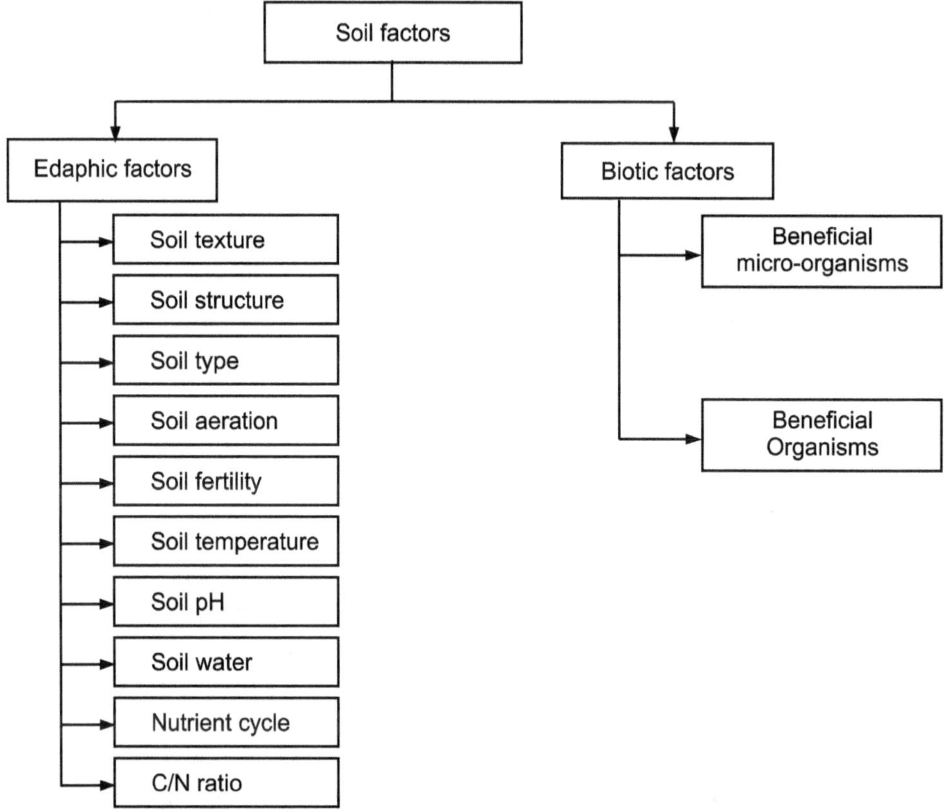

Fig. 2.4: Soil factors

2.3.2.1 Edaphic Factors

- **Soil texture:** It is a qualitative rather than a quantitative tool; it is a fast, simple and effective means to assess the physical characteristics of the soil. It can be determined by proportion of soil through sand, clay, slit and water holding capacity of the soil. This is used to determine crop suitability and to approximate the soils responses to environmental and management conditions such as drought or calcium (lime) requirements. Soil texture has an important role in nutrient management because it influences nutrient retention. For instance, finer textured soils tend to have greater ability to store soil nutrients. Knowing the soil texture alone will provide information about: (1) water flow potential, (2) water holding capacity, (3) fertility potential and (4) suitability for many urban uses like bearing capacity.

- **Soil structure:** Soil structure is the arrangement of soil particles into groupings. These groupings are called aggregates, which often form distinctive shapes typically found within certain soil horizons. For example, granular soil particles are characteristic of the surface horizon. Soil aggregation is an important indicator of the workability of the soil. Soils that are well aggregated are said to have "good soil tilth." The various types of soil structures are given below:

- **Soil aggregates:** Generally, only very small particles form aggregates, which include silicate clays, volcanic ash, minerals, organic matter and oxides. There are various mechanisms of soil aggregation.

Mechanisms of Soil Aggregation:

- Soil microorganisms excrete substances that act as cementing agents and bind soil particles together.

- Fungi have filaments, called hyphae, which extend into the soil and tie soil particles together.

- Roots also excrete sugars into the soil that help bind minerals.

- Finally, soil particles may naturally be attracted to one another through electrostatic forces, much like the attraction between hair and a balloon.

- The soil structure greatly depends on the soil profile.

Soil profile: The soil profile is an important tool in nutrient management. By examining a soil profile, we can gain valuable insight into soil fertility. As the soil weathers and/or organic matter decomposes, the profile of the soil changes. The soil profile is made up of distinct layers, known as horizons. They are natural layers of the soil, which vary in thickness, depending upon the location and have somewhat irregular boundaries (Fig. 2.5).

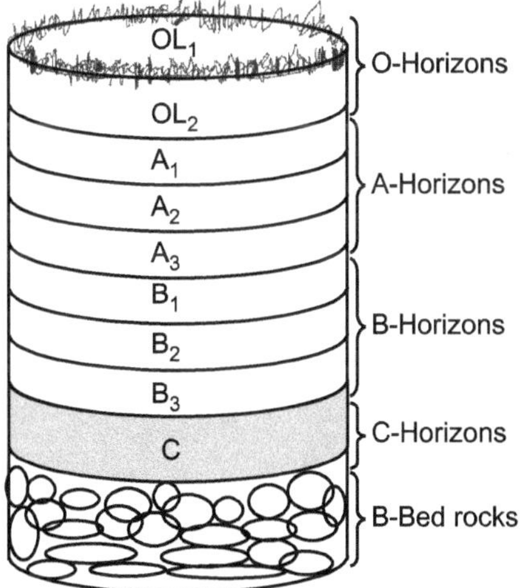

Fig. 2.5: Soil profile

O horizon: The "O" stands for organic. It is a surface layer dominated by the presence of large amounts of organic material in varying stages of decomposition. The O horizon should be considered distinct from the layer of leaf litter covering many heavily vegetated areas, which contains no weathered mineral particles and is not part of the soil itself. It contains high percentage of dead organic matter. This horizon is divided into OL_1 and OL_2 where OL_1 contains decomposed matter (on the surface of the soil) and OL_2 contains well decomposed organic matters which is not visible.

A horizon: The A horizon is the top layer of the soil horizons or 'top soil'. This layer has a layer of dark decomposed organic materials, which is called "humus". "A" Horizons may be darker in colour than deeper layers and contain more organic material or they may be lighter but contain less clay or sesquioxides. This layer is subdivided into A_1, A_2 and A_3. A_2 layer is known as washing out of clay. A_3 layer is intermediate layer between A and B. In this horizon most biological activity occurs. Soil organisms such as earthworms, potworms (enchytraeids), arthropods, nematodes, fungi and many species of bacteria and archaea are concentrated here, often in close association with plant roots. Thus the A horizon may be referred to as the biomantle.

B horizon: The B horizon is commonly referred to as "subsoil" and consists of mineral layers which may contain concentrations of clay or minerals such as iron or aluminium oxides or organic material moved there by leaching. Accordingly, this layer is also known as the "illuviated" horizon or the "zone of accumulation". This layer is also divided into three sub layers viz. B_1, B_2 and B_3. Plant roots penetrate through this layer, but it has very little humus. It is usually brownish or red because of the clay and iron oxides washed down from A horizon.

C horizon: The C horizon is simply named so because it comes after A and B within the soil profile. This layer is little affected by soil forming processes (weathering) and the lack of pedological development is one of the defining attributes. The C Horizon may contain lumps or more likely large shelves of unweathered rock, rather than being made up solely of small fragments as in the solum. "Ghost" rock structure may be present within these horizons. The C horizon also contains parent material. It forms the framework of the soil. The *A* and *B* layers are formed by this layer.

Bed rocks: This is the layer of partially weathered at the base of the soil profile. Unlike the above layers, this layer largely comprises continuous masses (as opposed to boulders) of hard rock that cannot be excavated by hand. Soils formed *in-situ* will exhibit strong similarities to this bedrock layer.

- **Soil types:** Soil type usually refers to the different sizes of mineral particles in a particular sample. Soil is made up in part of finely ground rock particles, grouped according to size as sand and slit in addition to clay and humus, organic material such as decomposed plant matter. The largest particles, sand, determine aeration and drainage characteristics, while the tiniest, sub-microscopic clay particles are chemically active, binding with water and plant nutrients. The ratio of these sizes determines soil type: clay, loam, clay-loam, silt-loam and so on.

Properties of Some Important Soils:

Sandy Soil:
- The soil is made of a greater proportion of big particles.
- They cannot fit closely together.
- There are large spaces between them. These spaces are filled with air.

- Water absorption is very high as the water passes quickly through these spaces.
- These soils are light, well aerated and dry.

Clay Soil:
- It is made of a relatively high proportion of fine particles.
- They have very less space between particles.
- Water can be trapped in the tiny gaps between them due to smaller size.
- Clay soils are heavy and hold more water.

Loamy Soil:
- It is a mixture of sand, soil and silt.
- Silt particles are present between the particles of sand and soil.
- This soil is considered the best for the growth of plants due to presence of humus.
- The percolation rate is between that of sandy soil and clay soil.

The different types of Indian soil are:

Alluvial Soils: This includes the deltaic alluvium calcareous alluvial soils, Coastal alluvium and Coastal sands. It is the most important soil group of India contributing the largest share to its agricultural wealth. This soil is derived from the deposition laid by the numerous tributaries of the Indus, Ganges and the Brahmputra systems.

Black Soils: These soils vary in depth from shallow to deep. The typical soil derived from Deccan trap is the "Regur" or black cotton soil. It is common in Maharashtra, Western parts of Madhya Pradesh, A.P., Gujarat and Tamil Nadu.

Red Soils: The ancient crystalline and metamorphic rocks on meteoric weathering have given rise to the red soils. The red colour is due to the wide diffusion of iron rather than to a high proportion of it. The soils comprise vast areas of Tamil Nadu, Karnataka, Goa, Daman and Diu, M. P., Orissa, Jharkhand, Bihar, West Bengal, U. P. etc.

Desert Soils: The most predominant component of this soil is quartz. Some of these soils contain high percentage of soluble salts, high pH, a very high percentage of calcium carbonate, but are poor in organic matter.

Problem Soils: These are the soils which owing to land and soil characteristics, cannot be economically used for the cultivation of crops without adopting proper reclamation measures.

Laterite Soil: The soil is mixture of hydrated oxides of aluminium and iron with small amount of manganese. This soil is poor in lime, magnesia and nitrogen but high in humus, P_2O_5.

Acid Soils: Soils having pH below 7 are considered to be the acidic, but those which have pH less than 5.5 and which respond to liming may be considered to qualify to be designated as acid soils. These occur widely in Himalayan region, Ganges delta and Peninsula.

- **Soil aeration:** Soil aeration is the mechanism of exchange of oxygen and carbon dioxide between soil pore space and the atmosphere in order to prevent the deficiency of oxygen and toxicity of carbon dioxide. Respiration by plant roots and microorganisms depletes oxygen and releases carbon dioxide and minute quantities of other gases into the soil atmosphere. The amount of carbon dioxide varies widely depending on temperature, organic matter and microbial respiration. A constant inflow of oxygen and out flow of carbon dioxide is essential for plant growth. Loosening a dense soil facilitates exchange of gases between soil air and atmosphere. Air filled pores commonly fluctuate from 15 to 30 per cent of the total volume depending upon water content, soil density and structure.

Causes of Poor Soil Aeration:
  (1) Compact soil.
  (2) Water logging.
  (3) Soils having excessive amount of readily decomposable organic matter.
  (4) Harmful effects of poor aeration.
  (5) Microbial activity is reduced, slow decomposition of organic matter.
  (6) Rhizobium cannot symbiotically fix atmospheric nitrogen.

• **Soil fertility:** Soil fertility is a complex process that involves the constant cycling of nutrients between organic and inorganic forms in the soil. As plant material and animal wastes decompose, they release nutrients to the soil solution. These nutrients may then undergo further transformations which may be aided or enabled by soil micro- organisms. Natural processes such as lightning strikes may fix atmospheric nitrogen by converting it to NO_2. Denitrification may occur under anaerobic conditions (flooding) in the presence of denitrifying bacteria. The cations, primarily phosphate and potash, as well as many micronutrients are held in relatively strong bonds with the negatively charged portions of the soil in a process known as cation exchange capacity. This helps in procuring the right fertilizers and choosing a suitable variety of seed in order to get the highest possible crop productivity.

Characters of Soil Fertility:
  ✓ It is rich in nutrients necessary for basic plant nourishment. This includes nitrogen, phosphorus and potassium.
  ✓ It consists of adequate minerals such as boron, chlorine, cobalt, copper, iron, manganese, magnesium, molybdenum, sulphur and zinc. These minerals promote plant nutrition.
  ✓ The soil fertility pH is in the range 6.0 to 6.8.
  ✓ It has a good soil fertility structure which results in well-drained soil fertility.
  ✓ It consists of a variety of microorganisms that support plant growth.

• **Soil temperature:** Soil temperature plays an important role in many processes, which take place in the soil such as chemical reactions and biological interactions. Soil temperature varies in response to exchange processes that take place primarily through the soil surface. These effects are propagated into the soil profile by transport processes and are influenced by such things as the specific heat capacity, thermal conductivity and thermal diffusivity. A denser and less reflective material increases the soil temperature by inhibiting evaporation. Soil temperature can serve as a useful guide for seeding operations. If the soil is too cool, germination is delayed, which results in seed damage and uneven or inadequate seeding emergence. Any thermometer that can measure temperature at a specific depth can be used to measure soil temperature.

Factors affecting Soil Temperature:
  ✓ **Solar radiation:** The amount of heat from the Sun that reaches the earth is $2.0 \text{ cal/cm}^2 \text{ min}^{-1}$. The amount of radiation received by the soil depends on angles with which the soil faces the Sun.

- ✓ **Condensation:** The heat increases whenever water vapour from soil depths or atmosphere condenses in the soil.
- ✓ **Evaporation:** The greater the rate of evaporation, the more the soil is cooled.
- ✓ **Rainfall:** Rainfall cools down the soil.
- ✓ **Colour of the soil:** Black coloured soils absorb more heat than light coloured soils. Hence, black colour soils are warmer than light coloured soils.
- ✓ **Moisture content:** A soil with a higher moisture content is cooler than dry soil.
- ✓ **Tillage:** The cultivated soil has greater temperature amplitude as compared to the uncultivated soil.
- ✓ **Soil texture:** Soil textures affect the thermal conductivity of soil. Thermal conductivity decreases with reduction in particle size.
- ✓ **Organic matter content:** Organic matter reduces the heat capacity and thermal conductivity of soil, increases its water holding capacity and has a dark colour, which increases its heat absorbability.

- **Soil pH:** The soil pH is a measure of the acidity or basicity in soils. pH is defined as the negative logarithm (base 10) of the activity of hydronium ions (H^+ or, more precisely, H_3O^+ aq.) in a solution. It ranges from 0 to 14, with 7 being neutral. A pH below 7 is acidic and above 7 is basic. The most common way of increasing soil pH is applying agricultural lime. Soil pH is considered a master variable in soils as it controls many chemical processes that take place. It specifically affects plant nutrient availability by controlling the chemical forms of the nutrient. The optimum pH range for most plants is between 6 and 7.5. Manganese (Mn) is an essential plant nutrient, so plants transport manganese into leaves but manganese toxicity symptoms are seen at pH below 5.6. In slightly to moderately alkaline soils, molybdenum and macronutrient (except for phosphorus) availability is increased, but P, Fe, Mn, Zn Cu and Co levels are reduced and may adversely affect plant growth. In acidic soils, micronutrient availability [except for Molybdenum (Mo) and Boron (Bo)] is increased. Concentrations of available N are less sensitive to pH than concentration of available Phosphorus (P). In order for P to be available for plants, soil pH needs to be in the range 6.0 and 7.5. If pH is lower than 6, P starts forming insoluble compounds with iron (Fe) and aluminium (Al) and if pH is higher than 7.5, P starts forming insoluble compounds with calcium (Ca). Most nutrient deficiencies are avoided between a pH ranges of 5.5 to 6.5. Soil pH is determined by using soil pH meter.

- **Soil water:** The rate of absorption is different for different types of soils. This phenomenon of absorption of water by soil is termed as percolation.

- **Percolation rate (mL/min):** Amount of water/percolation time.

- **Nutrient cycle:** The continuous recycling of nutrients into and out of the soil is known as the nutrient cycle. The cycle involves complex biological and chemical interactions. A simplified version of this cycle of plant growth has two parts: "inputs" that add plant nutrients to the soil and "outputs" that export them from the soil largely in the form of agricultural products. Nutrients are exported from the field through harvested crops and crop residues, as well as through leaching, atmospheric volatilization and erosion. The difference between the volume of inputs and outputs constitutes the nutrient balance.

Positive nutrient balances in the soils (occurring when nutrient additions to the soil are greater than the nutrients removed from the soil) indicate that farming systems are inefficient and, in the extreme, that they may be polluting the environment. Negative balances indicate that soils are being mined and that farming systems are unsustainable over the long term.

- **C/N ratio:** The C/N ratio (C : N) or carbon-to-nitrogen ratio is a ratio of the mass of carbon to the mass of nitrogen in a substance. It is used in analyzing sediments and compost. Carbon-to-nitrogen ratios are an indicator for nitrogen limitation of plants and other organisms. For practical agricultural purposes, compost should have an initial C/N ratio of 20-30 : 1. Examples: For soil microbes C/N ratio is 4 : 1 to 9 : 1; soil organic matter: 10 : 1 to 12 : 1 etc.

2.3.2.2 Biotic Factors

Biotic factor is defined as a factor created by a living thing or any living component within an environment in which the action of the organism affects the life of another organism. For example: a predator consuming its prey. A beneficial organism is any organism that benefits the growing process, including insects, arachnids, other animals, plants, bacteria, fungi, viruses and nematodes.

- **Beneficial soil microorganisms:** Microorganisms play a major role in the plant-soil relationship, particularly in the rhizosphere, i.e. the interface between root and soil. The majority of fungi and bacteria present in soils are considered to be beneficial to higher plants by: (a) direct association with roots (mycorrhizae, nodule forming bacteria); (b) breakdown and release of minerals from organic matter present in the soil resulting in essential element availability increased to higher plants; (c) parasitizing harmful or disease causing microorganisms or (d) suppressing growth, reproduction or activity of harmful disease causing microorganisms through other interactions such as chemical inhibition. They stimulate plant growth, help mineral nutrition and water uptake, fix nitrogen, protect plants against parasites. Mixed culture of beneficial microorganisms such as photosynthetic bacteria (*Rhodopseudomonas* sp), lactic acid bacteria (*lactobacillus* sp.), yeast (*saccharomyces* sp.) and fermenting fungi are positively improve the soil fertility as well as plant productivity.

- **Beneficial organisms:**

  Insects: Beneficial insects can include predators (such as lady bugs) of pest insects and pollinators (such as bees, which are an integral part of the growth cycle of many crops). Increasingly certain species of insects are managed and used to intervene where natural pollination or biological control is insufficient, usually due to human disturbance of the balance of nature. Brachonids, Chalcids and Ichneumon Wasps are small beneficial insects destroy leaf-eating caterpillars.

- **Nematodes:** Certain microscopic nematodes (worms) are beneficial in destroying and controlling populations of larvae that are damaging or deadly to crops and other plants. They are commonly used in organic gardening for their ability to kill various kinds of harmful larvae (fungus gnats, flea larvae, spider mites, weevils, grubs, rootworms, cutworms etc.).

Collection of Crude Drugs:

The collection of medicinal plants from wild populations can give rise to additional concerns related to global, regional and/or local over-harvesting and protection of endangered species. After cultivation of the plants it is essential to collect the plant parts for the next step of harvesting. Crude drugs are collected from wild or cultivated plants and hence proper selection of the plant parts and their proper collection give the improved quality of the plants. It even helps to increase the content of secondary metabolites in the plant parts. Hence drugs should be collected when they contain maximum amount of constituents in a highly scientific manner. Plant collections are important for:

1. Voucher specimens are the only verifiable record of the occurrence of a species in time and space.
2. The taxonomy of species is continually evolving. With herbarium specimens, species that have been subject to taxonomic change can be verified for an area without the expense of additional field work.
3. Even common species are sometimes misidentified in the field; less common species can be easily misidentified (lack of distinguishing features, lack of magnification, lack of time, large or difficult groups) or overlooked. Hence specimens should be collected and identified in a lab with all the tools and resources at hand.
4. The work of field professionals can be available to a wide audience through depositing specimens in a herbarium, as the specimens are available to many researchers, in many fields, the world over for hundreds of years to come.

There are several factors affecting the collection of plant parts (Fig. 2.6).

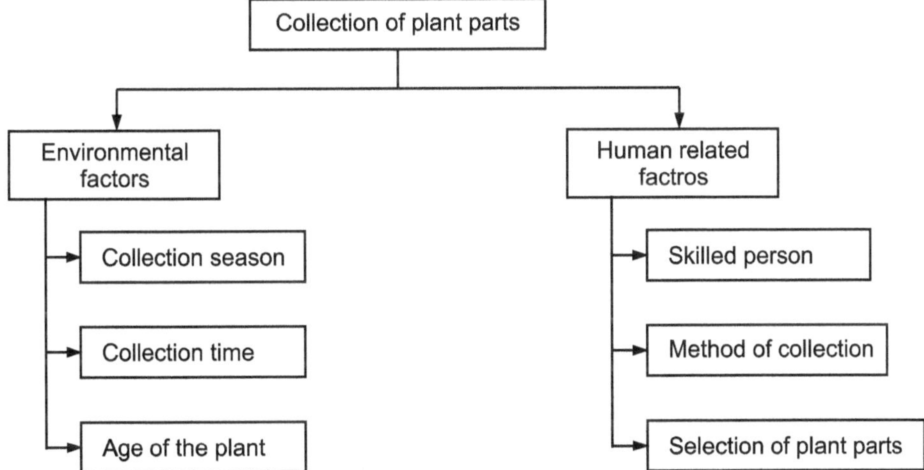

Fig. 2.6: Various factors affecting collection of crude drugs

Environmental Factors:

•   **Collection season:** Active constituents of herbs are affected by the seasons (due to climate, rainfall, day-length etc.). Medicinal plants should be therefore collected in the season in which their active constituents are highest. Example: Rhubarb (laxative) contains high anthranol in winter. This is then oxidized to anthroquinones in summer. Hence, it is collected in summer time. The entire plant of *Picrorrhiza kurroo* can be collected during July-August to March-April. Barks of Cinchona, Cinnamon, Cassia are collected either in spring or in autumn because the flow of sap is considered to be maximum at these times and barks readily detach from the wood. Sap is collected in the spring as it rises or as it tails in the autumn. e.g., *Betula pendula* produce huge quantities of sap during that time. Further the composition of a number of plant metabolites varies throughout the day and night due to interconversion is taking place at that time. Flowers are collected during spring or summer. Roots and rhizomes are collected during rainy season generally after three years of cultivation. Colchicum corm is free from bitterness and is devoid of the alkaloid colchicine in autumn. Bitterness starts to appear in spring and early summer when it is used as a drug.

- **Collection time:** The amount of a constituent is usually not constant throughout the life of a plant. The differences are sometimes not only quantitative but also qualitative. The stage at which a plant is collected is very important for maximizing the yield of the desired constituent. It is generally procured in the year or in the day. The composition of a number of secondary plant metabolites varies throughout the day and night due to some interconversion occurs in the plant body. The best time for collection (quality peak season or time of day) should be determined according to the quality and quantity of biologically active constituents rather than the total vegetative yield of the targeted medicinal plant parts. The best time to pick lavender, clove flowers are before the last blooms on each individual stalk has fully opened up.

Example: Cardiac glycosides of digitalis are present in their highest amount in the afternoon. Typically, for essential oil containing flower, dry days are chosen and the collection is carried out in the morning before sunlight has not evaporated too much of the essential oils present in the flowers. Even for essential oil containing leaves, they should be collected in the morning after the dew has dried from the plant, but before the heat of the sun has warmed the plant too much. This ensures that most essential oils are present in the leaves.

- **Age of the Plant:** The age of the plant governs not only the total quantity, but also relative proportion of the active constituents. Example: *Ammi visnaga* unripe fruits are richest in both khellin and visnagin. High proportion of pulegone (naturally occurring organic compound obtained from the essential oils) in young plants of Peppermint will be replaced by menthone and menthol and reduction in the percentage of alkaloids in Datura as the plant ages. Roots and rhizomes are collected after two-three years of plant growth. Secondary metabolites are more accumulated in *Agave americana* as the age is more. Even sap content is more if the leaves are mature and big for Aloe plant as age becomes more. Conium fruits contain coniin when fruits are mature and unripe. Santonica flowers are rich in santonin, when unexpanded; when it starts to open, the santonin content decreases.

Cleaning of Collected Plants:

- ✓ Underground organs should be freed from soil by shaking, brushing or washing under stream of water.
- ✓ Any diseased part or attacked by insects should be rejected.

- ✓ All large organs such as calumba roots should be sliced to facilitate drying.
- ✓ Some organs as ginger are usually peeled.
- ✓ The stalks are usually removed from leaves and fruits.

Human Related Factors:

- **Skilled person:** Collection practices should ensure the long-term survival of wild populations and their associated habitats. The population density of the target species at the collection sites is determined and species that are rare or scarce should not be collected. Local experts responsible for the field collection should have formal or informal practical education and training in plant sciences and have practical experience in fieldwork. They should be responsible for training any collectors who lack sufficient technical knowledge to perform the various tasks involved in the plant collection process. They are also responsible for the supervision of workers and the full documentation of the work performed. Field personnel should have adequate botanical training and should be able to recognize medicinal plants by their common names and by their scientific (Latin) names. The collection team should be familiar with good collecting techniques, transport and handling of equipment and medicinal plant materials, including cleaning, drying and storage. Training of personnel should be conducted regularly. The responsibilities of all those involved in collection should be clearly set out in a written document.

- **Method of collection:** Medicinal plants should not be collected in or near areas where high levels of pesticides or other possible contaminants are used or found, such as roadsides, drainage ditches, mine tailings, garbage dumps and industrial facilities which may produce toxic emissions. In addition, the collection of medicinal plants in and around active pastures, including riverbanks downstream from pastures, should be avoided in order to avoid microbial contamination from animal waste. In the course of collection, efforts should be made to remove parts of the plant that are not required and foreign matter, in particular toxic weeds. Decomposed medicinal plant materials should be discarded. When collecting roots of trees and bushes, the main roots should not be cut or dug up and severing the taproot of trees and bushes should be avoided. Only some of the lateral roots should be located and collected. Barks are collected by three methods like felling (bark is peeled off after cutting the tree at base), uprooting (the underground roots are dug out and barks are collected from branches and roots) and coppicing (plant is cut one meter above the ground level and barks are removed).

- **Selection of plant parts:** Collectors of medicinal plants and producers of medicinal plant materials and herbal medicines should prepare botanical specimens for submission to regional or national herbaria for authentication. The voucher specimens should be retained for a sufficient period of time and should be preserved under proper conditions. The name of the botanist or other experts who provided the botanical identification or authentication should be recorded. If the medicinal plant is not well known to the community, then documentation of the botanical identity should be recorded and maintained. Tubers, corns and bulbs are collected at the end of flowering or fruiting when all the aerial portions show signs of senescence. Leaves are collected just before flowering and flowers are collected just before pollination. Fruits are collected when they become fully mature and ripe.

Harvesting:

Medicinal plants should be harvested during the optimal season or time period to ensure the production of medicinal plant materials and is the most important step for finished herbal products of the best possible quality. The time of harvest depends on the plant part to be used. The best time for harvest (quality peak season/time of day) should be determined according to the quality and quantity of biologically active constituents rather than the total vegetative yield of the targeted medicinal plant parts. During harvest, care should be taken to ensure that no foreign matter, weeds or toxic plants are mixed with the harvested medicinal plant materials. The most important objectives of harvesting are (1) An economic point which needs focus with type of crude drug to be harvested (2) The Pharmacopoeial standards of which it needs to achieve (Fig. 2.7).

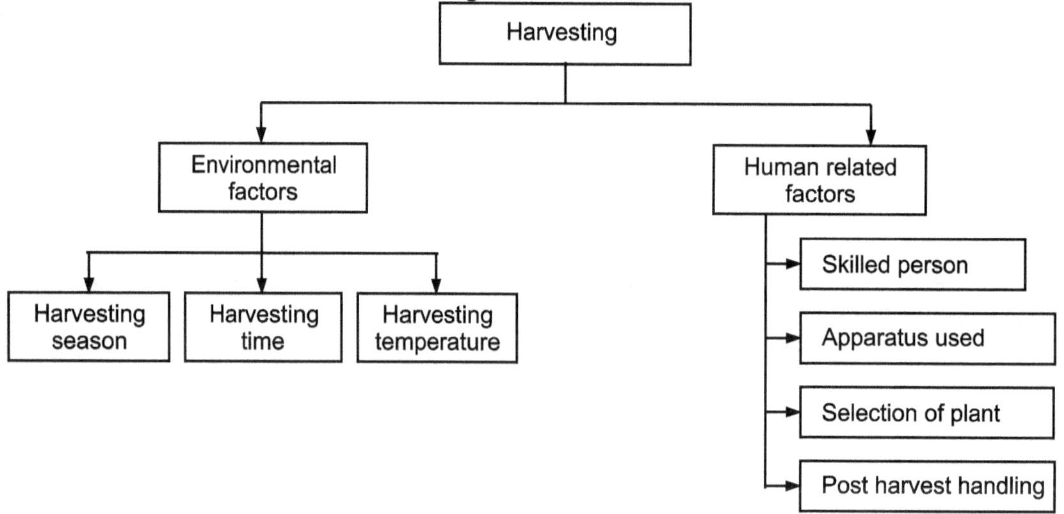

Fig. 2.7: Factor affecting Harvesting

- **Harvesting season:** Active constituents of herbs are affected by the seasons (due to climate, rainfall etc.). So medicinal plants should be collected in the proper season to get the high medicinal value as well as more chemical constituents. Medicinal plants should be harvested under the best possible conditions, avoiding dew, rain or exceptionally high humidity. If harvesting occurs in wet conditions, the harvested material should be transported immediately to an indoor drying facility to expedite drying so as to prevent any possible deleterious effects due to increased moisture levels, which promote microbial fermentation and mould. Generally roots and rhizomes are to be harvested during rainy season. Barks and flowers are harvested during autumn. Gums/Resins – harvested during dry weather.

- **Harvesting time:** It is also an important factor that reflects the quality of the plant parts. Determination of the right time for harvesting will vary from one species to another. Collection should be done at a time when the plants are in optimum condition with respect to required medical quality and efficacy. This also ensures the best possible quality of raw material and products. The concentration of biologically and medically active ingredients varies with the stage of plant growth and development. Roots and Rhizomes should be collected when aerial parts are dried down (if not – fleshy and difficult to dry) and harvested after sun sets. Bark is harvested in damp weather before noon. Aerial parts should be harvested during late noon season, around 4-5 O' clock. Flowers e.g., clove are harvested before they are fully expanded during sun sets.

1. **Harvesting of leaves:** The fresh leaves of herb can be picked at any time during the herb's growth. For harvesting herbal leaves for drying purposes, they should be collected in the morning after the dew has dried from the plant, but before the heat of the sun has warmed the plant too much. Generally leaves should be young. Leaves from the evergreen type herbs, such as rosemary and thyme, can be harvested just before flowering for the most flavor. When the entire herb plant is desired, the best time to harvest, is right before the plant is about to flower. If harvesting the whole plant from a wild growth of herbs, it is a good to harvest no more than 1/3 of the plants.

2. **Harvesting of flowers:** Flowers are the most delicate part of an herbal harvest. It is best to collect flowers during the middle of the day and especially on a day that is dry. Avoid any flowers that have any amount of damage or decay and do not collect spent flowers. Once picked, move the flowers from the harvest container to the drying area as quickly as possible to avoid bruising.

3. **Harvesting of seeds and fruits:** When harvesting herbal seeds, choose a dry day, just before the seed is ready to be dispersed. Seeds should no longer be green, brown or black as it is the signal that a seed has ripened enough. Seeds should also be hard and often have a dry pod surrounding the actual seed. It requires immense patience to not harvest too early.

4. **Harvesting of roots:** Herbal roots are harvested in the fall, when they are full of energy. Roots are some of the most powerful of the herbal parts and the gardener has to pay for them in effort. Roots are to be dug up whole. Fresh roots should be washed and cut while they are soft enough to work with. Dried roots can be tough as rocks (no exaggeration), when fully dried.

5. **Harvesting of barks:** Herbal bark is an important part of the herbal harvest. Since harvesting bark can result in the demise of the tree, it is imperative that the harvest is done correctly. Peeling of bark from any tree in a complete ring around the trunk should not be done as it will cut off the food supply to the tree and it will die. Bark is harvested during damp days and usually from young branches or young trees.

- **Harvesting temperature:** India has unique biogeographical positions having all known types of ecosystems ranging from coldest place, the dry cold desert of Ladakh (Nubra Valley with –57°C), to temperate, alpine and sub-tropical regions of north-west and trans-Himalayas; rain forests with high rainfall; wet evergreen humid tropics of western ghats and arid and semi-arid regions of peninsular India; dry desert conditions of Rajasthan and Gujarat to the tidal mangroves of Sunderban (West Bengal). Hence, medicinal plants should be harvested under the best possible climatic conditions for the specific species required to avoid either desiccation or fermentation and mould growths which minimize the deterioration of the material. It is having correlation between harvesting time and seasonal variations. During day and night time temperature variation occurs. Further seasonal changes will give more variation in the temperature. It is seen that day temperature below 23°C is suitable for roots and bark harvest, whereas leaf, flower and fruits are to be harvested during evening time when the temperature will be 25-28°C. The air temperature is kept at 20-40°C for thin materials such as leaves, but is often raised to 60-70°C for plant parts that are harder to dry e.g. roots and barks.

- **Skilled persons:** Growers and producers should have adequate knowledge of the medicinal plant concerned. This should include botanical identification, cultivation characteristics and environmental requirements (soil type, soil pH, fertility, plant spacing and light requirements), as well as the means of harvest and storage. All personnel (including field workers) involved in the propagation, cultivation, harvest and post-harvest processing stages of medicinal plant production should maintain appropriate personal hygiene and should have received training regarding their hygiene responsibilities. The person should be sure about the identity of the plants he intends to harvest without doubt; he should be able to distinguish clearly between the medicinal plant and its closely related relatives in order to avoid unwanted mixtures. He should choose healthy and well-developed plant material that should not be infested with fungal growth or insects, otherwise byproducts of these organisms will alter the ingredient profile and could even be poisonous. He should gather only plants that are abundant in that area. Special care has to be taken with leaves and flowers which are much more vulnerable to deterioration than roots due to the nature of their tissue. Unnecessary damage to the plant should be avoided i.e., exercise caution to enable that plant can re-grow. Further mechanical damage to the harvested material should also be avoided otherwise it can result in undesirable quality changes. Identification and discarding of unwanted plant materials during harvesting will ensure no foreign matter, weeds or toxic plants are mixed with the harvested medicinal plant materials.

- **Apparatus uses:** Special care should be taken before harvesting with the equipment. All equipment, when used, should be clean and free of remnants of previously harvested plants. All containers used during harvesting (cutting devices, harvesters and other machines) should be clean and free from contamination by previously harvested medicinal plants and other foreign matter. If plastic containers are used, then particular attention is given to any possible retention of moisture that would lead to the growth of moulds. Some of the examples are roots, rhizomes, tubers harvested by diggers or lifters. Small seeds are harvested with seed stripper. Seaweeds producing agar are harvested by long handled forks. Leaves are harvested by hand plucking, barks are harvested with an axe or bush knife etc.

Selection of the Plant Parts:

- **(a) Guidelines for root harvesting:** In many medicinal plants, the medically effective substances are found in the root. Thus, in many cases, the whole plant gets uprooted by the gatherers and never grow again. In order to ensure sustainable harvest of root material some of the rules are like:

(1)   Roots are dug at a considerable distance, at least 30 cm, from the main stem or tap root.

(2)   Severing of the tap root are avoided.

(3)   Only the lateral roots are collected.

(4)   After digging covering the hole will ensure protection against infection and invasion by pests.

(b) Guidelines for bark harvesting: The most common unsustainable practice is ring-barking where entire rings of bark are removed around the tree, inevitably leading to death of the tree and the plant can become endangered. For sustainable harvest of bark material some of the rules are:

(1)   The barks are peeled from the tree in small pieces leaving most of it intact on the trunk of the trees.

(2)   The barks are removed in long vertical strips using a thin flexible blade/bush knife.

(3)   Ring barking, which is the cut of off entire rings around the tree should be avoided.

(4)   The edges of the strip with an axe are not be cut as this causes the remaining bark to lift from the wood and dry out.

(5)   After harvesting of the barks, 'tree seal' are used, e.g., apply a piece of wet cow-dung to the bark wound.

(c) Guidelines for leaf harvesting: In order to ensure sustainable harvesting of leaves, some rules are followed:

(1)   Individual leaves are plucked instead of leaf striping and use of sharp pruning shears for leaves are avoided.

(2)   Regularly pruning branches will improve the quality and quantity of leaves.

(d) Guidelines for fruit harvesting: Fruits need to be extracted in a sustainable manner so that the biotic integrity of forests and woodlands is supported. In order to ensure sustainable harvesting of leaves, some rules are followed:

(1)   All healthy, high quality fruits are not collect but leave some on the ground so that more plants of good quality can germinate.

(2)   Fruits are collected from some trees and leave others completely.

(e) Harvesting of threatened species: Highly threatened species must not be harvested and collected at all in order to increase their prospects of survival. If this is not done, they are likely to be lost forever. There should be clear information on which plants are threatened. In such cases, the practitioners and communities are try to discover ways of using alternatives. Additionally, legislation should be put in place to ban not only the collection but the possession of and trade in those plants.

- **Post-harvest handling:** After harvest, the harvested fresh plant material undergoes a variety of processes which can be either desirable or undesirable. Through the harvesting process, the balance of substances within the plant is disturbed. Such processes are likely to alter the effectiness of some of the active ingredients. Once the harvesting is done, following rules and recommendations are to be followed in order to ensure a high quality of the harvested material and the products developed: (1) arriving at the place for drying or processing; unload and unpack the plant material as correctly as possible. (2) As soon as preliminary processing is to be started for unpacked plant materials.

Drying:

Drying is the most common and fundamental method for post-harvest preservation of medicinal plants because it allows for the quick conservation of the medicinal qualities of the plant material in an uncomplicated manner. Drying is defined as decreasing moisture content (MC) to preserve the product for extended shelf life. Factors such as scale of production, availability of new technologies and pharmaceutical quality standards are considered for medicinal plant drying in modern times. Natural drying, i.e. drying without auxiliary energy either in the field or in sheds, should only be considered for drying of small quantities. The active ingredients of different medicinal plants typically are concentrated in certain parts e.g. leaf, flower, fruit, bark or root and therefore, harvest and drying of plant parts is usually selective. As a result, the dryer design must correspond to the plant parts to be dried. For seed drugs, such as fennel or caraway, typical grain dryer types can be used. Drying of medicinal plant material directly on bare ground are avoided. If a concrete or cement surface is used, medicinal plant materials should be laid on a tarpaulin or other appropriate cloth or sheeting. Insects, rodents, birds and other pests and livestock, domestic animals are kept away from drying sites. For indoor drying, the duration of drying, drying temperature, humidity and other conditions are determined on the basis of the plant part concerned (root, leaf, stem, bark, flower, etc.) and any volatile natural constituents, such as essential oils.

Reason for Drying:

- To help in their preservation.
- To fix their constituents, by preventing reactions that may occur in presence of water.
- To prevent the growth of microorganisms such as bacteria and fungi.
- To facilitate their grinding.
- To reduce their size and weight.
- Insufficient drying favors spoilage by microorganisms and makes it possible for enzymatic destruction.

Factor affecting Drying:

- **Temperature:** The method and temperature used for drying may have a considerable impact on the quality of the resulting medicinal plant materials. To achieve increased dryer capacity, drying temperature is chosen as high as possible without reducing the quality of the product. If the plant requires enzymatic action, then slow drying at moderate temperature is necessary. For example, drying of Vanilla pods, cocoa seeds and Gentian root, enzymatic action is required. The characteristic colour and odour of vanilla are only developed as a result of enzyme action during the curing (Fermentation). Fermentation is mostly used to remove bitter or unpleasant-tasting substances or to promote the formation of aromatic compounds with a pleasant smell or taste. During this curing process the pods undergo fermentation and turn black in colour. If enzymatic action is not desired, drying is takes place as soon as possible after collection as in the case of Digitalis leaves. Absolute vapour content of the drying air is controlled by adjusting dew-point temperature. Temperature ranges from 30 to 90°C. The air temperature is kept at 20-40°C for thin materials such as leaves, but is often raised to 60-70°C for plant parts that are harder to dry e.g., roots and barks. By increasing temperature, drying time decreases exponentially. The reduction of drying time from increasing air temperature is desired in practice, because capacity of a dryer will be increased and allow for a considerable reduction of drying costs. Response of drying rate to temperature is a characteristic property of medicinal plant species. In similar experiments with flowers of *Chamomilla recutita*, drying time was reduced from 52 hours at 30°C to 1.6 h at 60°C. For roots of *Echinacea angustifolia*, the relation was 56 h at 30°C to 6.5 h at 60°C, for *S. officinalis*, drying time was reduced from 120 h at 30°C to 2 hours at 60°C. For glycoside species, a maximum temperature of 100°C is recommended, for mucilage species 65°C and for essential-oil species 35 to 45°C. The contents of metilchavicol and eugenol in *Ocimum basilicum* decreased during drying at 45°C, but the levels of trans-bergamotene, linalool and 1,8-cineole significantly increased.

- **Relative Humidity (RH):** Micro-organisms, like fungi, yeasts and bacteria, increasingly developed at RH > 70%. Since, the activity of decomposing enzymes is also enhanced by increasing water activity, a threshold of RH ≤ 60% is recommended to preserve the quality of medicinal plants during storage. Drying decreases the risk of external attack, e.g., by moulds. Living plant material has high water content: leaves may contain 60-90% water, roots and rhizomes 70-85% and wood 40-50%. The lowest percentage, often no more than 5-10%, is found in seeds. RH in a range from 30 to 70% is optimum.
- **Velocity:** The higher essential oil content (linalool) in *Ocimum basilicum* was obtained in the drying process with an air temperature at 60°C and air velocity of 1.9 m/s.

Drying Method:

Depending on the type of chemical constituents, a method of drying can be used for crude drugs (Fig. 2.8).

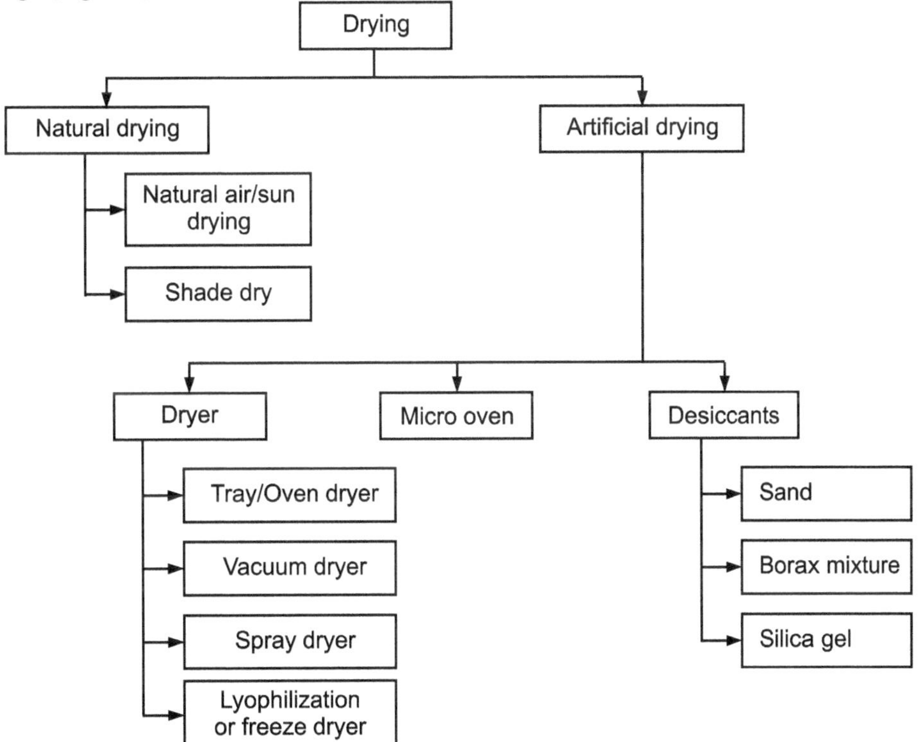

Fig. 2.8: Various drying methods

Natural drying: This is accomplished by natural air in sun or shade. The choice of sunshine or shade is determined by the sensitivity to light of the constituents. In the case of natural drying in the open air, medicinal plant materials should be spread out in thin layers on drying frames and stirred or turned frequently. In order to secure adequate air circulation, the drying frames should be located at a sufficient height above the ground. Efforts should be made to achieve uniform drying of medicinal plant materials and so to avoid mould formation. If the chemical constituents of the drugs are quite stable to the temperature and sunlight, such drugs can be dried directly in sunshine like gum, acacia, seeds and fruits. Further shade drying is preferred to maintain or minimize loss of colour of leaves (Digitalis, Senna) and flowers (Clove); and lower temperatures should be employed in the case of medicinal plant materials containing volatile substances (Peppermint). The drying conditions should be recorded. Herbs with high moisture content, such as mint and basil, need rapid drying or they will mold. To retain some green leaf colouring, dry in the dark by hanging plants upside down in bunches in paper bags. Hanging leaves down allows essential oils to flow from stems to leaves. The oil content of shade-dried Roman chamomile flowers was found to be larger (1.9% w/w) than that of sun-dried (0.4%) and oven-dried at 40°C (0.9%). General leaves are dried by tying whole stems very tightly in small bunches, then hanged in a dark, warm (21.1° – 26.7°C), well-ventilated, dust-free area. Individual stems will shrink and fall. Leaves are ready when they feel dry and crumbly in about 1 to 2 weeks.

Advantages of Air Drying:
    (a)   When herbs are not adversely affected by excessive sunlight.

Advantages of Shade Drying:
    (a)   When sunlight causes discolouration and warping/shriveling of the plant constituents.

Disadvantages of Natural Drying:
    (a)   Sometimes plants are placed by hand on drying frames or stands, to be air-dried in barns or sheds.
    (b)   This method of drying is labor-intensive and can take several weeks.
    (c)   The exact length of time for adequate drying depends on temperature and humidity.

Artificial Drying:
This is a rapid method performed at well-controlled temperature and is accomplished by direct fire, use of heated stones, hot water pipes, by use of stoves, drying chambers with controlled temperature and ventilation. Various methods like tray drying, vacuum drying, spray drying, freeze drying, microwave drying etc. are used.

Advantages:
    (a)   Generally the most acceptable form of drying herbs.
    (b)   Rapid (less exposure to heat that results in less chances of chemical alteration) method. Drying time can be reduced to hours or minutes.
    (c)   Control temperature (normally 40°C) and ventilation (allows dry air to replace wet air).
    (d)   Labour can also be greatly reduced.

Desiccants:
Sand: Sand is used as desiccant. Sand is least expensive and oldest method but still one of the best desiccants. It is dry, fine and almost salt free. A mixture of 2 parts borax to 1 part sand may be used, adding 1 tablespoon salt to each quart to speed drying.

Borax Mixtures: Pure borax may be used for rapid drying, but there is danger of burning and/or bleaching the flower parts, especially with delicate flowers. For a milder drying agent, borax is usually mixed with either white or yellow corn meal.

Salt or Silica Gel: Flowers dried in silica gel retain good colour because silica gel is the fastest-acting drying agent available. Silica gel is a blue crystal with a high water- absorbing capacity. It is an expensive desiccant, but can be used indefinitely, so it is worth the investment for people who continually collect and dry plant materials.

Storage:

Once drying is complete, plants are packaged for transportation and further processing. Dried herbaceous plants are generally compressed into bales weighing from 60 to 100 kg (13 to 220 pounds), which are then sewn into fabric bags or wrapped in plastic. Materials that cannot be baled, such as roots and bark, are placed in sacks. Smaller bags may be used for dense materials such as dried fruits or seeds. Very fragile materials, such as flowers, are packaged in crates. Dried plant materials tend to be hygroscopic (readily absorbing moisture) and must be stored under controlled humidity. Highly hygroscopic materials are generally packed in plastic. The crude drugs like roots, barks, large barks are packed in gunny bags. *Storage* is the main process to maintain the quality of the crude drugs and to protect the drugs from the insect attack. Dried leaves are stored whole in airtight containers, such as canning jars with tightly sealed lids. Seeds are stored whole and ground as needed. Leaves retain their oil and flavour if stored whole and crushed just before use. Dried drugs are protected from moisture during storage. Table 2.1 shows various storage conditions for various drugs.

Table 2.1: Storage condition of crude drugs

Name of the medicinal plants	Packing method
Aloe	Goat skin
Colophony and Balsam of tolu	Kerosene tin
Asafoetida	Well closed container to prevent loss of volatile oil
Cod liver oil	Brown coloured bottle to prevent light
Digitalis	Well closed container with desiccating agents to absorb excessive moisture from the drug
Opium seeds	Plastic sealed cover

Factor affecting Storage:

1. **Condition for storage materials:** Plant materials should be store in well aerated, dry and protected from light. Raw materials are supplied with air-conditioning and humidity control equipment as well as facilities to protect against rodents, insects and livestock whenever required.

2. **Condition for store house:** The floor should be tidy, without cracks and easy to clean. Plant materials are stored on shelves which keep the material a sufficient distance from the walls. Safety measures are taken to prevent the occurrence of pest infestation, mould formation, rotting or loss of oil. Regular inspections are carried out at regular intervals.

3. **Packaging:** Continuous in-process quality control measures are implemented to eliminate substandard materials, contaminants and foreign matter before and during the final stages of packaging. Processed medicinal plants are packaged in clean, dry boxes, sacks, bags or other containers as per standard operating procedures and national and/or regional regulations of the producer and the end-user countries. Packaging materials should be non-polluting, clean, dry and in undamaged condition. The fragile medicinal plant materials are packaged in rigid containers. Fresh plant materials are stored at appropriate low temperatures, ideally at 2-8°C whereas frozen products are stored at less than −20°C but wooden boxes and paper bags are not used for storage of crude drugs.

Processing:

The active principle of the plants are provides the medicinal qualities or therapeutic efficacy. Hence the active principles are required to separate from the plant constituents by means of extraction. The basic principle of extraction is the solubility of the constituents in the respective solvent. The phytoconstituents contained in every medicinal plant consist of a number of compounds, which individually or in groups can have a specific action on the human body. Different methods are used to extract these phytoconstituents in a crude extract form in which active principles are present, either sole or collectively. Mixtures of alcohols with water are the solvents with the greatest extractive power for almost all natural substances of low molecular weight like alkaloids, saponins and flavonoids. Ethyl alcohol is the solvent of choice for obtaining classic extracts such as tinctures and fluid, soft and dry extracts. Several types of machines are available for grinding crude drugs which increases the surface tension and reduce the size reduction that further helps in easy extraction. Some mills are used for size reduction of plant drugs namely,

- **Hammer mill:** A common type for grinding crude drugs like hard bark containing drugs.
- **Knife mill:** It is useful for production of low-dust powders of leaves, barks and roots for subsequent percolation or maceration.
- **Tooth mill:** It is used for production of very fine powders. Mills cooled with liquid nitrogen are available for heat sensitive compounds. Cold grinding is used for crude drugs containing volatile oils. All the plant materials are sifted to ensure the proper particle size and sifting can be performed according to two different principles.
- **Sieving:** In sieving the plant material is passed through a sieve of suitable mesh size giving two fractions. The fraction passing the sieve consists of particles with a size smaller than or corresponding to the mesh size. The remaining fraction consists of coarser particles which are returned to the mill for continued grinding.
- **Blast sifting:** In blast sifting the material to be classified is blown with compressed air into an apparatus which allows the particles to sediment according to their weight.

Various extraction procedures are available like infusion, maceration, percolation, digestion, decoction, continuous hot extraction, solvent-solvent precipitation, liquid-liquid extraction, distillation, specific procedures like microwave extraction, super critical fluid extraction, bioassay graded fractionation etc. for medicinal and aromatic plant extraction.

- **Infusion:** In this method, the plant material (herbal tea) is placed in a pot and wetted with cold water. Immediately afterwards, boiling water is poured over it, then left to stand, covered with a lid for about fifteen minutes, after which the tea is poured off.
- **Maceration:** This method is used frequently for water-soluble active constituents. It consists of macerating the plant material in cold water (15-20°) for several hours.
- **Percolation:** In this method, the ground plant material is subjected to a slow flow of fresh solvent.
- **Digestion:** This method is suitable for hard barks or woods which are difficult for water to penetrate. Digestion is also considered as maceration, but at a relatively elevated temperature. As a general rule the temperature of the extracting medium should be in the range of 35-40°C but not exceeding 50°C.
- **Decoction:** If the plant material is boiled for ten minutes or if boiling water is poured over it and allowed to stand for thirty minutes, the product is called decoction. The starting ratio of crude extract to water is fixed, e.g., 1 : 4 or 1 : 16; the volume is then brought down to one-fourth its original volume by boiling during the extraction process. Then the concentrated extract is filtered and used as such or processed further.
- **Continuous hot extraction method:** This procedure is considered as the most common method used for the extraction of organic constituents from dried plant tissue. It can be used both on laboratory and industrial scales. In the lab, the powdered material is continuously extracted in a Soxhlet apparatus with a range of solvents of increasing polarity.
- **Solvent-solvent precipitation:** (i) The extract dissolved in a suitable solvent is mixed with a less polar but miscible solvent causing the selective precipitation of the less soluble plant constituent e.g., the precipitation of triterpenoid saponins from the methanol extract of *Phytolacca dodecandra* by the addition of acetone and the precipitation of gum from aqueous extracts of *Olibanum* by addition of alcohol. (ii) By the addition of the extract to a solvent in which the constituents is insoluble or very sparingly soluble e.g. precipitation of resins from the alcoholic extracts by the addition of distilled or acidulated water.
- **Liquid-liquid extraction:** Liquid-liquid extraction is also known as solvent extraction and partitioning. It is a method to separate compounds based on their relative solubilies in two different immiscible liquids, usually water and an organic solvent. It is an extraction of a substance from one liquid phase into another liquid phase. It is performed using a separating funnel.
- **Counter current extraction:** This is a highly effective process whereby solvent flows in the opposite direction to plant material. Unlike maceration and percolation, which are batch processes, this method is continuous. Screw extractors and carousel extractors are two types of equipment used for counter current extraction.
- **Extraction with supercritical gases:** This is a method for extracting active ingredients using gases. An advantage of supercritical extraction is that it can take

place at low temperature, thus preserving the quality of temperature-sensitive components. The plant material is placed in a vessel that is filled with a gas under controlled temperature and high pressure. The gas dissolves the active ingredients within the plant material and then passes into a separating chamber where both pressure and temperature are lower. The extract precipitates out and is removed through a valve at the bottom of the chamber. The gas is then reused. Gases suitable for supercritical extraction include carbon dioxide, nitrogen, methane, ethane, ethylene, nitrous oxide, sulfur dioxide, propane, propylene, ammonia and sulfur hexafluoride.

- **Steam distillation:** Steam distillation is the method for extracting active ingredients from medicinal plants. The plant material is loaded onto perforated plates inside a cylindrical tank or still and steam is injected from below. The steam dissolves the desired substances in the plant and then enters a condenser where it is condensed back into a liquid. This condensate then passes into a flask, where the extract either rises to the top or settles to the bottom and is separated from the water. Distillation is complete when there is no more extract present in the condensate. The water may be reused and the extract is purified through centrifuging and filtering.

- **Phytonics process:** The products mostly extracted by this process are high quality natural fragrant essential oils, flavors and biological extracts which can be directly used without further physical or chemical treatment. The Phytonics process involves the use of a novel non-toxic solvent based on hydrofluorocarbon– 134a, having a boiling point of –25°C and a vapor pressure of 5.6 bar at ambient temperature and technology to optimize its remarkable properties in the extraction of plant materials.

2.4 PLANT HORMONES AND THEIR APPLICATIONS

Plant hormones or phytohormones are chemicals that regulate plant growth. Plant hormones are signal molecules produced within the plant and occur in extremely low concentrations. Hormones regulate cellular processes in targeted cells locally and when moved to other locations, in other locations of the plant. They affect gene expression and transcription levels, cellular division and growth. There are five major classes of plant hormones.

- **(1) Abscisic acid (ABA):** It is also called ABA and was discovered and researched under two different names *dormin* and *abscicin II* before its chemical properties were fully known. In general, it acts as an inhibitory chemical compound that affects bud growth, seed and bud dormancy. It mediates changes within the apical meristem, causing bud dormancy and the alteration of the last set of leaves into protective bud covers. In plants under water stress, ABA plays a role in closing the stomata. Induce seeds to synthesize storage protein.

- **(2) Auxins:** These are compounds that positively influence cell enlargement, bud formation and root initiation. They also promote the production of other hormones and in conjunction with cytokinins, they control the growth of stems, roots and fruits and convert stems into flowers. Auxins act to inhibit the growth of buds lower down the stems and also promote lateral and adventitious root development and growth.

The four naturally occurring (endogenous) auxins are IAA, 4-chloroindole-3-acetic acid, phenylacetic acid and indole-3—butyric acid and these were found to be synthesized by plants. Synthetic auxin analogs include 1-naphthaleneacetic acid and 2, 4-chlorophenoxyacetic acid (2,4-D).

(3) Cytokinins: They are a group of chemicals that influence cell division and shoot formation. They help delay senescence or the aging of tissues, are responsible for mediating auxin transport throughout the plant and affect internodal length and leaf growth. They have a highly synergistic effect in concert with auxins and the ratios of these two groups of plant hormones affect most major growth periods of plants. Cytokinins counter the apical dominance induced by auxins. They, in conjunction with ethylene, promote abscission of leaves, flower parts and fruits. There are two types of cytokinins:

(a) **Adenine-type:** They are represented by kinetin, zeatin and 6-benzyl-aminopurine.

(b) **Phenylurea-type:** They are like diphenylurea and thidiazuron (TDZ). Most adenine-type cytokinins are synthesized in roots.

(4) Ethylene: Ethylene is produced at a faster rate in rapidly growing and dividing cells, especially in darkness. It affects cell growth and cell shape; when a growing shoot hits an obstacle, while underground, ethylene production greatly increases, preventing cell elongation and causing the stem to swell.

(5) Gibberellins: Gibberellins or GAs include a large range of chemicals that are produced naturally within plants and by fungi. Gibberellins are important in seed germination, affecting enzyme production that mobilizes food production used for growth of new cells. GA3 was the first gibberellin to be structurally characterized. There are currently 136 GAs identified from plants, fungi and bacteria.

Other Known Hormones:

- **Brassinosteroids:** They are a class of polyhydroxy steroids, a group of plant growth regulators. They stimulate cell elongation and division, gravitropism, resistance to stress and xylem differentiation. They inhibit root growth and leaf abscission.

- **Jasmonates:** They are produced from fatty acids and seem to promote the production of defense proteins that are used to fend off invading organisms. They affect the storage of protein in seeds and seem to affect root growth.

- **Karrikins:** They are group of plant growth regulators found in the smoke of burning plant material that have the ability to stimulate the germination of seeds.

- **Stringolactones:** They are implicated in the inhibition of shoot branching. They are terpenoid lactones and are derived from carotenoids.

Plant growth retardants: They are most widely used group of bioregulators in agricultural and horticultural practice. They reduce the shoot growth of plants by inhibiting gibberellin biosynthesis. Plants treated with retardants are improved water use and less water stress due to reduction in leaf size. Examples: Paclobutrazol, uniconazole and flurprimidol.

2.5 POLYPLOIDY, MUTATION AND HYBRIDIZATION WITH REFERENCE TO MEDICINAL PLANTS

The method uses polyploidy, mutation and hybridization for improvement of the plant production.

2.5.1 Polyploidy

It is the process of genome doubling that gives rise to organisms with multiple sets of chromosomes. If the cell contains more than two haploid (n) sets of chromosomes, it called polyploidy. It occurs in the somatic cells. It is of two types autopolyploid (originated from spontaneous or induced duplication of the genome of a single species) and allopolyploid (originated from concurrent hybridization and duplication of the genomes of different species). In plant species, polyploidy mainly occurs in ferns (95%) as well as in angiosperms (around 50%). A chemical known as colchicine, derived from *Autumn crocus*, *Colchicum autumnale*, applied during cell division that disrupt mitosis creating copies of the chromosomes without dividing the cell and resulting in polyploid cells.

Applications:

- It provides significant information on the evolutionary history of plants which helps in better conservation of plant species.
- It helps in crop domestication as it found high in vegetative content.
- It also reveals information on how the plant genomes manage to succeed the effect of genome obesity.
- Flowers become larger with thicker petals resulting in longer lasting flowers.
- Increase fruits size than normal one.

2.5.2 Mutation

It is referred as sudden change in genetic sequences. It can be caused by copying errors in the genetic material during cell division and by exposure to radiation, chemicals or during meosis. Mutation can result in the morphological, anatomical and chemical changes in the plants with significant increase in the active constituents. The three types of changes in nucleotides and as per that it is classified as point mutation (cause by chemicals or malfunction of DNA replication), insertion (addition of one or more extra nucleotides into DNA) and deletion (deletion of one or more extra nucleotides into DNA). These changes occur with the help of mutagens. Mutagens are the agents that bring about a permanent alteration to physical composition of a DNA gene. There are two types namely chemical mutagens (Examples: Sulphur mustard, nitrogen mustard, Acridine yellow, 5-bromo Uracil etc.) and Physical mutagens (Examples: Alpha rays, Beta rays, UV radiation etc.).

Applications:

- This method is rapid method and cheap for development of new varieties.
- Induced mutagens are used for the induction of CMS (Congenital Myasthenic Syndrome), example: Ethidium bromide is used for induction of CMS in barley.
- It is effective for improvement of oligogenic chatachers (Qualitative characters are controlled by few genes).
- This method is quick, simple and best way when a new character is to be induced.
- It improves the disease resistance in crop plants.
- It is used to improve the specific characters of well adapted high yielding varieties.

2.5.3 Hybridization

It is the process through which hybrids are obtained. The cross between two genetically different parents is known as hybrid. The natural or artificial process that results in the formation of hybrid is known as hybridization. This method is used to create a variable population for the selection of types with desired combination of characters and to exploit and utilize the hybrid varieties. It results in progeny that differ qualitatively and quantitatively from the parents in the expression of secondary chemicals and morphological characters. Hence, it helps the breeders to transfer beneficial characteristics from wild plants to the cultivated crop species. There are three types of hybridization namely Intra-varietal hybridization (Crosses are made between the plants of the same variety), Inter-varietal or Intraspecific hybridization (Crosses are made between the plants belonging to two different varieties), Interspecific hybridization (Crosses are made between two different species of the same genus) and Introgressive hybridization (Transfer of some genes from one species into the genome of the other species).

Procedure:

It involves the following steps:

(i) **Selection of parents:** Parental plants must be selected from the local areas and are supposed to be the best suited to the existing conditions.

(ii) **Selfing of parents or artificial self-pollination:** Induce homozygosity for eliminating the undesirable characters and inbreeds forms.

(iii) **Emasculation:** It is the removal of stamens from female parent before they burst and shed their pollens. This method is essential in bisexual or self-pollinated plants.

(iv) **Bagging:** The emasculated flower or inflorescence is immediately bagged to avoid pollination by any foreign pollen. Butter paper or vegetable parchment bags are most commonly used.

(v) **Tagging:** The emasculated flowers are tagged just after bagging.

(vi) **Crossing:** The mature, fertile and viable pollens from the male parent are placed on the receptive stigma of emasculated flowers to bring about fertilization.

(vii) **Harvesting and storing the F, seeds:** Crossed heads of desirable plants are harvested and after complete drying they are threshed. Seeds are stored properly with original tags.

(viii) **Raising the F_1 generation:** The stored seeds are sown separately to raise the F_1 generation and these plants are progenies of cross seeds and therefore forms as hybrids.

Some examples of hybrid plants are Triticale (Wheat + Rye), Meyer lemon (True lemon tree + Mandarin Orange tree) etc.

Applications:

- This method improves yield and quality of crops.
- This method provides better resistance to diseases and insects.
- It improves hardiness of plants.
- It improves fruit sizes and quality.
- It improves storage capabilities of crops.
- It improves fall colours.
- It improves seedless varieties of crops.

2.6 CONSERVATION OF MEDICINAL PLANTS

Medicinal plant conservation strategies are based on an understanding of indigenous knowledge and practices. Conservation of medicinal plants in its bio-cultural perspective not only implies conservation of biodiversity but also provides conservation of cultural diversity. As per the world conservation strategy (1980), the conservation is defined as "the management of human use of the biodiversity so that it may yield the greatest sustainable benefit to present generation while maintaining its definitions invokes two complementary components conservation and sustainability". Many drugs contain herbal ingredients and it has been said that 80-90% of the world's population relies on some form of non-conventional medicine, but the market demand has led to an increased pressure on the natural resources that lend to the production of some of these plants. The most serious proximate threats when extracting medicinal plants generally are habitat loss, habitat degradation, global climate change and over harvesting. Hence highly threatened species must not be collected at all in order to increase their prospects of survival. There should be clear information on which plants are threatened. In such cases the practitioners and communities should try to discover ways of using alternatives. Additionally, legislation should be put in place to ban not only the collection but the possession of and trade in those plants. The practitioners should be involved in the processes of conserving the threatened plants concerned. The regulation should also draw on the harvesting practices observing ethical, legal and social rights of all those concerned in the communities where the plants are native. As per recent statistical reports, about 17,000 species of medicinal and aromatic plants are well documented and about 50,000 plant species are used globally. About 3,000 species are traded internationally and about 900 species are commercially cultivated in world wide. According to WWF (World Wide Fund for Nature) about 30 – 45% of medicinal plant species may be threatened with extinction in the wild, which means around 4000 to 10,000 plants are may be at risk. Various national and international agencies have formulated various policies and strategies for the conservation of the medicinal plants. According to these strategies, the primary goals are:

    (a)   Maintenance of essential ecological processes and life support systems for human survival.
    (b)   Preservation of species and genetic diversity.
    (c)   Sustainable use of species and ecosystems which supports rural communities and also the industries.
    (d)   Maintenance and assessment of germplasm for future use.

Some agencies are:

- IUCN (The International Union for Conservation of Nature and Natural Resources): Founded in 1948.
- WWF (World Wide Fund for Nature): It is established in 1961.
- UNDP (United Nations Development Programme): It is established in 1965.
- UNEP (United Nations Environment Programme): It is established in 1972.
- WRI (World Resources Institute): It is founded in 1982.
- FRLHT (Foundation for Revitalization of Local Health Traditions): It is established in 1993.

NMPB (National Medicinal Plants Board): It is established in 2000 by the Government of India has the primary mandate of coordinating all matters relating to medicinal plants and support policies and programmes for growth of trade, export, conservation and cultivation. The Board is located in the Department of Ayurveda, Yoga & Naturopathy, Unani, Siddha & Homeopathy (AYUSH) of the Ministry of Health & Family Welfare. According to IUCN, the number of endangered plant species is about 8500 worldwide, in which more than 250 plant species are in India. Some of the important endangered plant species are *Rauwolfia serpentine, Taxus baccata, Taxus brevifolia, Santalum album* etc. Guidelines on The Conservation of Medicinal Plants (IUCN, WWF, 1993), WHO (World Health Organization) Guidelines on good agricultural and collection practices (GACP) for medicinal plants (WHO, 2003) have been established where the significance of ecology, identification and traditional use of plants, as well as cultivation and conservation of plants both *in situ* and *ex situ* are strongly emphasized. The mission for the conservation of plants and their habitats are:

(a) To preserve wild populations of different plants species with their inherent intra-specific diversity for further evolution.

(b) Revitalization of social processes for transmission of traditional knowledge of health care for its wider use and applications.

The objectives are to:

(a) Establish a system of protected areas where special measures needs to be taken to conserve biological diversity;

(b) Promote the protection of ecosystems, natural habitats and the maintenance of viable populations of species in natural surroundings; and

(c) Develop necessary regulatory provisions for the protection of threatened species and populations.

The states like Karnataka, Tamil Nadu, Kerala and UP are involved in the conservation of medicinal plants.

The most widely accepted scientific technologies of biodiversity conservation are the *in-situ* and *ex-situ* methods.

In-situ Conservation:

This process is also known as on site conservation. This is the process of protecting the existing biological and genetic diversity at best and cost effective way. In this technique wild species or stock of a biological community or endangered plant is preserved in its natural habitat either by protecting or cleaning up the habitat.

(a) **Medicinal plant conservation areas:** During 1997 FRLHT (Foundation for Revitalization of Local Health traditions) Bangaluru, Karnataka, in collaboration with State Forest Departments established a coordinated network of in-situ medicinal plants conservation areas (around 30 Nos.) located within the protected areas of Kerala, Tamil Nadu and Karnataka.

(b) **Sacred Groves:** These are the combinations of forest whose entire biodiversity along with other natural resources is conserved by the forest village communities. This method provides the conservation of forest biodiversity, conservation of threatened taxa etc.

(c) **Conservation of Ethnomedicinal plants:** There are more than 6000 plant species are exist with their medicinal values but not have scientific evidences, is traditionally passed on orally through generations. Those plants are requires to conserve for future uses and to know their therapeutic activities through scientific research.

Ex-situ Conservation:

It is a process of protecting endangered plants from threatened habitat and placing in a new location which are in wild area or within them of humans i.e., by cultivating and maintaining plants in biotic gardens, parks, other suitable sites.

(a) **Ethno medicinal plant gardens:** It is an important process for creating a network of regional and sub-regional ethno medicinal plant gardens which contain all the ethnic communities' medicinal plants from the different regions of India. These gardens provide ethno medicinal history and their detailed knowledge and also act as regional repositories of our culture.

(b) **Gene banks:** Gene banks are a type of bio-repository which preserves genetic material. In plants, this is by freezing cuts from the plant, or stocking the seeds. In plants, it is possible to unfreeze the material and propagate it. Gene banks are used to store and conserve the plant genetic resources of major crop plants and their crop wild relatives that results in conservation of agricultural biodiversity. Various types of gene banks include seed bank, tissue bank, Cryo bank, pollen bank, field gene bank etc.

(c) **Nursery or demonstration plots:** This is one of the important methods for conservation of traditional medicinal plants and to get the proper idea about the history of the medicinal plants. These nurseries are the primary sources of supply of the plants, seed materials etc. The forest departments, agricultural extension agencies, various non Governmental Organizations (NGOs) should be encouraged to establish various nurseries and allot plots for growing medicinal plants in existing ones.

Some of the important National institutions for Agricultural Research:

- Central Arid Zone Research Institute (Czari), Jodhpur-3, Rajasthan.
- Central Plantation Crops Research Institute, Kasaragod, Kerala. Central Research Institute for Dryland Agriculture, Hyderabad, A.P.
- Central Rice Research Institute, Cuttack, Orissa.
- Central Soil and Water Conservation Research and Training Institute, Dehradun, Uttaranchal.
- Central Soil Salinity Research Institute, Karnal, Haryana.
- Central Tobacco Research Institute, Rajamundry, AP.
- Indian Agricultural Research Institute, New Delhi.

There some legal protection and conservation rules for medicinal plants by which farmers are benefited in India such as:

Plant Variety Protection Act 1970 (PVPA): It is an intellectual property statute in the USA. The PVPA gives breeders up to 25 years of exclusive control over new, distinct, uniform and stable sexually reproduced or tuber propagated plant varieties. It is a right for limited period of legal control to breeders of sexually reproduced or tuber propagated plant varieties.

Farmer's Right Act 2001: The Protection of Plant Variety and Farmers Right Act, 2001 (PPVFR Act) is an Act of the Parliament of India. This act enacted to provide for the establishment of an effective system for protection of various plant varieties, the rights of farmers and plant breeders and to encourage the development and cultivation of new varieties of plants. Farmers are entitled to save, use, sow, re-sow, exchange or sell their farm produce including seed of a registered variety in an unbranded manner. Farmers are totally exempted from payment of any fee in any proceedings under this Act. Annual fee is required to pay every year for maintaining the registration and renewal fee is also to pay for the extended period of registration.

Duration of Registration:
- **For trees and vines** (Perennials): 18 years from the date of registration of the variety.
- **For other crops** (Annuals): 15 years from the date of registration of the variety.
- **For extant varieties:** 15 years from the date of notification of that variety by the Central Government under section 5 of the Seeds Act, 1966.

Exemptions provided by the Act:
- **Farmers' Exemption**: Farmer shall be entitled to produce, save, use, sow, re-sow, exchange, share or sell his farm produce including seed of a variety protected under this Act.
- **Researcher's Exemption**: (i) the use of registered variety for conducting experiment. (ii) the use of variety as an initial source of variety for the purpose of creating other varieties.

EXERCISE

Long Essays:
1. Define cultivation. Explain various factors affecting cultivation.
2. Explain various types of cultivation. Note on soil factors affecting cultivation.
3. Explain various factors affecting collection and harvesting of crude drugs.
4. Explain processing of medicinal and aromatic plants.
5. Explain various methods for crop improvement technologies.

Short Essays:
1. Write a note on Exogenous factors of cultivation.
2. Write a note on Endogenous factors of cultivation.
3. Write a note on biotic factors of cultivation.
4. Write a note on soil structures for effective cultivation.
5. Write a note on collection of crude drugs.
6. Write a note on harvesting of crude drugs.
7. Write a note on drying methods for crude drugs.
8. Write a note on storage of crude drugs.
9. Explain the role of various plant hormones in growth of medicinal plants.
10. Note on conservation of Medicinal plants.

Multiple Choice questions (MCQs):

1. Exogenous factor for cultivation is ......

    (a) Transport   (b) Fertilizers

    (c) Soil nature   (d) Chemical race

2. Endogenous factor for cultivation is ......

    (a) Transport   (b) Fertilizers

    (c) Soil nature   (d) Chemical race

3. During rainy season alkaloid content in Datura is ......

    (a) Less   (b) More

    (c) Same   (d) Varies

4. Optimum temperature for propagation is ......

    (a) 25-35°C   (b) 18-28°C

    (c) 30-35°C   (d) 10-20°C

5. With altitude, the bitter content in Gentiana lutea is ......

    (a) Decrease   (b) Increase

    (c) Same   (d) Varies

6. On the basis of reaction to the photoperiod, Tobacco plant is ......

    (a) Short day plant   (b) Intermediate day plant

    (c) Long day plant   (d) Very long day plant

7. *Pythium spinosum* is ......

    (a) Fungal pest   (b) Viral pest

    (c) Bacterial pest   (d) Insect

8. Hey fever is caused by ......

    (a) Parthenium   (b) Insect

    (c) Virus   (d) Rag weed

9. Bordeaux mixture is ......

    (a) Insecticide   (b) Rodenticide

    (c) Herbicide   (d) Fingicide

10. Parathion is ......

    (a) Insecticide   (b) Rodenticide

    (c) Herbicide   (d) Fingicide

11. Humus decomposed in soil layer ......

    (a) O-Horizon   (b) A-Horizon

    (c) B-Horizon   (d) C-Horizon

12. In soil layer B- horizon is known as ......
    (a) Washing out   (b) Washing in
    (c) Zone of accumulation   (d) Weathering

13. "Dead organic matter" contains in soil layer of ......
    (a) A-horizon   (b) B-horizon
    (c) C-horizon   (d) O-horizon

14. Washing out of clay is known for soil layer of ......
    (a) A-horizon   (b) B-horizon
    (c) C-horizon   (d) O-horizon

15. Quartz containing soil is known as ......
    (a) Red soil   (b) Acid soil
    (c) Desert soil   (d) Alluvial soil

16. Laterite soil contains ......
    (a) High humus low magnesia   (b) High nitrogen low humus
    (c) High humus high nitrogen   (d) High magnesia high nitrogen

17. Soil pH required for available phosphorus in plant is ......
    (a) 5 to 8   (b) 6 to 7.5
    (c) 7 to 8   (d) 2 to 4

18. Phosphorus forms insoluble compound with calcium at pH ......
    (a) > 10 but < 15   (b) < 7
    (c) > 7.5 but < 10   (d) <4

19. For soil microbes C/N ratio is ......
    (a) 4 : 1 to 9 : 1   (b) 5 : 1 to 8 : 1
    (c) 6 : 1 to 10 : 1   (d) 3 : 1 to 8 : 1

20. Chalcids acts as ......
    (a) Beneficial fungi   (b) Harmful fungi
    (c) Beneficial insect   (d) Harmful insect

21. Plants are cut few meter above the ground level and barks are removed. This method is
    known as ......
    (a) Uprooting   (b) Coppicing
    (c) Cutting   (d) Felling

22. Harvesting time for aerial parts of plants is ......
    (a) 9 to 10 am   (b) 2 to 3 pm
    (c) 4 to 5 pm   (d) 4 -5 am

23. Temperature required for root harvesting is ......
    (a) Above 25°C   (b) Below 23°C
    (c) Below 35°C   (d) Above 35°C

24. Small seed are harvested with ......
    (a) Digger   (b) Forks
    (c) Seed stripper   (d) Hand plucking

25. Flowers are packed in ......
    (a) Plastic bag   (b) Crates
    (c) Small bag   (d) Air tight containers

26. Agar is harvested by ......
    (a) Lifter   (b) Stripper
    (c) Long handled fork   (d) Bush knife

27. Barks are harvested with ......
    (a) Bush knife   (b) Lifter
    (c) Forks   (d) hand pluck

28. Enzymatic action is required for drying of drug like ......
    (a) Nux vomica   (b) Digitalis
    (c) Cocoa seed   (d) Liquorice

29. Clove flower buds are dried under ......
    (a) Sun light   (b) Tray dryer
    (c) Shade   (d) Vacuum

30. Acacia is dried under ......
    (a) Shade   (b) Sun light
    (c) Vacuum   (d) Tray dryer

31. Aloe is store in ......
    (a) Kerosene   (b) Gunny bag
    (c) Goat skin   (d) Plastic sealed cover

32. Kerosene tin is used for storage of drug like ......
    (a) Digitalis   (b) Opium
    (c) Cinchona   (d) Colophony

33. Tooth mill is used for production of ......
    (a) Low dust powder   (b) Coarse powder
    (c) Very fine powder   (d) Medium coarse powder

34. Plant materials are extracted by using slow flow of solvent, is known as ......

    (a) Maceration   (b) Decoction

    (c) Percolation   (d) Infusion

35. Soxhlet apparatus is an example of ......

    (a) Digestion   (b) Percolation

    (c) Continuous hot extraction   (d) Maceration

36. Counter current extraction method is used by ......

    (a) Carousel extractor   (b) Soxhlet

    (c) Reflux   (d) Bioguided fractionation

37. Suitable gas used as solvent in Super critical fluid extraction is ......

    (a) CO_2 (b) NO_2

    (c) O_2 (d) NH_4OH

38. Under stressed water, ABA hormone is acts as ......

    (a) Opening of stomata   (b) Closing of stomata

    (c) Both   (d) None

39. Natural occurring Auxin is ......

    (a) IBA   (b) 2,4-D

    (c) NAA   (d) 3-Acetic acid

40. Synthetic auxin analog is ......

    (a) IBA   (b) 2,4-D

    (c) NAA   (d) 3-Acetic acid

41. Cytokinins are used for ......

    (a) Root formation   (b) Shoot formation

    (c) Root inhibition   (d) Shoot inhibition

42. 6-BAP is an example of ......

    (a) Phenyl urea type cytokinin   (b) Adenine type cytokinin

    (c) Amine type cytokinin   (d) Phenyl ketone cytokinin

43. Thidiazuron is an example of ......

    (a) Phenyl urea type cytokinin   (b) Adenine type cytokinin

    (c) Amine type cytokinin   (d) Phenyl ketone cytokinin

44. Stringolactones are derived from ......

    (a) Fatty acids   (b) Carotenoids

    (c) Smoke of burning plant   (d) Steroidal compound

45. Colchicine is induced ......
    (a) Polyploidy   (b) Mutation
    (c) Chemical race   (d) Hybridization
46. Crosses are made between two different species of the same genus is known as ......
    (a) Introgressive hybridization   (b) Interspecific hybridization
    (c) Intra vaietal hybridization   (d) Intra specific hybridization
47. Crossing are made between the same variety of plants ......
    (a) Intravarietal hybridization   (b) Inter varietal hybridization
    (c) Introgressive hybridization   (d) Intra specific hybridization
48. Removal of stamen from female flowering plant is known as ......
    (a) Bagging   (b) Emasculation
    (c) Tagging   (d) Crossing
49. Triticale is the hybrid of ......
    (a) Wheat + Rice   (b) Rye + Rice
    (c) Wheat + Rye   (d) Only Rye variety
50. FRLHT is established in ......
    (a) 1990   (b) 1993
    (c) 2001   (d) 1983
51. Farmers Right Act in ......
    (a) 2001   (b) 2004
    (c) 2000   (d) 1970

ANSWERS

1. (b)	2. (a)	3. (a)	4. (b)	5. (b)	6. (a)	7. (a)	8. (d)	9. (d)
10. (a)	11. (b)	12. (c)	13. (d)	14. (a)	15. (c)	16. (a)	17. (b)	18. (c)
19. (a)	20. (c)	21. (b)	22. (c)	23. (b)	24. (c)	25. (b)	26. (c)	27. (a)
28. (c)	29. (c)	30. (b)	31. (c)	32. (d)	33. (c)	34. (c)	35. (c)	36. (a)
37. (a)	38. (b)	39. (a)	40. (b)	41. (b)	42. (b)	43. (a)	44. (b)	45. (a)
46. (b)	47. (a)	48. (b)	49. (c)	50. (b)	51. (b)			

PLANT TISSUE CULTURE AND ITS APPLICATIONS

♦ LEARNING OBJECTIVES ♦

After completing this unit, reader should be able to:

❖ Know definition of plant tissue culture and its historical development.

❖ Know various types of culture, technique used for tissue culture and laboratory requirement of tissue culture.

❖ Know requirement of sub-culture and their maintenance.

❖ Know various applications of plant tissue culture.

❖ Know edible vaccines.

3.1 PLANT TISSUE CULTURE

Plant cell and tissue culture technique has a great significance in the field of plant biotechnology especially in the crop improvement strategies. Plant tissue culture is defined as the process of *in-vitro* culture of explants (pieces of living differentiated tissues) in nutrient medium either in solid (Agar medium) or liquid (suspension culture) media under aseptic conditions for the growth of cells, tissues, organs or plantlets. It is one of the most beneficial of all the sciences and has immense interest to the molecular biologists, plant breeders and industrialists for the product development as well as helps in improving the plants of economic importance.

3.2 HISTORICAL DEVELOPMENT OF PLANT TISSUE CULTURE

A, German botanist, Gottlieb Haberlandt, cultured fully differentiated plant cells isolated from different plants in the year 1902. This was the very first step or concept for the beginning of plant cell and tissue culture. Cell Doctrine further admitted that a cell is capable of showing totipotency. Totipotency is the regeneration capacity of the parenchyma cells. Thereafter Scientist Hannig cultured embryos from several cruciferous species in 1904. Scientist Kolte and Robbins cultured root and stem tips respectively in 1922. Scientist Went discovered first plant hormone Indole Acetic Acid (IAA) in 1926. In 1932, Prof. White developed plant tissue culture medium for *in-vitro* culture of meristematic cells of Tomato. The composition of medium was salt, yeast extract, sucrose and three vitamins namely pyridoxine, thiamine and nicotinic acid. Thereafter Prof. White introduced vitamin B as growth supplement in tissue culture media for tissue culture of tomato root tip in 1934. Scientists Gautheret, White and Nobecourt are also made valuable contributions to the development of plant tissue culture techniques through proliferation of callus culture in 1939 of tobacco tumor tissues from interspecific hybrid of *Nicotiana glaucum* and *Nicotiana longsdorffi*. The first true plant tissue cultures were obtained by Gautheret from cambial tissue of *Acer pseudoplatanus*. With the identification of a variety of plant growth regulators such as cytokinin, auxin, other hormones, vitamins, etc. and their role in affecting cell division and differentiation, the methods of plant tissue culture developed in a proper manner. Further in 1941, Van Overbeek discovered nutritional value of liquid endosperm of coconut for culture of isolated carrot embryo. Scientist White and Braun together experimented on crown gall and tumor formation in plants, growth of bacteria free crown gall tissues in 1942. Scientist Caplan and F C Stewart together applied coconut milk and 2, 4-D for proliferation of cultured carrot and potato tissues in 1948.

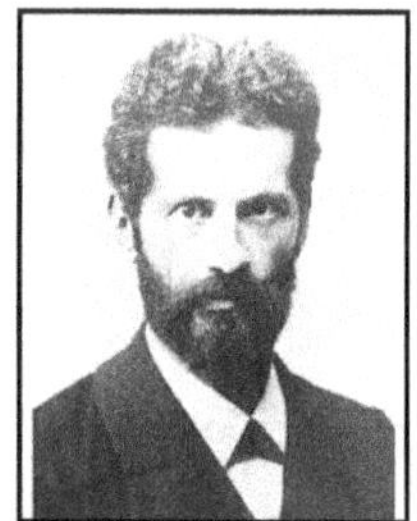

Gottlieb Haberlandt

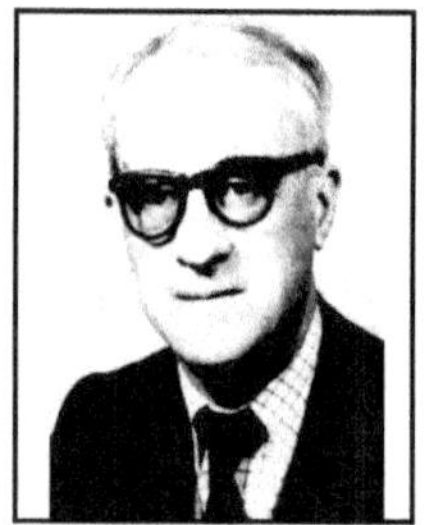

Roger J. Gautheret

Some of other important discoveries of Prof. Gautheret are explained in Table 3.1.

Table 3.1: Some discoveries related to tissue culture

Year	Discovery
1932	Developed root tip and root fragment culture.
1934	Developed cambium culture of woody plants.
1937	Discovered Indole Acetic acid promotes root growth.
1939	Discovered carrot explants develops undifferentiated mass and that can be maintained by repeatedly subculturing.

Embryo culture also had its beginning early in the first decade of the last century with barley embryos. Scientist Ball discovered whole plant from shoot tip and organ regenerated on callus in 1950. In 1954, Scientist Muir, discovered plant from single cell. Scientist Miller in 1955, discovered Kinetin hormone. In 1957, Miller and Skoog proposed that root and shoot differentiation is regulated by Auxin and cytokinin ratio.

The first plant from a mature plant cell was regenerated by Braun in the year 1959. Foundation of commercial plant tissue culture was laid in 1960 with the discovery for a million fold increase in the multiplication of an orchid which was accomplished by G.M. Morel. Some other discoveries related to plant tissue culture are tabulated in Table 3.2.

Table 3.2: Some discoveries related to tissue culture by famous scientists

Year	Discovery	Scientist
1960	Development of planting technique for isolation of single cell	Bergmann
1962	Developed new medium for plant tissue culture	*Murashige and Skoog*
1970	Successful protoplast fusion	Power
1970	Successful Anther culture	Shri S.C. Maheshwari and Sipra Guha
1971	Plant regenerated from protoplast	Takabe
1974	Biotransformation in plant tissue culture	Reinhard
1978	Production of somatic hybrid pomato	Melchers

Terms Used in Tissue Culture:

- **Explant:** An excised piece of differentiated tissue or organ is regarded as an explant. The explant may be taken from any part of the plant body e.g., leaf, stem, root.

- **Callus:** The unorganized, autonomus, uncontrolled and undifferentiated mass of plant cells is known as callus. Generally, when plant cells are cultured in a suitable medium, they divide to form callus i.e., a mass of parenchymatous cells.

- **Differentiation:** It is the process by which meristem cells are converted into two or more types of cells or tissues that are different from each other.

- **Dedifferentiation:** The phenomenon of mature cells reverting to meristematic state to produce callus, means the process of formation of unorganized tissues from the highly organized tissues. Dedifferentiation is possible since the non-dividing quiescent cells of the explant, when grown in a suitable culture medium revert to meristematic state.

- **Re-differentiation:** The ability of the callus cells to differentiate into a plant organ or a whole plant is regarded as re-differentiation, that means the dedifferentiated cells lose the capacity of division and becomes mature to form specific functions.

- **Totipotency:** The ability of an individual cell to develop into a whole plant is referred to as cellular totipotency. The inherent characteristic features of plant cells namely dedifferentiation and re-differentiation are responsible for the phenomenon of totipotency.

- **Plasticity:** It is the condition of the adaptability of a plant species to change in its environment or differences between its various habitats.

- **Organogenesis:** The development of adventitious organs or primordia from undifferentiated cell mass in tissue culture by the process of differentiation.

- **Synthetic seed:** It is the condition where artificial encapsulation of somatic embryos, shoot bud or aggregates of cell of any tissues done by a hydrogel which have the ability to form a plant in *In-vitro* or *Ex-vivo* condition.

- **Somoclonal variation:** The genetic variations found in the *In-vitro* cultured cells are known as somaclonal variations. It occurs due to change in chromosome number and/or structure in plant tissue cultures.

- **Micropropagation:** The production of a large number of individual plants from a small piece of plant tissue cultured without formation of callus in an aseptic nutrient medium.

3.3 TYPES OF CULTURES

The plant growth and development occur in two different ways namely determinate growth where plant growth occurs with certain shape and size like leaves, fruits, flowers etc., and indeterminate growth where plant growth occurs in the roots and stem part which is proliferate continuously. Types of cultures are depends on the type of explant used. Hence, plant tissue culture broadly classified in to eight types viz.

1.	Seed Culture	2.	Embryo Culture
3.	Meristem Culture	4.	Bud Culture
5.	Callus Culture	6.	Cell Suspension Culture
7.	Anther Culture	8.	Protoplast Culture
9.	Hairy root culture	10.	Immobilized cell culture

Seed culture:

Seeds are cultured *in-vitro* to generate seedlings or plants in aseptic condition for raising the sterile seedling. The seed culture is done to get the different kinds of explants from aseptically grown plants that help in better maintenance of aseptic tissue (Fig. 3.1).

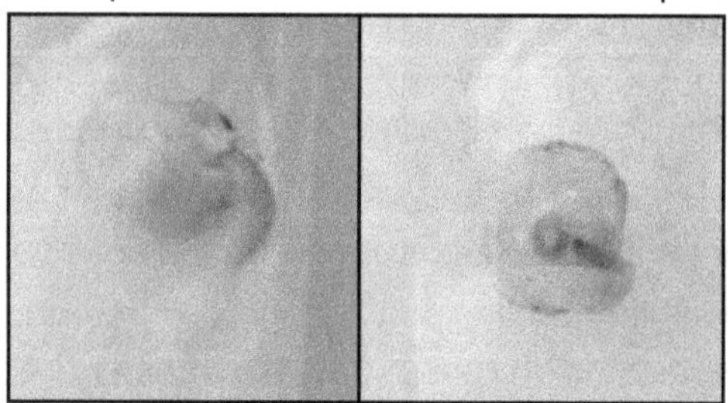

Fig. 3.1: *In-vitro* Seed culture

Importance:

- Increasing efficiency of germination of seeds.
- It is possible to independent on asymbiotic germination.
- It is important in production of Orchids.

Embryo culture:

Embryo culture is the sterile isolation and growth of an immature or mature embryo *in-vitro* for procurement of a viable plant. Embryo developed (initially white in colour) from wide hybridization between two different species may not mature fully due to embryo-endosperm incompatibility. The whole process is known as Embryogenesis (Fig. 3.2).

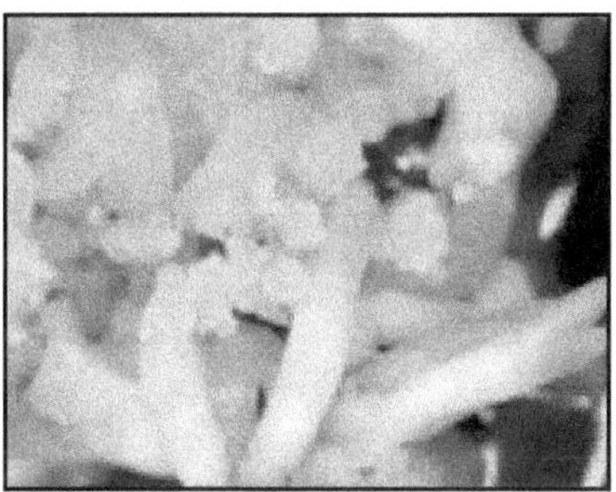

Fig. 3.2: *In-vitro* **embryo culture**

Importance:

- It is useful in production of haploids.
- It helps in prevention of seed dormancy.
- It helps in shortening of breeding cycle.
- It helps in prevention of embryo abortion with early ripening stone fruits.

Meristem Culture:

It is the culture technique by which the apical meristem of shoots of angiosperms and gymnosperms are cultured to get the disease free plants. Generally meristem tips, between 0.2-0.5 mm, most frequently produce virus-free plants and this method is referred to as meristem-tip culture (Fig. 3.3). These explants are cultured on a medium containing cytokinin (plant hormone).

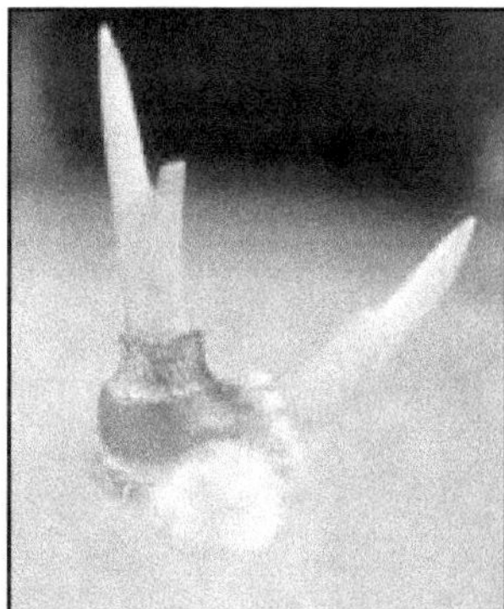

Fig. 3.3: *In-vitro* **meristem culture**

Importance:

- It helps in production of virus free plants.
- It helps in Germplasm conservation.
- It helps in production of transgenic plants.
- It helps in rapid clonal multiplication.
- The method is successful in case of herbaceous plants than woody plants.
- It helps in culture of Potato, Banana, Cardamom, Sugar cane, sweet potato etc.

Bud culture:

Buds contain active meristems in the leaf axils, which are capable of growing into a shoot. Each node of the stem is cut and allowed to grow on a nutrient media to develop the shoot tip from the axil which ultimately develops into new plantlet. In axillary bud method, where the axillary buds are isolated from the leaf axils and develop into shoot tip under little high cytokinin concentration (Fig. 3.4).

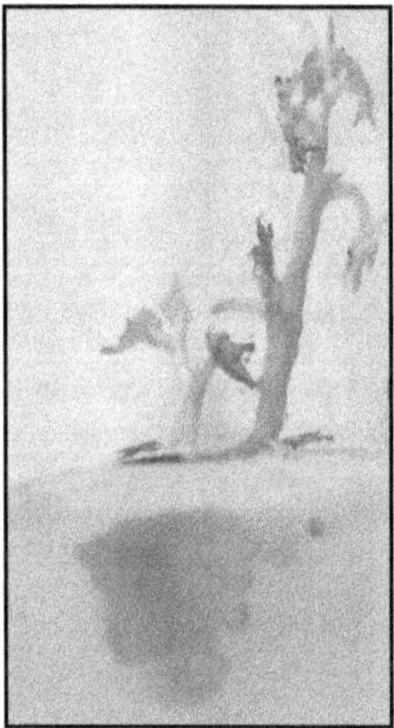

Fig. 3.4: *In-vitro* bud culture

Importance:

- Easy step for micropropagation.
- Easy method for production of disease free plants.
- Isolation of phytoconstituents is easy.

Callus culture:

It is culture of undifferentiated mass of parenchyma cell produced from an explant of a seedling or other plant part in agar medium under aseptic condition is known as callus culture. Callus is densely aggregated, uncontrolled, undifferentiated, unorganized, aerated homogenous parenchymatous mass (Fig. 3.5).

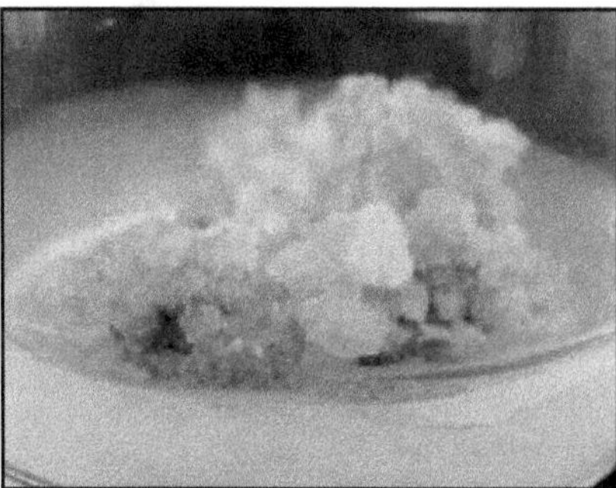

Fig. 3.5: *In-vitro* callus culture

Importance:

- It is the source of tissue for plant regeneration. The whole plant can be regenerated in large number from callus tissue through manipulation of the nutrient and plant hormones in the culture medium. This phenomenon is known as plant regeneration or organogenesis or morphogenesis.

- Chromosomal variation occurs genetically or epigenetically in the cells of callus tissue.
- Increased amount of secondary metabolites are obtained by extraction of the particular callus tissue.
- This method is the source of Tissue for Cell Suspension Culture.
- Several biochemical assays are performed from callus culture.

Principles:

- Aseptic preparation of plant material.
- Selection of suitable nutrient medium supplemented with appropriate ratio of plant growth regulators such as auxins and cytokinins or only appropriate auxin.
- Incubation of culture under controlled physical condition.

Steps involved:

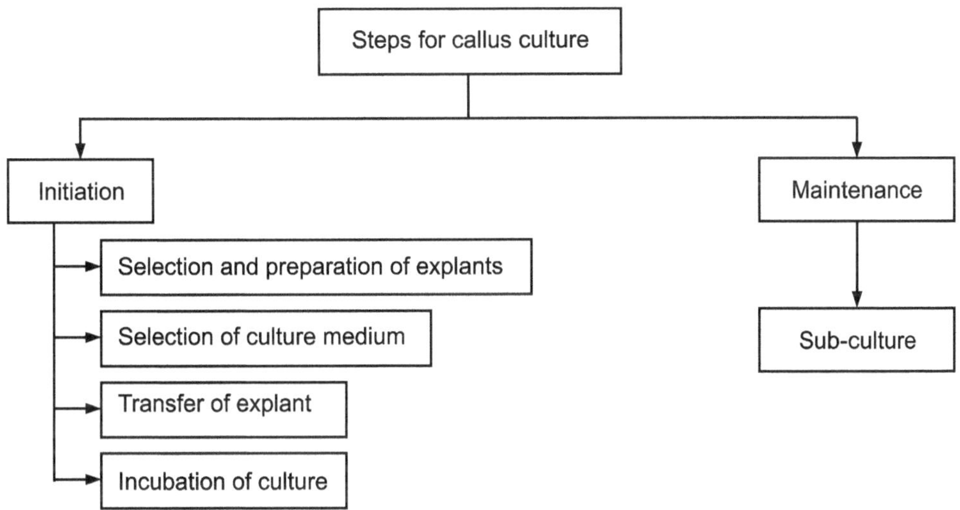

Fig. 3.6

Preparation of explants: Based on the totipotency of the explants, they are selected in young parts. After selection they are surface sterilized with the help of various steps such as washing under running tap water for several times, 1% bavistein treatment, followed by 70% alcohol, 1% sodium hypochlorite, 0.1% mercuric chloride and finally cleaned with double distilled water.

Selection of culture medium: Plant growth hormone such as auxin and cytokinin in the ratio of 10 : 1 to 100 : 1 induces roots whereas 1 : 10 to 1 : 100 induces shoots. Furthermore 1 : 1 ratio helps in callus growth. Mainly solidified agar gel containing MS medium is favorable for callus culture. Media are autoclaved at 15 psi pressure for 15-20 mins at 121°C. The pH is adjusted to 5.7 using 0.1 M HCl or NaOH. Generally agar is used at 0.8 to 1.0% concentration and widely used gelling agent. Agar is resistant to enzymatic hydrolysis at incubation temperature and also neutral to media constituents hence do not react with any other ingredients. Due to these properties, agar is used as solidifying media.

Transfer of explant: Sterilized explants are aseptically transferred media containing agar nutrients with the help of sterile forceps in laminar air flow cabinet.

Incubation of culture: Explant containing culture vessels are aseptically incubated under controlled physical conditions viz. temperature is to maintain 25 ± 2°C, photoperiod should maintain 16 hours day and 8 hours dark conditions, light intensity 2000 to 3000 Lux, relative humidity 55% to 60%. Generally BOD incubator is used for incubation. During this period callus is formed through three stages likely, induction (where metabolic activities of the cell increases), cell division (where active cells are divided) and cell differentiation (where secondary metabolites formed through morphological and physiological differentiation).

BOD incubator: It is the most versatile and reliable low temperature incubator which is designed to maintain at 20°C for Biological Oxygen Demand or Biochemical Oxygen Demand (BOD) determination. It provides controlled temperature conditions for accelerated tests and exposures. It is based on the principle of thermo-electricity. The incubator has a thermostat which maintains a constant temperature by creating a thermal gradient.

Conditions:

Temperature: Standard temperature range: 2°C to 50°C.

Temperature control: ± 0.5°C, 24 hours light and temperature programming. Automatic digital temperature recorder.

Light: Adjustable fluorescent light up to 10,000 Lux.

Relative humidity: 20 to 98%.

Relative humidity control: ± 3%, uniform air circulation.

Attached with shaker for agitation in suspension culture.

Maintenance: Maintenance of callus is possible by sub-culturing callus in fresh medium. This is vital stage for the further growth of the Callus because in the same medium nutrient and water content are reduced as a result metabolic toxins are accumulated. Hence, sub-culturing is necessary in the fresh medium which is repeated after every 4-5 weeks. During the growth period callus appears as yellowish, white, green, or pigmented with brown and purple. Pigmentation is sometimes uniform throughout the callus or some regions remain unpigmented. If callus grown is dark, due to lack of chlorophyll it showed white, if grown in light, then callus formed as green, if carotenoid pigments are more, then callus formed as yellow, purple pigmentation of callus indicated the formation of Anthocyanins whereas more phenolic content indicates the callus is brown in colour.

Cell Suspension Culture:

Suspension culture is defined as a uniform suspension of separate cells in liquid medium where agar is not used. In this medium, callus fragments are transferred to liquid medium and agitated continuously to keep the cell alive and separate. Agitation is also achieved by rotary shaker attached within the BOD incubator at a rate of 50 to 160 rpm. This culture technique is used to study the morphological and biochemical changes during their growth and developmental phases.

Importance:

- Suspension culture is consists of only single cells which are physiologically and biochemically uniform.

- This culture is capable of contributing significant information about cell physiology, biochemistry, metabolic events etc.
- It is important for plant biotransformation and plant genetic engineering.
- No toxic products are formed with this culture technique.
- It helps for induction in somatic embryos and shoots.
- It helps in *in-vitro* mutagenesis and selection of mutants.
- It helps in production of secondary metabolites.
- Shorter duration and continuous process.

Growth pattern:

Under appropriate light, temperature, aeration and nutrient medium the growth of suspension culture is monitored very easily by simply counting the cell number per unit volume of culture in relation to days of culture and follows a growth curve which consists of lag phase, logarithmic phase or exponential phase, linear phase, stationary phase and death phase (Fig. 3.7).

Lag phase: The cells adjust themselves to the nutrient medium and undertake all the necessary synthesis prior to cell division in this phase.

Logarithmic phase or exponential phase: After lag phase the next phase is called as logarithmic phase. As the population size of plant cell approaches one half of the carrying capacity, the growth of culture per time unit increases.

Linear phase: A further period of rapid cell division results in a linear increase in number and the phase is called linear phase which is also a part of exponential phase.

Stationary Phase: As nutrients are depleted and some of the cells of the culture being to show senescent characteristics. If the cells are removed just before or just after the entry into stationary phase in each growth cycle and are sub-cultured to fresh medium, then identical patterns of growth of the cell line is maintained in each sub-culture.

Death phase: The rate of cell division within the culture declines and it passes through the stationary phase. At this time the growth rate slowly decreases due to limitation of nutrients. If sub-culture is not carried out then cell death occurs.

For experimental studies on growth of cell suspension, the inoculum or cell density is an important factor. Very low density or high density of cells in liquid medium is unable to grow. For cell growth, an initial density of 2×10^6 cells/ml to 2×10^8 cells/ml is inoculated in liquid medium.

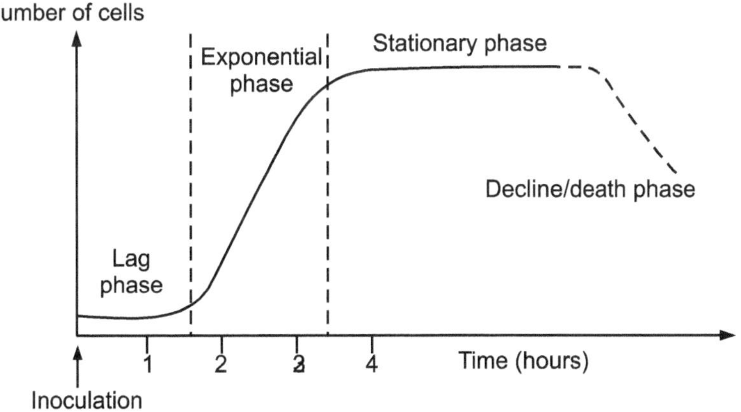

Fig. 3.7: Growth pattern in the suspension culture

Types (Fig. 3.8):

Batch culture: In this type of culture cell material grows in a finite volume of agitated liquid medium. These cultures are maintained by continuous sub-culturing. It is commonly maintained in conical flasks incubated on orbital shakers at 80 to 120 rpm. It is a close system with no addition or removal of nutrient during incubation period.

The biomass growth follows sigmoid curve of growth consisting of lag phase, log phase and stationary phase. Cells are transferred when they reacts with early stage of stationary phase. There is constant change in growth pattern and metabolism of cells.

Continuous culture: Steady state of cell density is maintained by regular replaced a portion of used medium by fresh medium. As a result, physiological states of growing cells are stabilized. In this system, nutrition depletion does not occur due to continuous flow of nutrients and the cells are always in steady growth phase.

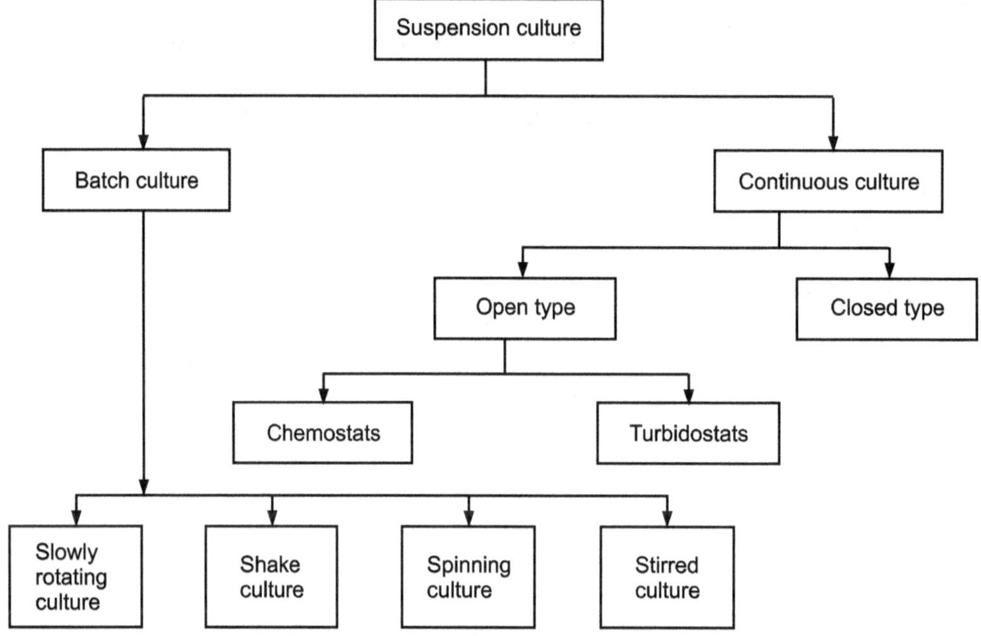

Fig. 3.8: Types of suspension culture

Importance of Single Cell Culture:

Single cell culture technique is very important and it has a wide industrial application.

- Single cell culture is used successfully to obtain single cell clones.
- Plants are regenerated from the callus tissue derived from the single cell clones.
- Produced high degree of spontaneous variability in the cultured tissue.

Measurement of Cell Growth:

The cells in suspension culture grown by cell division and the number of cells increases. Growth in such cultures can be monitored by determination of cell number, cell dry weight, packed cell volume, etc.

Viability of Cell:

The most frequently used staining method for assessing cell viability is fluorescein diacetate (FDA). FDA dissolved in 5 mg/ml of acetone is added to cell population at 0.01%

final concentration. Dead cells fluoresce red. Evans blue also used at a final concentration of 0.01% is specific for dead cells. The non-viable cells stain blue and the viable cells remain unstained. Further 1% 3-[4,5-dimethyltiazol-2-yl]-2,5- diphenyltetrazolium bromide (MTT) is added in the single cells and viable cells are formed Pink and red coloured whereas dead cells does not take any colour.

Anther Culture:

It is the *in-vitro* culture technique of anther containing microspores from unopened flower bud or immature pollen grains (Pollen culture) on a suitable nutrient medium under aseptic condition for the purpose of development of haploid plantlets. By this culture technique haploid cells are obtained which is known as Androgenesis (Fig. 3.9).

Steps:

The young flower buds are collected and washed under running tap water. Surface sterilized by immersing in 70% ethanol or 2.0% sodium hypochlorite solution. Then washed in sterile water and transferred into a sterile petridish. With the help of sterile sharp scalpel the buds are split open and anther lobes are taken out. One of the anther lobes of each bud is checked by crushing into acetocarmine stain under microscope for the proper stage of microspore development. The filament portions are removed from the selected anther lobes. The intact anther lobes are placed into proper media and then incubated at 24°-28°C in dark for 3-8 weeks. The haploid embryos or plantlets develop, come out by bursting the anther lobes.

Importance:

- It is used to study genetic recombination in higher plants.
- It is used to study mode of differentiation from single cell to whole organisms.
- It is used to study of factor controlling pollen embryogenesis of higher plants.
- It is used for mutation studies.
- It is used for hybrid development.
- It is used for genome mapping.
- It is used for formation of double haploid that are homozygous and fertile.

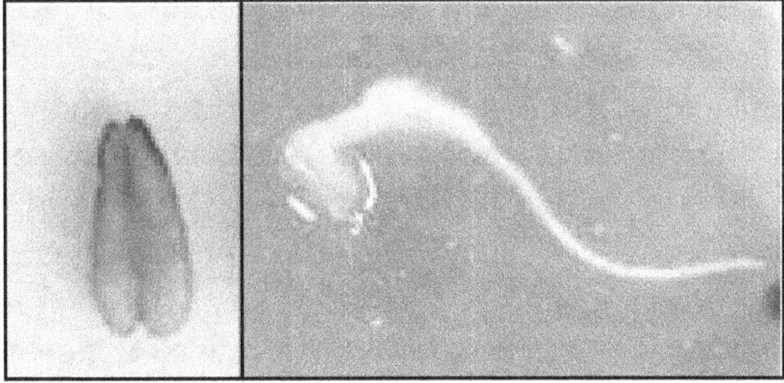

Fig. 3.9: Anther culture

Protoplast Culture:

In this culture method, isolated protoplasts are cultured either in a liquid medium or semisolid agar medium in a thin layer or as small drops of nutrient medium in sterile petridish. Protoplast cells are having cell membrane without cell wall (Fig. 3.10). They are isolated either by enzymatic method or by mechanical method. Mechanical method is manual method and there is a possibility of loss of protoplast cell due to friction force in motor and pestle. This method is avoided by following technique likely a small piece of epidermis is selected from the explants then the cells are subjected to plasmolysis. This causes protoplasts shrinking and finally the tissue is dissected to release the protoplasts from the cell wall. In enzymatic method, enzymes such as cellulase, hemicellulase and pectinase are used. At first, pectinase is used to breaks up the cell aggregates into individual cells by degrade middle lamella then these free cells are exposed to cellulase to release protoplasts from the cell wall. This enzymatic method is used widely to get more yields of protoplast cells as well as minimal or less damage to the protoplast cells.

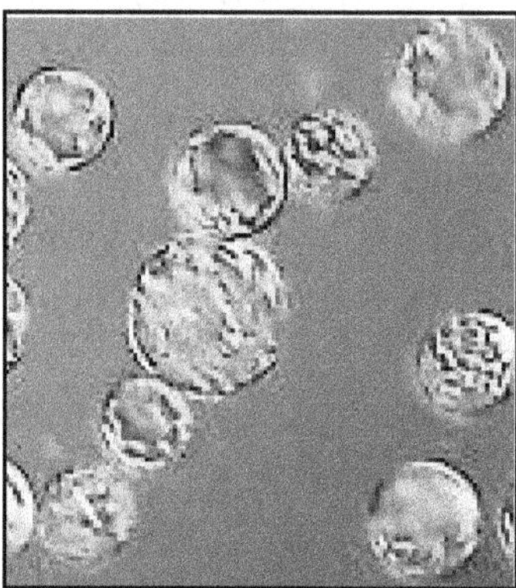

Fig. 3.10: Protoplast culture

Methods of culture:

Protoplast culture is carried out in liquid culture, agar culture, droplet culture, co-culture, hanging droplet culture, immobilised/bead culture and feeder layer technique. In liquid culture, protoplasts easily get divide in liquid media and osmotic pressure of the medium is regulated. In agar culture, agarose is most frequently used to solidify protoplast culture media. Protoplast suspension is taken at double density and mixed with melted agar medium at 45°C and mixed well and plated in small petridish. In droplet culture technique, suspending protoplasts in liquid culture media are placed on petridishes in the form of droplet, the cultured protoplasts clump together at the centre of droplets. In co-culture technique, the newly isolated protoplast suspension is mixed with an authentic fast growing protoplast suspension and mixed protoplasts are plated for development of the isolated protoplast. By hanging drop technique, protoplasts are cultured in an inverted droplet on the inner surface of the lid of petridish. In bead culture, the protoplasts suspension is mixed with polymers such as alginate, carrageenan, etc. and then small beads are made by dripping into the liquid medium and then cultured into liquid medium. In Feeder layer technique, protoplast cell suspensions are exposed to X-rays (to inhibit cell division) and then plating them in a thin layer on agar plates for the isolated less number of protoplasts.

Importance of Protoplast Culture:

- This technique is used to study Morphogenesis.
- This technique is used to study Photosynthesis.

- It helps in gene transfer.
- It helps in study of cell wall formation and their osmotic behaviour.
- It helps in crop improvement through somatic hybridization.
- Protoplast cells also can regenerate into whole plants.
- It develops novel hybrid plants through protoplast fusion.

Hairy Root Culture:

This technique is also known as transformed root culture. It is a culture produced after the infection of explants or cultures by anaturally occurring soil bacterium *Agrobacterium rhizogenes* that contains root-inducing plasmids (Ri plasmids) are infect plant roots and cause them to produce an opines (food source for the bacterium) and abnormally very fast growth. It grows by increasing the rate of cell division and cell elongation. Hairy roots are induced in most of the dicot plants by genetic transformation (through T-DNA, transfer DNA) with *A. rhizogenes*. Hairy root culture shows very high growth rate in the absence of the growth regulator and do not require conditioning of the medium (Fig. 3.11).

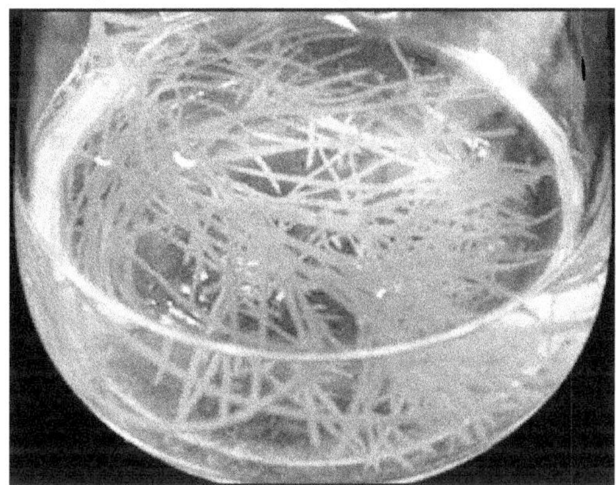

Fig. 3.11: Hairy root culture

Importance:

- It helps in production of high secondary metabolites.
- The culture grows under phyto-hormone free conditions.
- The culture shows fast growth that reduces culture time and easy handling.
- It helps in functional analysis of gene.
- It also used for regeneration of whole plants.
- The culture expresses foreign proteins.
- The culture is genetically and biosynthetically stable.

Immobilized Cell Culture:

It is the technique which confines the cells to a definite region in a space, known as matrix. During that condition, the catalytic activity of the cells retains and prevents its entry into the mobile phase. Immobilization is achieved by binding these cells onto or within a solid support. Some of the important materials are used as matrix like gelatin, polylysine, agarose, alginate etc.

The cells are immobilized by covalently, adsorbed, cross linked, encapsulated and entrapment methods (Fig. 3.12).

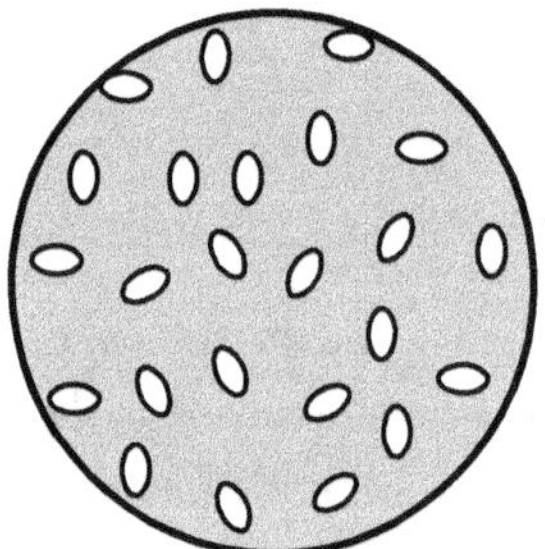
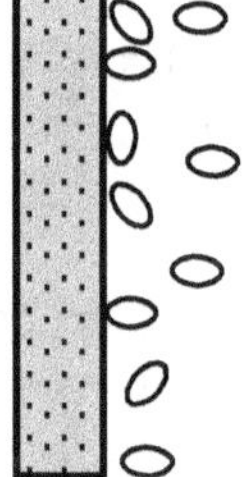
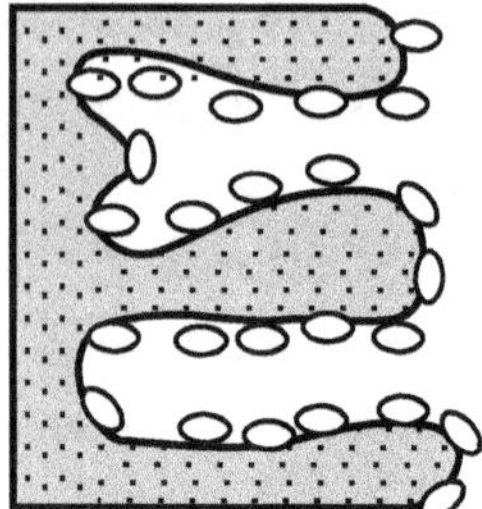

Entrapment method   **Attachment and adsorption method**

Fig. 3.12: Immobilized cell culture

Importance:
- Encapsulation method protects cells from mechanical damage in large fermenters.
- It is used in synthetic seed technology.
- It is used for transfer of protoplast.
- It is cultured as single cell for longer period.
- It helps in conservation of rare cells for further growth into whole plant.
- It helps in production of higher amount of plant secondary metabolites.
- It helps in biotransformation.

Basic Requirement for Plant Tissue Culture Laboratory:
- Equipment and apparatus
- Washing and storage facilities
- Media preparation, sterilization and storage room
- Transfer area
- Culture rooms or incubators for maintenance of cultures
- Observation or data collection area
- Transplantation area

Equipments and Apparatus: Culture tubes as well as culture bottles are required for *in-vitro* culture of explants. All the culture bottles should be made up of Borosil glass. In addition, glassware like graduated pipettes, measuring cylinders, beakers, filters, funnel and petridishes are required for preparations. Glasswares should be made up of pyrex (Fig. 3.13).

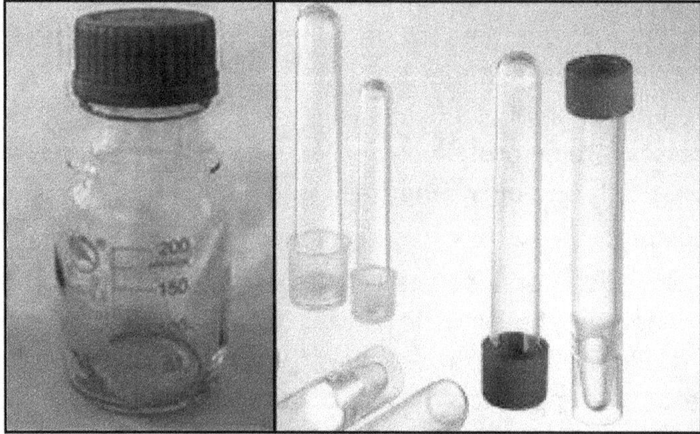

Fig. 3.13: Culture tubes and bottle

Various equipments such as scissors, scalpels, and forceps are required for explants preparation and transfer. Gas burner is required for flame sterilization of equipments. An autoclave to sterilize the media and Hot air oven is required for the sterilization of glass wares. pH meter is required to adjust the medium pH. Weighing balance is used for weighing various nutrients, laminar airflow with UV light fitting cabinet is required for aseptic transfer the explants into the medium. BOD incubator is required for incubation where growth is observed.

Washing and Storage Facilities: Area should be with large stainless steel sink, water facility for running water, draining-boards or racks and ready access to a deionizer, distilled and double-distilled apparatus. Space should also be available to set up drying ovens, washing machines, plastic or steel buckets for soaking lab ware, acid or detergent baths, pipette washers, driers and cleaning brushes. For storage of washed and dried lab ware, the laboratory is provided with dustproof cupboards or storage cabinets.

Media Preparation Room or Space:

This room should be spacious where most of the activities are performed i.e., media preparation and sterilization of media and glassware's needed for culture. There should be sufficient working bench as well as storage space. In this room, various apparatus and equipments are placed such as different types of Glassware, Different kinds of balances, required chemicals, Hot plates and Stirrer, Water bath, pH meter, Autoclave and Hot air oven, Microwave oven, Vortex, Shaker, Centrifuge, Refrigerator and Freezer and Dust free storage cabinet.

Sterilization room:

In this room sterilization of culture media is carried out using autoclave whereas glasswares and other metallic equipments are sterilized with hot air oven. The interior of the cabinet is sterilized with the ultraviolet (UV) germicidal light and wiping the floor of cabinet with 70% alcohol.

Transfer Area:

Transfer of culture into sterilized media i.e. whole tissue culture techniques are carried out in a very clean laboratory having dry atmosphere with contamination free environment. Hence, a sterile dust-free room or cabinet is needed. The 'laminar air flow cabinet' (Fig. 3.14) is the most common accessory used which is designed with horizontal air flow or vertical air flow where the air is forced into the cabinet through a bacterial HEPA (High Efficiency Particulate Air) filter (particle size 0.3 µm). The air flows over the working bench at a constant rate which prevents the particles (microorganisms) from settling on the bench. Furthermore inoculation chamber, a specially designed air tight glass chamber fitted with UV light, is also used as transfer area. Inside cabinet, there is arrangement for Bunsen burner.

Culture Room or Incubation Room:

Plant tissue cultures should be incubated under conditions of well-controlled tempe-rature, illumination, photoperiod, humidity and air circulation because environmental factors have significant effect on the growth as well as on differentiation of cultured tissues. Incubation culture room is essential for incubation under well controlled environmental conditions. BOD incubator is used for the incubation of all cultured explants (Fig. 3.15). Culture rooms are constructed with proper air-conditioning; perforated shelves to support the culture vessels, fitted with fluorescent tubes having a timing device to maintain the photoperiod. For the suspension cultures, rotary shakers are used to fit with BOD incubator. Air conditioners and heaters are used to maintain the temperature around 25 ± 2°C and humidity is maintained by uniform forced air-ventilation, ranged of 20 to 90%. The lighting is adjusted up to 10,000 Lux.

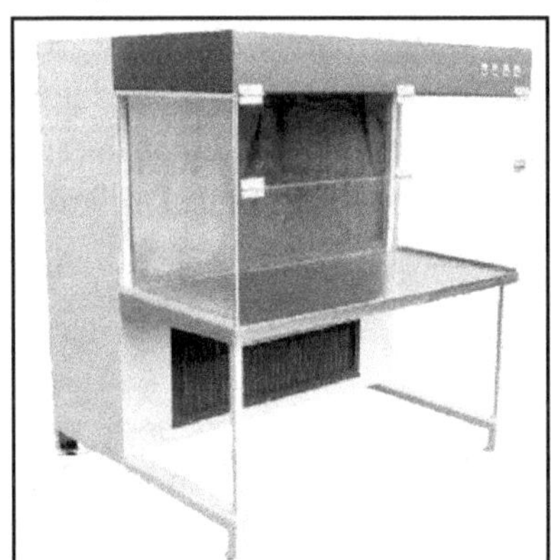

Fig. 3.14: Laminar air flow cabinet

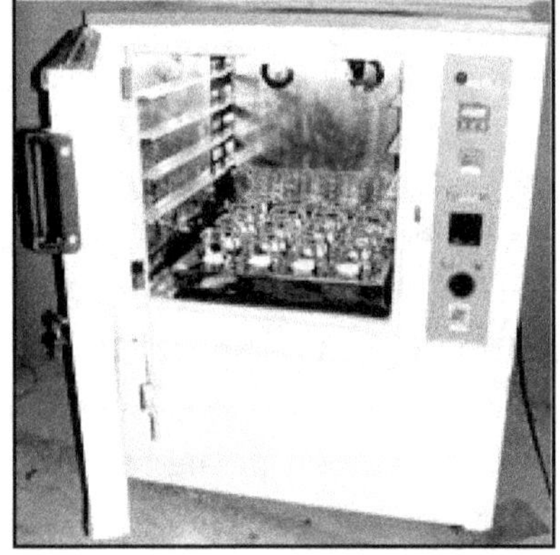

Fig. 3.15: BOD incubator

Data Collection Area:

The growth and development of tissues cultured *in-vitro* are generally monitored by observing cultures at regular intervals in the culture room. All data is to be feeded in computer. Arrangement should be there where the observations are carried out under aseptic conditions using microscope. Special facilities are required for germplasm conservation i.e., cryopreservation accessories should be there.

Transplantation Area:

Plants regenerated from *in-vitro* tissue culture are transplanted to soil in pots. Then they are transferred to greenhouse after acclimatization under well humid condition and controlled temperature and under controlled entry of sunlight.

3.4 NUTRITIONAL REQUIREMENTS, GROWTH AND THEIR MAINTENANCE

General procedure involve in plant tissue culture:

- **Sterilization of glasswares and vessels:** All the required glasswares are kept overnight dipped in sodium dichromate – sulphuric acid solution for removal of dirt, or any microorganisms or any waxy materials. Then further cleaned with running tap water followed by double distilled water. Then placed inverted position in plastic bucket for removal of extra water. Drying of glasswares are carried out in hot air oven at temp about 121°C for 30 minutes. For plastic materials, sterilization is carried out with non-abrasive detergent followed by cleaning under running tap water finally then rinsed with acetone for drying. All the cleaned materials are stored in dust proof cupboard for further use. All the stainless steel equipments, scalpels, forceps are sterilized with flame sterilization followed by wrapped with aluminium foil after cooling and kept in dust free cupboard.

Other glasswares are also kept in sterile conditions by wrapped in aluminium foil with cotton pads for prevention of dust particles.

- **Preparation and sterilization of explants:** It is very important step for the plant tissue culture. Explants are selected as per the totipotency and is selected from any part of the plants such as young leaves, roots, flowers, stems, cambium, anthers etc. After selection, the young part is removed with sharp knife and sterilization is carried out. Various types of sterilants are used for sterilization such as chromic acid (3-5 min), 0.1% mercuric chloride (3-10 min), 1-2% sodium or calcium hypochlorite (5-15 min) and 70% alcohol for 3 to 10 sec followed by washing with double distilled water. Generally, leaves are sterilized with 0.1% mercuric chloride solution followed by sterile water. Stems are sterilized with 2% sodium hypochlorite solution for 15-20 minutes followed by washing with sterile double distilled water. Seeds are sterilized by ethanol for 10 second followed by rinsed with purified water and then 10% calcium hypochlorite solution for 15 minutes. Fruits are cleaned with ethanol followed by 2% sodium hypochlorite solution for 10 minutes and finally sterile double distilled water washing for 15 minutes.
- **Production of callus from explants:** Sterile explants further transferred aseptically in to the sterilized medium and incubated into BOD incubator for necessary growth. Temperature is maintained at 25°C ± 2°C kept for 2-3 weeks.
- **Proliferation:** Developed callus further cut into small pieces with sterile scalpel and transferred into another fresh medium for further proliferation. This process is also known as sub-culturing. This method is carried out at an interval of 4-5 weeks based on the growth of the callus.
- **Suspension culture:** It contains a uniform suspension of separate cells in liquid medium. For this callus is transferred in to liquid medium and agitated continuously (80-150 rpm) in BOD incubator for cells separate. After cell growth, again sub-culturing is carried out.

Culture media:

Culture media plays a vital role for the *in-vitro* growth and morphogenesis of plant tissues because it should contain the same nutrients for growth as required by the whole plant. The composition of the culture media is primarily dependent on two parameters viz. the particular species of the plant and the type of material used for culture. The media used are solid (solid medium) or liquid (liquid medium) in nature which is dependent on the better response of a culture. There are several culture media developed such as White's medium, Murashige and Skoog (MS) medium, B-5 medium, N-6 medium, Nitsch's medium etc.

- (a) **White's medium:** This culture media is developed for root culture of tomato. This is one of the earliest media with low salt formulation.
- (b) **Murashige and Skoog (MS) medium:** Murashige and Skoog (MS) originally formulated a medium to induce organogenesis and regeneration of plants in cultured tissues. MS medium is widely used for many types of culture systems.
- (c) **B-5 Medium:** Developed by Gamborg, B-5 medium is prepared for cell suspension and callus cultures. At present with certain modifications, this medium is used for protoplast culture.

(d) N-6 medium: Chu formulated this medium and it is used for cereal anther culture. This medium is used to improve the formation, growth and differentiation of pollen callus in rice.

(e) Nitsch's medium: This medium was developed by Nitsch and Nitsch for anther cultures. This medium is used in the production of haploid plants of various species of Nicotiana raised from pollen grains. Some pollen grains proliferate into embryo-like structures that develop in stages similar to those of zygotic embryos.

Table 3.3: Composition of Culture Media

Components	Amount (mg l^{-1})				
	White's	Murashige and Skoog (MS)	Gamborg (B5)	Chu (N6)	Nitsch's
Macronutrients					
$MgSO_4 \cdot 7H_2O$	750	370	250	185	185
KH_2PO_4	–	170	–	400	68
$NaH_2PO_4 \cdot H_2O$	19	–	150	–	–
KNO_3	80	1900	2500	2830	950
NH_4NO_3	–	1650	–	–	720
$CaCl_2 \cdot 2H_2O$	–	440	150	166	–
$(NH_4)_2 \cdot SO_4$	–	–	134	463	–
Micronutrients					
H_3BO_3	1.5	6.2	3	1.6	–
$MnSO_4 \cdot 4H_2O$	5	22.3	–	4.4	25
$MnSO_4 \cdot H_2O$	–	–	10	3.3	–
$ZnSO_4 \cdot 7H_2O$	3	8.6	2	1.5	10
$Na_2MoO_4 \cdot 2H_2O$	–	0.25	0.25	–	0.25
$CuSO_4 \cdot 5H_2O$	0.01	0.025	0.025	–	0.025
$CoCl_2 \cdot 6H_2O$	–	0.025	0.025	–	0.025
KI	0.75	0.83	0.75	0.8	–
$FeSO_4 \cdot 7H_2O$	–	27.8	–	27.8	27.8
$Na_2 \cdot EDTA \cdot 2H_2O$	–	37.3	–	37.3	37.3
Sucrose (g)	20	30	20	50	20
Organic supplements **Vitamins**					
Thiamine HCl	0.01	0.5	10	1	0.5
Pyridoxine (HCl)	0.01	0.5	1	0.5	0.5
Nicotinic acid	0.05	0.5	1	0.5	5
Myoinositol	–	100	100	–	100
Others					
Glycine	3	2	–	–	2
Folic acid	–	–	–	–	0.5
Biotin	–	–	–	–	0.05
pH	**5.8**	**5.8**	**5.5**	**5.8**	**5.8**

Table 3.4: Functions of Elements in Plant Tissue Culture

Elements	Functions
Nitrogen	It is essential component for proteins, nucleic acid.
Calcium	Important for synthesis of cell wall and cell functioning
Potassium	It regulates osmotic potential
Magnesium	It is component of chlorophyll
Phosphorus	It is component of nucleic acid
Sulphur	It is component of amino acids
Manganese	It is cofactor for certain enzyme and helps in cell elongation
Iron	It helps in electron transfer reaction
Copper	It involves in electron transfer reaction
Cobalt	It is component of vitamin-B_{12}
Zinc	It requires for chlorophyll biosynthesis
Molybdenum	It is component of certain enzymes and helps in cell elongation
Chlorine	It helps in photosynthesis
Boron	It is used for retardation of cell division and cell elongation

Culture Media contains the following Constituents:

Inorganic Nutrients:

Mineral elements are very important for growth of a plant. The inorganic nutrients consists of macronutrients (concentration >0.5 mmol//l) and micronutrients (concentration <0.5 mmol/l). The inorganic salts in water undergo dissociation and ionization. Essentially about 15 elements found important for plant growth. There are broadly two types of nutrients namely macronutrients and micronutrients. Macronutrients such as nitrogen, phosphorus, potassium, calcium, magnesium and sulphur are present as salts in the medium. Nitrogen concentration should be 2-20 mmol/l whereas calcium, magnesium, sulphur and phosphorus concentration should be in the range of 1-3 mmol/l. Micronutrients such as iron, copper, manganese, zinc, boron, molybdenum are essential for plant growth. In addition certain media are also enriched with cobalt, iodine and sodium. In MS medium, K^+ ions are contributed by KNO_3 and KH_2PO_4 while NO_3^- ions come from KNO_3 and NH_4NO_3.

Organic nutrients:

Optimum growth of plants is also achieved by proper application of vitamins and amino acids. Among the vitamins thiamine (Vitamin B_1), pyridoxine (vitamin B_6), nicotinic acid (vitamin B_3) and ionositol are essential ingredients for growth of plants. Apart from that casein hydrolystate, coconut milk, corn milk, malt extract, yeast extracts are used for growth of plant tissue culture.

Sucrose at concentration of 2-5% is used as carbon source. During the course of sterilization (by autoclaving) of the medium, sucrose gets hydrolyzed to glucose and fructose. Glucose and fructose are also used for growth of tissues. The plant cells in culture first utilize glucose and then fructose. The hydrolyzed products of sucrose are efficient sources of energy.

Amino acids are also plays important role in the growth of plant tissues. Organic nitrogen (in the form of amino acids such as L-glutamine, L-asparagine, L- arginine, L-cysteine) is more readily taken up than inorganic nitrogen by the plant cells.

Activated charcoal supplemented in the medium also stimulates the growth and differentiation of certain plant cells (carrot, tomato, orchids). Some toxic/inhibitory compounds (e.g. phenols) produced by cultured plants are removed (by adsorption) by activated charcoal which facilitates efficient cell growth.

Growth regulators (Fig. 3.16):

Plant hormones are a group of natural organic compounds that promote growth, development and differentiation of plants. Four broad classes of growth regulators or hormones are used for culture of plant cells viz. auxins, cytokinins, gibberellins and abscisic acid which promote growth, differentiation and organogenesis of plant tissues in cultures. Auxins induce cell division, cell elongation, and formation of callus in cultures. At a low concentration, auxins promote root formation while at a high concentration callus formation occurs. They are dissolved in ethanol or in dilute sodium hydroxide then concentration made up as per require amount with water. Some examples are Indole 3-acetic acid (IAA), 2, 4-dichlorophenoxy acetic acid (2,4-D), Indole-3 butyric acid (IBA), 1-naphthyl acetic acid (NAA). 2, 4-dichlorophenoxy acetic acid is most effective and is widely used in culture media.

Cytokinins are derivatives of a purine namely adenine. These adenine derivatives are involved in cell division, shoot differentiation and somatic embryo formation. Cytokinins promote RNA synthesis and thus stimulate protein and enzyme activities in tissues. Some examples are kinetin and benzyl-amino purine which are frequently used in culture media.

The concentrations of auxins and cytokinins are very important for the morphogenesis of culture systems. When the ratio of auxins to cytokinins is high, embryogenesis, callus initiation and root initiation occur whereas for proliferation of axillary and shoots, the ratio of auxins to cytokinins is low. It is considered that the formation and maintenance of callus cultures require both auxin and cytokinin, while auxin is needed for root culture and cytokinin for shoot culture. But the actual concentrations of the growth regulators in culture media are varied on the type of tissue explant and the plant species.

Gibberellins:

About 20 different gibberellins are identified as growth regulators. Of these, gibberellin A_3 (GA_3) is the most commonly used for tissue culture. GA_3 promotes growth of cultured cells, enhances callus growth and induces dwarf plantlets to elongate. Gibberellins are capable of promoting or inhibiting tissue cultures, depending on the plant species. They usually inhibit adventitious root and shoot formation.

Abscisic acid (ABA):

The callus growths are stimulated or inhibited by ABA which is largely depends on the nature of the plant species. It is an important growth regulation for induction of embryogenesis.

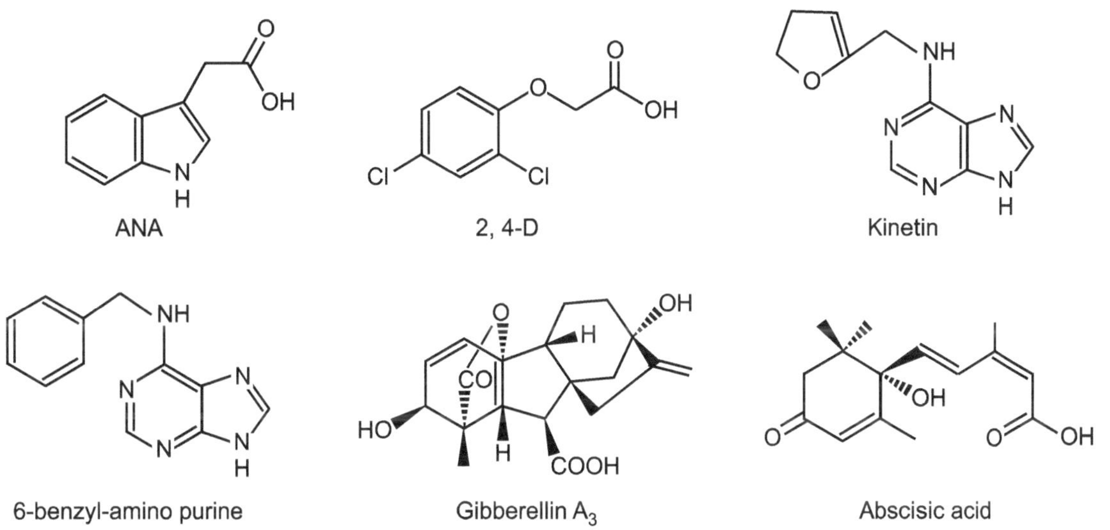

Fig. 3.16: Structures of various growth regulators

Solidifying Agents:

For the preparation of semisolid or solid tissue culture media, solidifying or gelling agents are required that provides support to tissues growing in the static conditions.

Agar:

Agar, a polysaccharide obtained from seaweeds, is most commonly used as a gelling agent for the following reasons:

1. It does not react with media constituents.

2. It is not digested by plant enzymes.

3. It is stable at culture temperature.

Agar at a concentration of 0.5 to 1% in the medium can form a gel. Gelatin is also used as gelling agent at 10% concentration but generally not used in tissue culture because gelatin melts at low temperature (25°C), and consequently the gelling property is lost.

pH of medium:

The optimal pH for most tissue cultures is in the range of 5.0-6.0. The pH generally falls by 0.3-0.5 units after autoclaving. At a pH higher than 7.0 and lower than 4.5, the plant cells stop growing in cultures. In general, pH above 6.0, the medium became hard whereas pH below 5.0 does not allow gelling of the medium.

3.5 APPLICATIONS OF PLANT TISSUE CULTURE IN PHARMACOGNOSY

1. Development of Clonal and Micro-Propagation through multiplication of genetically identical plants or crops. It is very used in horticulture, in the crops which have long seed dormancy, tree species, orchids and many fruit plants.

2. Production of biomass energy which is useful in forestry.

3. Increased production of secondary metabolites which helps in isolation of the constituents for drug discovery as well as various Pharmaceutical formulations.

4. Procurement of Genetic Variability which is due to cells of various ploidy levels and genetic constitution of the initial explant or also may be developed due to different cultural conditions. It helps for production of hybrid plants by polyploidy, mutation and hybridization techniques. It is a great application in the field of horticulture as well as in Agronomy. It helps in development of useful characters such as resistance to a particular disease, herbicide resistance and stress tolerance.

5. Somatic Embryogenesis and Synthetic Seed development by which the mass production of adventitious embryos occurs that ultimately develop into complete plantlet in maturing media. This method is useful for production of disease free propagules as well as production of asexually propagating plants. It is innovative technique in agriculture field.

6. Breaking Dormancy is a further challenging for hard coated seeds. By this culture technique the seed dormancy period is reduced and the breeding cycle is shortened which improve early growth of plants.

7. Propagation of haploid Plants through anther or pollen culture (androgenesis) or through ovaries or ovule culture (gynogenesis).

8. Establishment of Somatic Hybrids through Somatic hybridisation, i.e., the asexual hybridization. It is carried out by fusion of protoplast cells by hybridization. Products of fusion between two protoplasts (heterokaryon) are cultured to regenerate a new somatic hybrid plant of desired genotype.

9. Development of Transgenic Plants by carrying genes for different traits like insect resistance, herbicide tolerance, delayed ripening, increased amino acid and vitamin content, improved oil quality, etc.

10. Germplasm Conservation through *in-vitro* method is gaining importance. The storage collection provides a cost effective alternative to growing plants under field conditions, nurseries or greenhouses. Recently, pollen preservation is very important for endangered plant species.

3.6 EDIBLE VACCINES

Vaccines are proved to be boon for the prevention of infectious diseases. A vaccine is a biological preparation that provides active acquired immunity to a particular disease. Vaccine consists of dead pathogens or live but attenuated organisms. They induce immunity against pathogen either by production of antibodies or by activation of T-lymphocytes. Edward Jenner first produces live vaccine for small pox from cow pox virus in the year 1796. The process of administrating vaccines is known as vaccination. There are three types of traditional vaccines namely, inactivated or killed vaccines (examples: Typhoid, Cholera, Plague, Rabies etc.), live attenuated vaccines (examples: BCG, Typhoid oral, Oral polio, Measles, Mumps etc.) and toxoids (examples: Diptheria, tetanus). Some properties of vaccines are like they should cheap, should not be toxic, low level of side effect, should not cause any problem in any individual, should not contaminate the environment, vaccination technique should be simple. The uses of vaccines in many countries are limited due to high cost hence an alternate cost effective vaccines are introduced which is known as edible vaccines. These vaccines are easily administrable, storable and widely acceptable as bio-friendly in all developing countries. Oral administration of edible vaccines proves reduction of the incidence of various diseases like hepatitis, diarrhoea etc., which face the problem of storing and administering vaccines. Edible vaccines are obtained by incorporating a particular gene of interest into the plant, which produces the desirable encoded protein. This process is known as transformation, and the altered plants are known as transgenic plants. They are specific to provide mucosal activity along with systemic immunity. Various foods that are used as alternative agents for injectable vaccines include cereals (wheat, rice, corn), fruits (bananas) and vegetables (lettuce, potatoes, tomatoes). The main advantages for edible vaccines that syringes and needles are also not required which reduces the incidence of various infections. Thereafter elimination of contamination with animal viruses-like the mad cow disease, which is a hazard in vaccines developed from cultured mammalian cells, as plant viruses cannot infect humans. They act by stimulating the mucosal as well as systemic immunity, as soon they meet the digestive tract lining. They produce antibody mediated immune response and cell mediated immune response. Edible vaccines enable the process of seroconversion in the presence of maternal antibodies, so they play a vital role in protecting children against diseases like group-B *Streptococcus*, respiratory syncytial virus (RSV), etc. They are produced for various human and animal diseases (measles, cholera, foot and mouth disease and hepatitis B, C and E) and are also used to prevent dengue, hookworm, rabies, etc. by combining with other vaccination programmes enabling multiple antigen delivery.

Examples: The first successful human trial for an edible vaccine was conducted in year 1997 in which volunteers were fed transgenic potatoes, which possessed the b-subunit of the *E. coli* heat-labile toxin, responsible for diarrhoea. But it has a major drawback that it needs to be eaten as raw because cooking causes denaturation of protein and makes it ineffective. Plants used for edible vaccines are like Tobacco, Potato, Banana, Tomato, Rice, Carrot, Corn, Muskmelon, Soybean etc.

Preparation:

Live attenuated vaccines are prepared by grown disease causing organism under special laboratory conditions that causes loss of virulence or disease causing properties. The attenuation is obtained by heat or by passage of the virus in foreign host like tissue culture cells or embryonated eggs. Cell culture is required for the viral vaccines because viruses are replicated inside the living cells. Example: Sabin polio vaccine is produced by attenuated with high inocula and rapid passage in primary monkey kidney cells.

Inactivated vaccines are produced by killing the disease causing microorganism with heat or by chemicals. Vaccines are also produced by gene techniques where single gene is expressed in a foreign host by cloning.

Advantages of Edible Vaccines:

1. Edible vaccines have efficient mode of action for immunization.
2. They are comparatively cost effective, as they do not require cold chain storage.
3. They do not need sophisticated equipments and machines as they are easily grown on rich soils.

4. They are widely accepted as they are orally administered unlike traditional vaccines that are injectable.

5. They are safe as they do not contain heat-killed pathogens.

6. The production process is scaled up rapidly by breeding.

Importance:

- It is used for cancer therapies like colon cancer and cervical cancer.
- It is used for autoimmune diseases like Type-I diabetes and multiple sclerosis.
- It is applied for many infectious diseases like AIDS, tetanus, small pox, measles, plague, foot and mouth disease, tuberculosis, influenza etc.

EXERCISE

Long Essays:

1. Define Plant tissue culture. Explain lab requirement and general method involves in plant tissue culture.
2. Explain the detail history of plant tissue culture.
3. Explain various types of plant tissue culture.
4. Explain callus and suspension cultures.
5. Explain the role of nutrients and plant growth regulators in *in-vitro* culture technique.

Short Essays:

1. Explain the general composition of culture media.
2. Explain the role of culture media in plant tissue culture.
3. Explain the basic requirement of plant tissue culture lab.
4. Explain hairy root culture and immobilized cell culture.
5. Explain growth pattern of suspension culture.
6. Explain lab requirement for plant tissue culture.
7. Explain protoplast culture.
8. Explain anther culture and seed culture.
9. Explain callus culture.
10. Explain suspension culture.
11. Explain the term: Organogenesis, Totipotency, Synthetic seed, Differentiation, De-differentiation, Re-differentiation.
12. Explain nutrient requirement for preparation of media.
13. Explain plant growth regulators in plant tissue culture.
14. Explain application of Plant tissue culture.
15. Explain edible vaccine.

Multiple Choice Questions (MCQs):

1. Embryo culture is carried out in 1904 by ......

   (a) Hannig   (b) Kolte

   (c) Robbins   (d) Haberlandt

2. First differentiated plant cell was isolated by ......
    (a) Hannig   (b) Kolte
    (c) Robbins   (d) Haberlandt

3. Scientist "Went" first discovered plant hormone ......
    (a) NAA   (b) IBA
    (c) IAA   (d) Kinetin

4. Prof. White was first developed plant tissue culture medium for ......
    (a) Callus of leaves   (b) Meristem cells of tomato
    (c) Callus of carrot   (d) Meristem cells of tobacco

5. Liquid endosperm of coconut for culture of isolated carrot embryo was developed by Scientist ......
    (a) Gautheret   (b) Van Overbeek
    (c) Caplan   (d) White

6. Coconut milk and 2,4-D is used for proliferation of cultured carrot was applied by Scientist ......
    (a) White   (b) Van Overbeek
    (c) Caplan   (d) Nobecourt

7. First cambium culture of woody plant was discovered in ......
    (a) 1932   (b) 1934
    (c) 1939   (d) 1937

8. Plant from single cell was discovered by Scientist ......
    (a) White   (b) Miller   (c) Muir   (d) Caplan

9. Anther culture was discovered by Scientist ......
    (a) Takebe   (b) Sipra Guha
    (c) Maheshwari and Sipra Guha   (d) Melchers

10. Scientist Reinhard has discovered ......
    (a) Somatic hybrid
    (b) Biotransformation in plant tissue culture
    (c) Protoplast fusion
    (d) Single cell isolation

11. The process by which meristem cells are converted into more cells are known as ......
    (a) Differentiation   (b) De-differentiation
    (c) Re-differentiation   (d) Plasticity

12. Regeneration capacity of plant cells are known as ......
    (a) Plasticity   (b) Totipotency
    (c) Micropropagation   (d) Differentiation

13. Synthetic seed is known as ......
    (a) Encapsulation of somatic seeds
    (b) Encapsulation of somatic embryos
    (c) Encapsulation of stem
    (d) Encapsulation of anthers

14. The process of formation of unorganized tissues from organized tissues is known as ......
    (a) Organogenesis
    (b) Re-differentiation
    (c) De-differentiation
    (d) Differentiation

15. Embryo culture helps in ......
    (a) Production of Orchids
    (b) Increasing germination of seeds
    (c) Prevent seed dormancy
    (d) Increase breeding cycle

16. Rapid clonal multiplication is possible through ......
    (a) Anther culture
    (b) Seed culture
    (c) Protoplast culture
    (d) Meristem culture

17. BOD incubator is ......
    (a) Biological Oxygen Demand
    (b) Bio fuel Oxygen Demand
    (c) Basic Oxygen Demand
    (d) Biological Oxygen Depositor

18. Adjustable fluorescent light in BOD is ......
    (a) 10000 Lux
    (b) 100000 Lux
    (c) 5000 Lux
    (d) 50000 Lux

19. Purple pigmentation of callus indicates ......
    (a) More Phenolic
    (b) More flavonoids
    (c) More anthocyanin
    (d) More quinones

20. The colour of dead single cells in fluorescent diacetate is ......
    (a) Red
    (b) Blue
    (c) Pink
    (d) Unstain

21. The viable single cells are taking pink colour with reagent ......
    (a) Fluorescent diacetate
    (b) Evans Blue
    (c) MTT
    (d) Bromine water

22. Haploid cells are obtained by anther culture is also known as ......
    (a) Organogenesis
    (b) Androgenesis
    (c) Somoclonal variation
    (d) Plantagenesis

23. Protoplast cells are ......
    (a) Cells with cell wall
    (b) Cells with cell membrane without cell wall
    (c) Cells with cell wall without cell membrane
    (d) Hybrid cell

24. Break up of cell aggregates is possible through ......
    (a) Pectinase   (b) Cellulase
    (c) Lygase   (d) Isomerase
25. Agrobacterium is required for culture of ......
    (a) Protoplast   (b) Hairy root
    (c) Anther   (d) Seed
26. Matrix used in immobilized cell culture is ......
    (a) Agarose   (b) Pectinase
    (c) Cellulose   (d) Guar gum
27. Biotransformation is possible through ......
    (a) Protoplast culture   (b) Immobilized cell culture
    (c) Organ culture   (d) Micropropagation
28. HEPA filter removes particle size of ......
    (a) 0.03 µM   (b) 0.3 µM
    (c) 0.003 µM   (d) 3 µM
29. Example of sterilants is ......
    (a) 2% NaCl   (b) 2% Sodium hypochlorite
    (c) 1% sodium sulphate   (d) 2% Sodium sulphate
30. Root culture of Tomato is well established in ......
    (a) B-5 medium   (b) MS medium
    (c) White's medium   (d) N-6 medium
31. B-5 medium is also known as ......
    (a) MS medium   (b) Nitsch's medium
    (c) Gamborg Medium   (d) White medium
32. Cereal Anther culture is suitable in ......
    (a) N-6 medium   (b) Nitsch's medium
    (c) B-5 medium   (d) MS medium
33. High concentration of auxin promotes ......
    (a) Root   (b) Callus
    (c) Shoot   (d) Both shoots and roots
34. Medium pH is optimum for tissue culture is ......
    (a) 4.5   (b) 7.0
    (c) 5-6   (d) 6-8
35. Live attenuated vaccine is ......
    (a) Typhoid   (b) Oral Polio
    (c) Plague   (d) Rabies

ANSWERS

1. (a)	2. (d)	3. (c)	4. (b)	5. (b)	6. (c)	7. (b)	8. (c)	9. (c)
10. (b)	11. (a)	12. (b)	13. (b)	14. (c)	15. (c)	16. (d)	17. (a)	18. (a)
19. (c)	20. (a)	21. (c)	22. (b)	23. (b)	24. (a)	25. (b)	26. (a)	27. (b)
28. (b)	29. (b)	30. (c)	31. (c)	32. (a)	33. (b)	34.(c)	35. (b)	

✱✱✱

TRADITIONAL SYSTEM OF MEDICINES AND PLANT SECONDARY METABOLITES

◆ LEARNING OBJECTIVES ◆

After completing this unit, reader should be able to understand:

❖ Role of Pharmacognosy in Allopathy as well as various traditional system of medicines such as Ayurveda, Siddha, Unani, Homeopathy and Chinese medicines.

❖ General introduction about various Traditional System of Medicines.

❖ Plant secondary metabolites and their role in human.

❖ Various plant secondary metabolites, their classification, properties and identification tests.

❖ Various methods for extraction of plant secondary metabolites.

(A) PHARMACOGNOSY IN VARIOUS SYSTEMS OF MEDICINE

4.1 ALLOPATHY

Allopathy is derived from the Greek word **allos** means "other or different" and **pathos** means disease or suffering. In combination it means "other than the disease." The term Allopathy was given by Samuel Hahnemann in early 19th century. Allopathy medicine is basically a part of Western medical system. This system is spread all over the world and adopted by many countries over the world due to effectiveness in emergency. This system is drug oriented methodology which depends on three things viz. hypothesis, experimentation and result of the experiment. The main methodology of this system is experimentation. In this system, doctors treat a disease based on the symptoms not based on causes. This system is also known as evidence based or modern medicine. The main drawback is most of the drugs have side effects and for being out of poor people due to the high cost of drugs and also treatments.

In this system, the drugs are manufactured using synthetic chemicals or chemical derived from natural products like plants, animals or mineral sources. Various drugs like tablets, capsules, injections, tonic etc. It also uses modern equipments for diagnosis, analysis and surgery.

4.1.1 Role of Pharmacognosy in Allopathy

Pharmacognosy plays a diverse role in the discovery, characterization, production and standardization of these drugs. It is used by pharmaceutical companies to screen, characterize and produce new drugs for the treatment of multiple human diseases. Naturally occurring drugs are not produced in mass quantities hence they are studied in order to develop synthetic biosimilars. Producing these compounds synthetically allows through modifications viz. increases in bioavailability, altered pharmacokinetics and increased efficacy. These modifications transform a crude inactive plant extract into a powerful drug. Some examples are like anticancer drugs, CVS drugs. Thus, natural compounds provide excellent models to discover novel drugs. **Digitalis**, the most important medicinal plant, is directly used in Allopathy medicine as cardio protective action. Likewise, the importance of medicinal plants are studied in other countries in order to fight currently untreatable, life-threatening diseases such as Alzheimer's, HIV, chronic pain, and malaria. Many natural drugs are under investigation in clinical trials for new drug discovery.

4.2 AYURVEDA, SIDDHA, UNANI AND HOMEOPATHY

In the suktas of Rigveda and Atharwaveda medicinal property of plant is written with their uses (around 5500 years ago). A plenty of medicinal plants are described in old Ayurveda Books, Charak samhita and Sushrut samhita. But it is not so easy to find all those medicinal plants as when required. Hence in 1978, the department of AYUSH (Department of Ayurveda, Yoga and Naturopathy, Unani, Siddha and Homoeopathy) has set up research organization so called "Central Council for Research in Ayurveda and Siddha (CCRAS)" under ministry of Health and Family Welfare, Government of India to co-ordinates and promotes research in the fields of Ayurveda and Siddha medicine. Furthermore in 1971, The Central Council of Indian Medicine (CCIM), a statutory body established under AYUSH, to monitor higher education in areas of Indian medicine, including Siddha. Thereafter in 2001, The Government of India, set up the Traditional Knowledge Digital Library as a repository of 223,000 formulations of various systems of Indian medicine, such as Ayurveda, Unani and Siddha to fight against biopiracy and unethical patents.

4.2.1 Ayurveda

Ayurveda is originated from Sanskrit, composed of "*ayus*" and "*veda*." "*Ayus*" stands for life and "*Veda*" is knowledge of science. Ayurveda is in combination, 'the knowledge of life' or 'the science of life'. According to Charaka (the ancient Ayurvedic scholar), "ayu" means the mind, body, senses and the soul.

Ayurveda is an intricate medical system which is one of the oldest forms of healthcare system, originated in India thousands of years ago. The fundamentals of Ayurveda are found in the *Vedas* (Hindu scriptures) — the ancient Indian books of wisdom. The *Rig Veda* (written over 6,000 years ago), contains a series of prescriptions to overcome various ailments of human.

The aim is to prevent illness, heal the sick and preserve the life as follows:

- "*Swasthyas swasthya rakshanam*": This indicates prolong life with health protection.
- "*Aturasya vikar prashamanamcha*": This indicates elimination of diseases and dysfunctions of the body.

Basic Principles:

The Universe is made up of five elements: air, fire, water, earth and ether as per Ayurveda. All these together are known as "Panchabhuta" (Fig. 4.1). These elements are interconnected with the human body by three "*doshas*" namely *Vata, Pitta* and *Kapha*. Any of the *doshas* accumulate beyond the desirable limit in the body; the body loses its balance. Every individual is depends on getting a right balance of these three *doshas* ("*tridoshas*"). Ayurveda suggests healthy lifestyle and nutritional guidelines to help the body to reduce the excess *doshas* (Fig. 4.2).

Sushrut Samhita said a healthy person is one who works on Ayurveda, with the balance of *doshas*, appetite is good, all tissues of the body and all natural urges are properly functioning and whose mind, body and spirit are cheerful.

Tridosha or the Theory of Bio-energies:

The three *doshas* that are found in our body:

- *Vata* pertains to air and ether elements that act as the force. It directs nerve impulses, circulation, respiration, and elimination.
- *Kapha* pertains to water and earth elements. *Kapha* is responsible for growth and protection. Examples: The mucosal lining of the stomach, the cerebral-spinal fluid etc.
- *Pitta* pertains to fire and water elements deals with metabolism, e.g., the transformation of foods into nutrients. It helps in metabolism in the organ and tissue systems.

'Panchakarma' or the Therapy of Purification:

Panchakarma is recommended to purge these unwanted toxins if any present inside the body. It is also known as cleansing process which is much more pure. These specialized procedures consist of the following:

- **Vaman:** It indicates therapeutic vomiting or emesis.
- **Virechan:** It indicates Purgation.
- **Basti:** It indicates Enema.
- **Nasya:** It indicates elimination of toxins through the nose.
- **Rakta moksha:** It indicates bloodletting or detoxification of the blood.

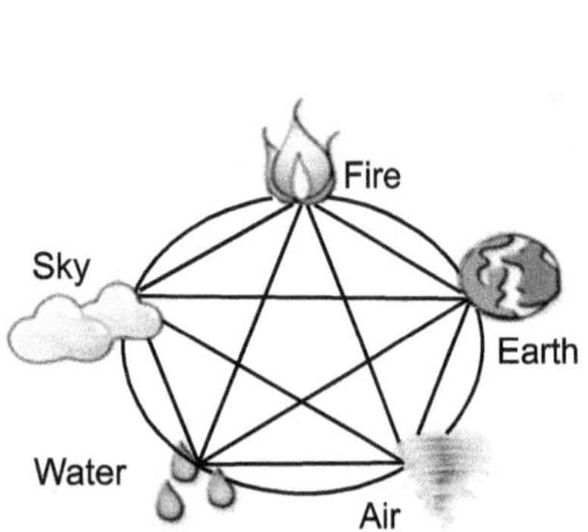

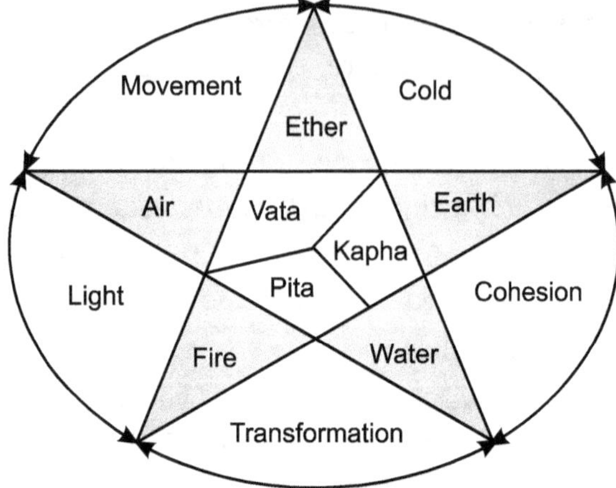

Fig. 4.1: Panchabhuta in Ayurveda   **Fig. 4.2: Principle of Ayurveda medicine system**

Treatment in Ayurveda:

Ayurveda has eight different techniques to diagnose illness, namely Nadi (pulse), Mootra (urine), Mala (stool), Jihva (tongue), Shabda (speech), Sparsha (touch), Druk (vision), and Aakruti (appearance). The treatments are carried out using plant based products procured from roots, leaves, fruits, bark, or seeds.

Ayurvedic Dosage Forms and their Evaluation Methods:

Ayurvedic dosage forms can be grouped into four types depending on their physical nature. A) Solid dosage forms like Vatika, Gutika B) Semisolid dosage forms like Kalka, Aveleha, C) Liquid dosage forms like Arista, Asava, Taila, D) Powder dosage forms like Churna.

All the Ayurvedic preparations consists of two words. The first word may indicate either the disease for which the preparation is used (Jwarantaka Vati) or the property of the preparation (Kaameshwara-Modaka) or the drug contained (Arjuna Aristha) or the name of some God or Saint (Narayana Taila) and the second word always indicates the type of preparations (Aristha, Vati, Taila etc.).

Standardization of Ayurvedic Preparations:

Ayurvedic medicines are manufactured under different pharmaceutical process to result in various dosage forms such as extracts, tinctures, decoctions, pills, powders, tablets, capsules, semisolid pastes, jellies, syrups etc. The general standardization protocols to determine the percentage of active medicaments could not be followed for Ayurvedic herbal preparations. The procedures have to be modified in order to make the preparation safe. This is because of few reasons like:

(i)   Ayurvedic preparations are polyherbal or herbomineral preparations.

(ii)   Even a single herb is used in the preparation, the single herb will contain multiple constituents.

(iii) Bioactive chemical constituents are not known in the herbal preparation and even if it is known and compare with the markers, it does not necessarily reflect its connection with biological effects

(iv) The principle of holistic approach does not permit assaying a single marker.

So the approach has to be made from raw materials to finished products for the successful outcome.

Role of Pharmacognosy in Ayurveda Medicine System:

Herbal drugs play a major role in formulation of Ayurvedic medicines. Many medicinal plants that used in Ayurveda are selected based on plenty availability, low cost, less side effect, effective therapeutic efficacy and also low toxicity. Ayurvedic formulations that are available in market composed of more than 5 to 10 medicinal plants either from leaves or roots or bark or flower parts as sources. A vast number of crude drugs that are used in Ayurvedic preparations, procured from the plant sources which are belongs to the Pharmacognosy. Pharmacognosy helps in development of Pharmacopoeial standard for herbal drugs with respect to identification followed by characterization. Hence, correct authentication of crude drugs is the preliminary source for Ayurvedic medicine system for combined formulation. Thereafter Pharmacognosy helps in identification of drugs through morphology and microscopy examinations that further helps in detection of adulterants as well as substituents. Hence authenticated drugs are used for the formulations which give proper therapeutic actions with less side effects. Furthermore Pharmacognosy helps in identification, detection and isolation of the phytochemicals which gives idea for root level curing of the diseases. Seventy percent of the population in the rural India is dependent on the ayurvedic system of medicine which is of plant origin.

Ayurvedic products in Indian market are projected to register a CAGR of 16% during 2016-2021. It is predicted that many Ayurvedic formulations viz. Ayurvedic nutraceuticals and dietary supplements, Ayurvedic cosmetics and skin care products are likely to boost the market over the years. Awareness of side-effects of allopathy and health concerns is few of the major factors driving consumer preference for Ayurvedic products in the country. There are more than 5000 plants which are used in Ayurveda among that some of the major plants are namely Ashwagandha, Ashoka, Triphala, Amla, Arjuna, Turmeric, Shatavari, Tulsi, Haridra, Neem, Rauwolfia, Gymnema, Pudina, Hibiscus, Lemon grass, Henna, Black pepper, Clove, Cinnamon, Ginger etc.

4.2.2 Siddha

Siddha medicine is also one of the oldest traditional medicines. This healing system is originated in South India. This system is based on ancient medicinal practices as well as spiritual disciplines. It also includes alchemy and mysticism. This system is thought to have developed between 2500 and 1700 BC.

Siddha medicine originated in Tamil Nadu, India as evident in the earliest Tamil writings (Tamil is one of the principal Dravidian languages). There are references in literature of Tamil shangam (1st–4th century CE), in the *Tolkappiyam* ("Ancient Literature"), a treatise on grammar and poetics, and in *Tirukkural* ("Sacred Couplets"), a work attributed to the Tamil poet-saint Tiruvalluvar about this system.

Principle:

The concepts of the Siddha medicine system is also allied to the Ayurveda system. The only difference is that the siddha medicine based on the concept of *Vaadham*, *Pitham* and *Kabam* in childhood, adulthood and old age, respectively, whereas in ayurveda, it is totally reversed, as said Kabam is dominant in childhood, Vaatham in old age and Pitham in adults.

According to the Siddha medicine, various psychological and physiological functions of the body are made up of the combination of seven elements namely:

(a) *ooneer* (plasma) is responsible for growth, development and nourishment;

(b) *ischeneer* (blood) is responsible for nourishing muscles, imparting colour and improving intellect;

(c) *oon* (muscle) is responsible for shape of the body;

(d) *koluppu/Kozhuppu* (fatty tissue) is responsible for lubricating joints as well as oil balance;

(e) *elumbu* (bone) is responsible for body structure and posture and movement;

(f) *elumbu majjai* (bone marrow) is responsible for formation of blood corpuscles; and

(g) *sukkilam* (semen) which is responsible for human reproduction.

In this medicine system, the physiological components of the humans are classified as *Vaadham* (air), *Pitham* (fire) and *Kabam* (earth and water) as like as Ayurveda system.

The Five Elements:

According to this medicine system, the five elements that exist in nature are earth, water, fire, air, and ether, all of which form the original basis of all corporeal things. Traditionally, it believed that there is an intimate connection between the macrocosm of the external world and the microcosm of the corporeal being. As per the system the element of earth is present in the human bone, flesh, nerves, skin and hair; water, as element, is present in bile, blood semen, glandular secretions, and sweat; the fire element is present in hunger, thirst, sleep, beauty, and indolence; the air is present in contraction, expansion, and motion; and the ether is present in stomach, heart, neck and head.

Role of Pharmacognosy in Siddha System:

The *siddhars* did extensive research on plants and devised methods by which plants are used to control many diseases and also cures medicinally. There are many plants that are also described by them which are poisonous in nature as well as some plants are also used as antidotes for them. Therefore, plants are classified based on the way they affected the body.

Siddha medicine gives importance to the multiple uses of plants and minerals. For simple ailments, herbs are used as preliminary treatment in this system. According to Siddha theory, it is believed that mercury preparations provided immunity to the body from decay, enabling it to conquer disease. Mercury and sulfur are used as supreme curatives even though those minerals are extremely toxic to the human body. Siddha medicines are used for the management of chronic diseases and degenerative conditions, such as autoimmune conditions, rheumatoid arthritis, collagen disorders, and conditions of the central nervous system but the effectiveness are varied as per the situations. Some examples are like the leaf extract of *Adhatoda vasica* is used to cure bronchial asthma, eosinophilia, seeds and leaves of *Apium graveolens* are used in the treatment of asthma and bronchitis as well as liver and spleen diseases, roots of *Boerhavia diffusa* is used for the treatment of asthma etc.

4.2.3 Unani

Unani medicine system is also known as Unani tibb, Arabian medicine or Islamic medicine. This system is a traditional system of healing and health maintenance. It is believed that the system is originated in South Asia which is found in the doctrines of the ancient Greek physicians Hippocrates and Galen (460-377 BC). As per their literature, this medicine system is originated in Greece and Aesculapius is credited as originator of this Unani system. Unani system is written in Unan or Yunan in Arabic language. Hence, Unani medicine is also known as Arabian or Islamic medicine. This medicine system is so popular that it developed in the four time periods each in a different geographical location such as Greek period, Arab-Persian period, Spanish period and Indian period.

Unani medicine first came in India around 12th or 13th century with establishment of Delhi Sultanate (1206-1527) and Islamic rule over North India. Subsequently, the system is flourished under Mughal Empire. Alauddin Khilji was famous Unani physicians (Hakim) during that time. In India, Ajmal Khan was the man who contributed almost single handedly for this medicine system and made available some of the great benefits of traditional medicine.

Principle:

This medicine system is based on two theories namely Hippocrates theory (Humour theory) and Pythogoras theory (Four Proximate qualities). The four humours namely Phlegm, Blood, Yellow bile and Black bile. Phlegm means Balgham, Blood is Dam, Yellow bile is Safra and Black bile is Sauda. The proximate qualities are like Hot, Cold, Moist and Dry. All the humours are entered into the body and due to their balance or imbalance, healthy and illness are occurred respectively. It believes that the medicine system has originated at *Circa* 1025 AD and the evidence is given in the book *The Canon of Medicine* in Persia, written by Avicenna, after influenced by Greek, Islamic medicine and Indian medical teaching of Sushruta and Charata.

Treatments:

There are six external or physical factors in Unani medicine, known as *asbab-e-sittah-zarooriah*. All these factors are essential in establishing a synchronized biological rhythm and thus living a balanced existence. The six *asbab-e-sittah-zarooriah* are:

- *Hawa:* It indicates air, in which the quality of the air a person breathes is thought to have a direct effect on human temperament that gives impact on health.

- *Makool-wo-mashroob:* It indicates food and drink, in which the nutritional value and the quality and quantity of one's food and drink are believed to ensure physical fitness by strengthening *tabiyat*.

- ***Harkat-wo-sakoon-e-jismiah:*** It indicates exercise and repose, which emphasizes the positive effects of balanced physical exercise on an individual's internal resistance and *tabiyat*.

- ***Harkat-o-sakoon nafsaniah:*** The mental work and rest, which emphasizes the simultaneous engagement of the human mind in numerous emotional and intellectual activities. This medicine system believes that the human mind and brain need adequate stimulation and proper relaxation as well.

- ***Naum-o-yaqzah:*** It is sleep and wakefulness, in which an individual's health and alertness are understood as being dependent on a specific amount of sound sleep.

- ***Ihtebas* and *istifragh*:** It indicates retention and excretion, which considers the metabolism of food and liquid as both affecting and being regulated by *tabiyat*. Unani medicine system believes that assimilation of food and liquid facilitates the elimination from the body of excessive and noxious substances. That means to maintain a harmonic and synchronized *tabiyat*, certain beneficial end-products of *kaun-o-fasad* (genesis and lysis) are retained and harmful substances are expelled out from the body.

These six factors are directly affecting the harmony of the human mind and body. Socioeconomic, geographic, and environmental factors are considered secondary factors (*asbab-e-ghair-zarooriah*) which indirectly influence *tabiyat*. But both the primary and the secondary factors are considered in the Unani process of treatment.

Role of Pharmacognosy in Unani System of Medicine:

Medicinal plants are rich resources of ingredients which are used in drug development either pharmacopoeial, non-pharmacopoeial or synthetic drugs. It cures very critical diseases like Bars (vatiligo), Dau sadaf (psoriasis), Iltehab-e-kabid (Infective Hepatitis), Hasat-ul-kulya wa masana (Renal and Bladder calculus) etc. with the help of medicinal plants. Rural as well as some urban people are dependent for their health care on Unani system of Medicine due to low cost, low side effect and safe health care solution.

Some medicinal plants that are abundantly used in Unani system,

(a) *Aristolochia indica, Artemisia vulgaris, Cannabis sativa, Carica papaya, Celastrus paniculatus;*

(b) *Momordica charantia* are used for abortifacient and emmenogogues;

(c) *Berberis aristata, Butea monosperma, Hibiscus rosa-sinensis* and *Saraca asoca* are used for emmenagogues (stimulates or increases menstrual flow) and also have depressant action on uterine muscles;

(d) *Allium sativum, Cinnamomum zeylanicum* and *Sesamum orientale* are used as stimulant action on the uterine muscles;

(e) *Punica granatum* are used for abortifacient and have depressant action on the uterine muscles.

4.2.4 Homeopathy

Homeopathic medicine system works on the principle of 'like cures like' (Similia Similibus Curanter). This medicine system of healing was coined by Dr. Samuel Hahnemann, a German physician. He has translated a book on the medicinal properties of drugs. During that time he read the properties of the medicine *Cinchona* and saw *Cinchona* cures malaria, because of its bitter taste. After that he named his new healing science by combining the two Greek words **homeo-**, meaning "same," and **pathy**, meaning "disease." Materia Medica is a book where the properties of medicines are listed on healthy individuals. Homeopathy system relies on this book.

Theory:

Homeopathic medicine believes, various materials found in nature contain an energy field that can exert a healing effect on the body. This energy field is amplified, or "**potentiated**," by a series of dilutions. It is noticed that dilution enhanced the medicinal power of the drugs. The more the "mother tincture" is diluted, the healing effect will be stronger. It is based on the Dynamization theory by which the quality of the medicines is improved by vigorous shaking. This method is also helps to remove the poisonous properties of the drugs. The materials used in homeopathic formulations can come from natural herbs, from minerals, or from animal parts. Homeopathic preparations are written as 2X, 4X, 6X etc., "X" indicates potency. These indicate the number of times the mother tincture is diluted and potentiated. The higher number indicates more dilute with stronger healing effect.

Principle:

Homeopathy is based on the principle of "like with like", that is a substance which causes symptoms when taken in large doses, can be used in small amount to treat those same symptoms. The treatment is based on the concept of proving and prover. Prover is the healthy person whereas proving is the symptoms that are caused in prover by the various potencies of medicines. Like, drinking too much coffee can cause sleeplessness and agitation, so according to this principle, it could be used to treat people with these symptoms. Homeopathic medicines are prepared by specialist pharmacies using a careful process of dilution and a specific form of vigorous shaking.

Role of Pharmacognosy in Homeopathy Medicine System:

Traditional medicines are used by people about 60% of the world's population for their primary health care system. Most of the drugs used in modern medicine and ancient Indian medicinal system are of plant origin. Dilutions of the drugs are prepared uniform drug strength which is represented by the dry crude drug as the unit strength. In case of mother tincture, it is made from dried substances and the plant juice as the unit from the fresh plant. Homoeopathy uses animal, plant, mineral, and synthetic substances in its remedies. *Arsenicum album* (arsenic oxide), *Natrum muriaticum* (sodium chloride), opium (plant), and thyroidinum (thyroid hormone) are some of the homoeopathic medicines extracted from different sources.

Some important medicinal plants used in Homeopathic medicine systems are:

(a) *Rhus toxicodendron*, used in treating paralysis of the lower extremities,

(b) *Aconite napellus* and *Gelsemium sempervirens* are used in homeopathic for treatment of paralysis.

(c) *Agaricus muscarius, Cocculus indicus, Solanum dulcamara,* and *Hypericum perforatum* which are all poisonous sources, are used in Homeopathic medicine system.

(d) *Arnica* Montana, *Strychnos* and *Nux-vomica* are another well-known plants source, used in pain relief as well as antacid respectively in homeopathy medicine.

(e) Belladona liquid from *Atropa belladonna* is used for running nose and any cold conditions in Homeopathic medicine.

4.2.5 Chinese Systems of Medicine

Chinese medicine (CM) is a broad range of medicine practices that developed in China. It is based on a tradition of more than 2,000 years, including various forms of herbal medicine, acupuncture, massage, exercise and dietary therapy. The medicine practitioners used herbal medicines and various mind and body practices, such as acupuncture and tai chi, to treat or prevent health problems. The traditional Chinese medicine is based on 5,000 years of practice and experiences. This medicine system provides a complete assessment based on a unique cultural, diagnostic, and therapeutic approach. Chinese medicine system consist of three parts namely theory, treatment and prevention.

Theory: Chinese Medicine system is based on two systems viz. Yin and Yang theory, and five element theory. Yin and Yang Theory is based on the "Principle of Chi" that promotes biological activities by energy generation. This Yin and Yang theory represent positive and negative side of the energy which are opposite to each other. Health reflects the balance between Yin and Yang. If Yin principle predominates the body then weakness, exhaustion are the result. Excess Yang causes irritability and excitement. When the Yin and Yang elements in a person's body are balanced the person is in good health. The five element theory is based on vital five organs namely heart, liver, spleen, lungs and kidney are related to five elements such as earth, wood, metal, fire and water. They all are interlinked and together they are known as "Wu Xing" (Fig. 4.3).

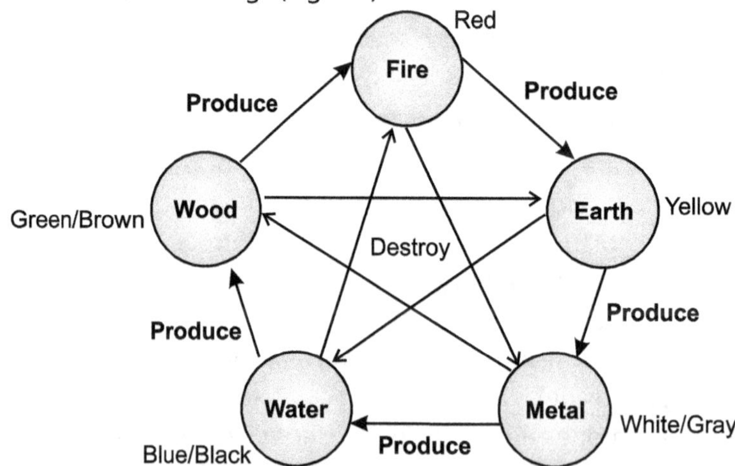

Fig. 4.3: Five element theory

Principle:

The Eight Principles are in this system as follows:

1. **Yin:** Yin is cold. Yin with Yang is indicates for pattern diagnosis and describes the relationship between other three pairs of Principles.

2. **Yang:** Yang with Yin describes relationship between the other three pairs of the Principles. Like heat is Yang.

3. **Interior:** Interior describes diseases at manifest themselves in deep inside the body (Zang-fuorgans), such as *qi*, blood, and bone marrow.

4. **Exterior:** Exterior describes diseases that manifest themselves on surface of the body namely hair, skin, nails, and meridians. Its clinical features include body chills, fever, a weak pulse, headache etc.

5. **Heat:** Heat describes the absence of Cold. Its symptoms are rapid pulse, fever, body chills, dehydration, and a sore throat when it combines with exterior pattern but in combination with an interior pattern, its symptoms are cold drinks, clear urine, and a slow pulse.

6. **Cold:** Cold describes the absence of heat. With combination of Exterior pattern, its symptoms are body aches, a tense pulse, fever, body chills, and headaches but with an Interior pattern, its symptoms show nausea, stomach pain, vomiting, and diarrhoea.

7. **Deficiency:** Deficiency is used to describe a vacuity in *qi*, blood (*Xue*), or body fluids (Jinye) but it depend on the relation to Interior/Exterior and Cold/Heat, it can manifest as constipation, having a small appetite, dizziness, and slow pulse.

8. **Excess:** Excess is classified as any disease that cannot be identified as a Deficiency pattern. It means that one of the six excesses is present. Depending on how it relates to Interior/Exterior and Cold/Heat and show quick pulse, sweaty palms, and sharp stomach pains.

Treatment:

It aims to restore harmony between Yin and Yang with the patients as well as between patients to the World. Treatments are carried out with help of Herbalism, Acupuncture, Moxibustion, Cupping and Massage therapy.

Role of Pharmacognosy in Chinese Medicine:

Chinese herbal medicines are mainly plant based and they packaged as powders, pastes, lotions or tablets forms, based on uses of herbs. In this system, herbs are sometimes combined in formulations and given as teas and other various dosage forms. The system believes that herbs help boost *Qi* (Life force) and balance Yin and Yang in formulated drugs where many herbs are used in combinations that have scientific validation of their effectiveness as tonics or remedies for specific illness. Herbs restore energy balance to the opposing forces of energy i.e. Yin and Yang which run through invisible channels in the body. More than 300 herbs are traditionally used in Chinese medicine system. Some of important herbs are like Ginseng (*Panax notoginseng*), Wolfberry (*Lycium barbarum)*, Dong quai (*Angelica sinensis*), Astragalus (*Astragalus membranaceus*), Atractylodes (*Atractylodes lancea*), Bupleurum (*Bupleurum chinense*), Cinnamon (*Cinnamomum cassia*), Datura (*Datura metel*), Ginger (*Zingiber officinalis*), Coptis (*Coptis chinensis*), Ginkgo (*Ginkgo biliba*), Mushroom (*Macrohyporia cocos*), Hoelen (*Pachyma hoelen*), Licorice (*Glycyrrhiza inflata*), Ephedra (*Ephedra sinica*), Rhubarb (*Rheum palmatum*), Rehmannia (*Rehmannia glutinosa*), Red yeast rice, Gotu kola (*Centella asiatica*), Salvia (*Salvia miltiorrhiza*).

Differences between Ayurveda and Homeopathy:

Ayurveda	Homeopathy
1. The system believes in preventing a disease.	1. The system believes in curing a disease.
2. Ayurvedic medicines complement the allopathic medicines.	2. Homeopathy is against allopathic medicines.
3. The system believes: the health and well-being of a person depend on the balance of three key components, the wind, bile, and phlegm.	3. The system believes: in the "vitalist" philosophy, i.e. some internal or external factors disturb the vital force of the body which affects the health of a person.
4. The system uses some surgical procedures such as "**Kshar sutra**" or purification techniques like "**Panchkarma**" for treating diseases.	4. The system is not uses any surgical procedures.
5. This system uses herbs, minerals like sulfur, copper, lead, arsenic, gold, vegetable drugs, and animal products such as milk, gallstones, and bones to make the medicines.	5. This system uses various plants, synthetic materials, mineral substances which are diluted in alcohol or distilled water. The final medicine contains only a small percentage of the substance.
6. The medicines may incorporate a small amount of toxic materials such as lead, mercury, arsenic	6. The medicines contain water and alcohol. The use of toxic materials is very rare.

Differences between Homeopathy and Allopathy:

Homeopathy	Allopathy
1. The study involves long consultation or discussion regarding all aspects of patient's illness and life.	1. The studies and outcome of studies are purely empirical.
2. The system seeks to embrace the body's natural response system by either attacking the root cause of the illness or by encouraging the symptoms of healing.	2. The system fights the body's natural response system by attacking the symptoms of healing.
3. It is a method of treating disease with remedies that produce effects similar to those caused by the disease itself.	3. It is a method of treating disease with remedies that produce effects different from those caused by the disease.

Homeopathy	Allopathy
4. This treatment generally takes time to show results as it focuses on hitting the root cause of the disease.	4. This treatment show results very quickly, as it immediately suppresses the symptoms of a disease, leaving out with another problem in the form of a side-effect.
5. The treatment show permanent results, i.e. once a disease is completely treated over a course of time, it will not occur again.	5. The treatment provides a partial and quick relief from a disease which may not be permanent.

Differences between Ayurveda and Allopathy:

Ayurveda	Allopathy
1. It focuses on the wellness as a complete package, be it physical, psychological, spiritual or social wellness.	1. It is a system of physical health and it believes in the replacing/changing of the organs or systems for treatment and not much worried about the cure.
2. It takes the body as a whole and the physician has knowledge of all the systems of medicines.	2. It takes the body in pieces, is objective and incomplete in nature.
3. This system provides natural cure in which scope of side effects is very less or mild.	3. This system provides side effects either in external or internal.
4. The medicines decontaminate the whole body.	4. The medicines partially cleanse the body.
5. The system considers that until a body has the disease-causing factors, diseases will keep hitting again and again. It considers the detoxification as a primary part of the treatment.	5. The system focuses on suppressing the signs and symptoms of a disease and never appreciates to remove the disease causing factors completely.

(B) INTRODUCTION TO SECONDARY METABOLITES

Plants produce a vast number of different chemical compounds which are broadly categorized by primary metabolites and secondary metabolites. Primary metabolites are essentials for the plants for their survival likely: sugar, proteins, amino acid etc. Thereafter secondary metabolites are the products that are considered as waste substances of plants. These secondary metabolites are not essential, but stored in various parts of the plant bodies and provide protections to the plants from attacks of microorganisms, attractors for pollinators etc. They are produced by the plants are extremely diverse. These secondary metabolites are relatively produced in low quantities in plants but have significant economic and medicinal value to the humans. High concentration of secondary metabolites present in plants indicates more resistant plants. They are categorized based on chemical structure (like presence of sugars, different rings), composition, their solubility in various solvents and the various biosynthesis pathways. A simple classification includes three main groups: the terpenes (made from mevalonic acid, composed almost entirely of carbon and hydrogen), phenolics (made from simple sugars, containing benzene rings, hydrogen, and oxygen), and nitrogen-containing compounds. Furthermore various scientific research evidences proved that the therapeutic efficacy and pharmacological actions are mainly by the action of secondary metabolites and hence plant secondary metabolites are gaining importance to natural product chemists. Based on the characterization, secondary metabolites of few plants are described in this section.

4.3 ALKALOIDS

Alkaloids are a large and complex group of highly diverse natural products. In early days plant derived alkaloids are used as ingredients in poison. The name "alkaloids" (Derived from Alkali) was introduced in 1819 by the German chemist Carl Friedrich Meissner. They are cyclic compounds group of compounds contain one or more basic nitrogen atoms in a heterocyclic ring. They have low molecular weight. About 25% higher plants are produce alkaloids and they are procured from various parts of the plants such as all parts (E.g. Datura), Bark (E.g. Cinchona), Seeds (E.g. Nux vomica), Roots (E.g. Aconite), Leaves (E.g. Tobacco), Fruits (E.g. Black pepper), Latex (E.g. Opium) etc. Apart from this alkaloids are also obtained from animal sources like Muscopyridine from a musk of a deer, Castoramine from North America Rodent, Canadian beaver (*Castor canadensis*), and from bacteria sources like Pyocyanine from *Pseudomonas aeruginosa*. As per **Ladenburg** in the late 1880, Alkaloid is defined as: plant derived compounds having a nitrogen based heterocylic ring within their molecules with basic nature. They are highly poisonous but in low dose give therapeutic activities.

Physical Properties:
- Alkaloids are crystalline in nature but few are amorphous solid (Example: Emetine). Solid nature due to presence of O-atom in the ring structure.
- Alkaloids are insoluble in water but soluble in most of the organic solvents. Caffeine, cocaine, codeine, nicotine are slightly soluble in water, Morphine, yohimbine are very slightly water-soluble.
- Alkaloids are optically active. Most of the alkaloids are laevo-rotatory but few are dextro-rotatory (e.g. Coniine) and few are even optically inactive, viz. papaverine.
- Alkaloids are bitter in taste and have pronounced physiological activity.
- They have molecular weight in between 100-900.
- They are sometime non-volatile liquids (Examples: Hyoscine, Pilocarpine), sometime volatile liquids (Examples: Nicotine, Coniine).
- They are generally colourless (Few are coloured such as Colchicine and Berberine are yellow, Betanidine is orange, Salt of Sanguinarine is cupper red).

Chemical Properties:
- Alkaloids are naturally occurring organic compound.
- They mostly contain basic lone pair electron on nitrogen, hence they are basic in nature (Some compounds like theobromine, theophylline are amphoteric in nature).
- Alkaloids react with acids to form salts. These salts are usually freely soluble in water (Example: Quinine sulfate is water soluble but Quinine mono-sulphate is insoluble in

water) and alcohol but poorly soluble in most organic solvents (Exceptional: Scopolamine hydrobromide is soluble in organic solvents). Strong bases form salt with weak acid and vice versa. Very weak bases form unstable salts like Caffeine, nicotine etc.

- They form precipitate with heavy metal iodides.
- Naturally alkaloids exist either in free state (as amine) or as salt with acid or alkaloid N-oxides.
- They contain one or more nitrogen in their structure and forms primary amines ($R-NH_2$; Example: Norephedrine), Secondary amines (R_2-NH; Example: Ephedrine), Tertiary amines (R_3-N; Example: Atropine) and Quaternary ammonium salt (R_4-N; Example: d-Tubocurarine).
- They decomposed by heat but some are undergoes for sublimation (E.g. Caffeine, Strychnine).
- They decomposed at temperature above 70°C for long time.

4.3.1 Classification

Broadly Alkaloids are classified in mainly four types (Fig. 4.4).

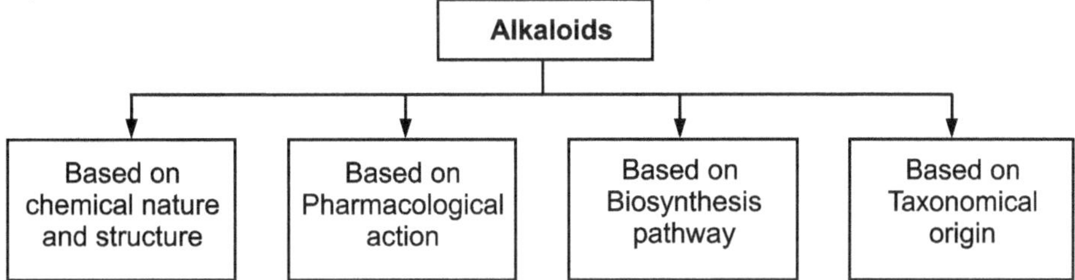

Fig. 4.4: Major classification of Alkaloids

(A) Based on Chemical Nature and Structure:

They are further classified into several types (Fig. 4.5).

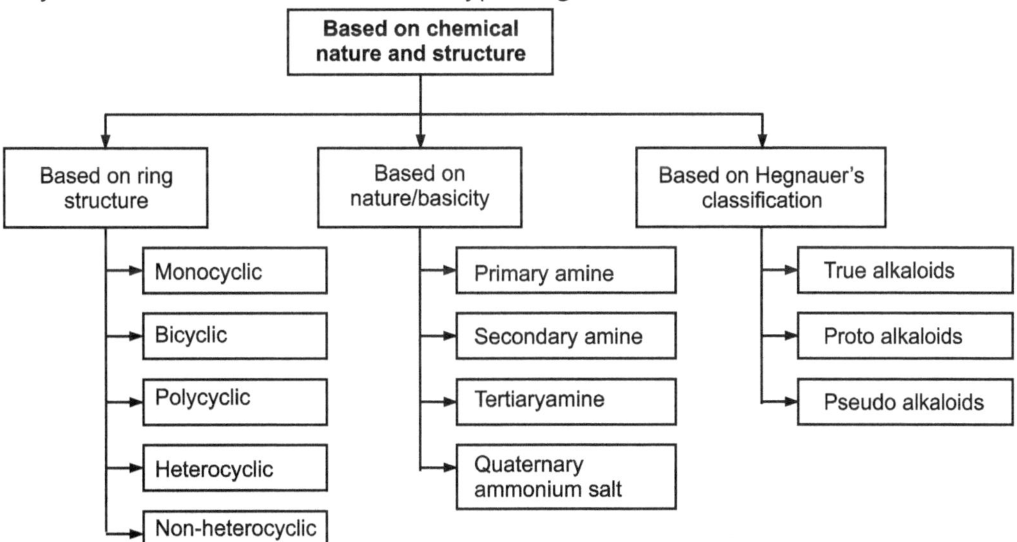

Fig. 4.5: Classification of Alkaloids based on Chemical nature and structure

Monocyclic alkaloids: They contain a single, unfused ring. Example: Nicotine.

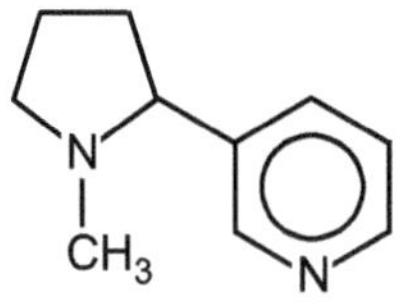

Nicotine

Bicyclic alkaloids: They consist of molecules with a 1,4 nitrogen bridged cycloheptane structure. Examples: Atropine, Cocaine.

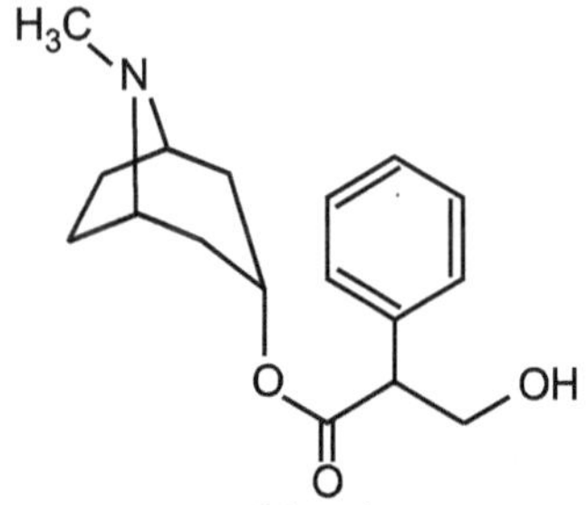

Atropine

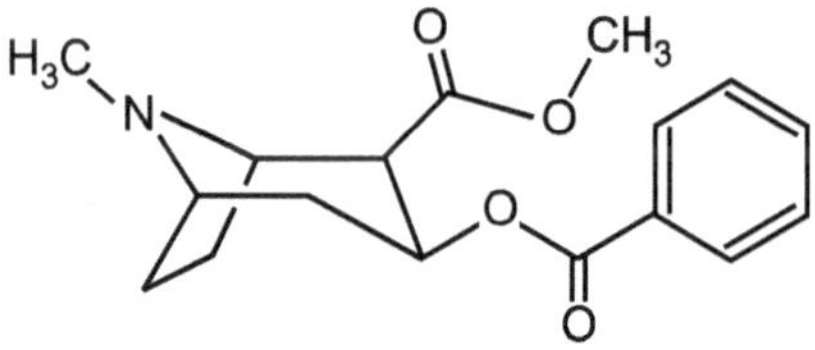

Cocaine

Polycyclic alkaloids: They are having more than two rings. Examples: Strychnine, Cannabinol, Morphine, Codeine etc.

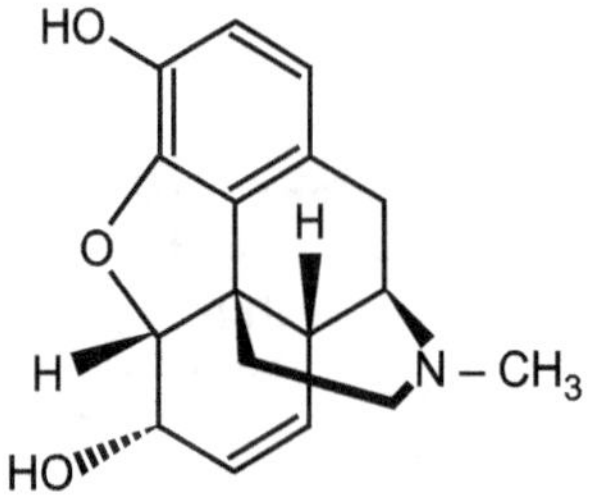

Morphine

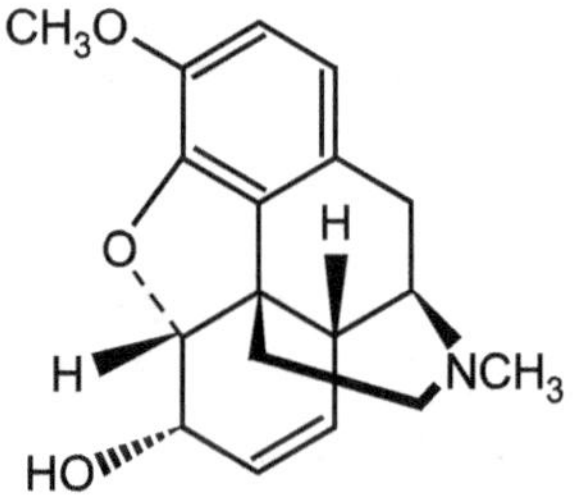

Codeine

Heterocyclic Alkaloids:

Types of alkaloids, structures, examples, biological sources, family and uses of some heterocyclic alkaloids are shown in Table 4.1.

Table 4.1

Types of alkaloids	Structure	Example	Biological source and Family	Uses
Pyrrole	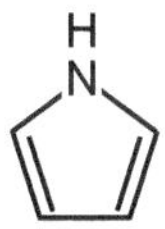	Hygrine from Coca	*Erythroxylum coca* Family: Erythroxylaceae	Analgesic
Pyrrolidine	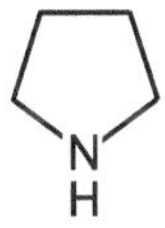	Nicotine from Tobacco	*Nicotiana tabacum* Family: Solanaceae	Stimulant
Pyridine	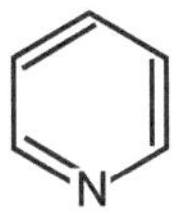	Lobeline from Lobelia	*Lobelia inflate* Family: Campanulaceae	Use in Asthma
Piperidine	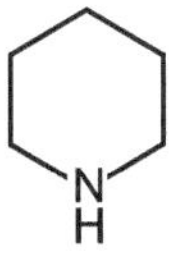	Piperine from Black pepper	*Piper nigrum* Family: Piperaceae	Anti-inflammatory activity
Imidazole	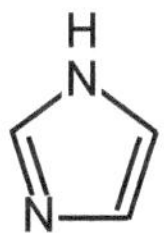	Pilocarpine from Pilocarpus	*Pilocarpus microphyllus* Family: Rutaceae	Treating glaucoma
Quinoline	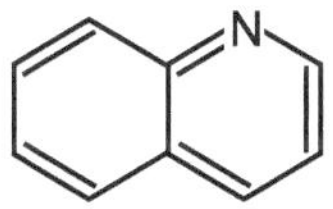	Quinine from Cinchona	*Cinchona officinalis* Family: Rubiaceae	Antimalarial
Isoquinoline	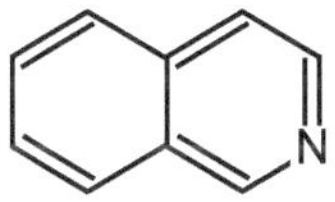	Morphine from Opium	*Papaver somniferum* Family: Papveraceae	Analgesic
Indole	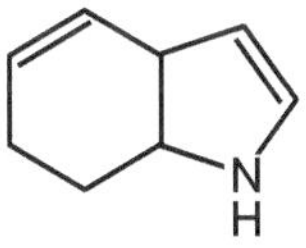	Reserpine from Rauwolfia	*Rauwolfia serpentine* Family: Apocyanaceae	Antihypertensive
Purine	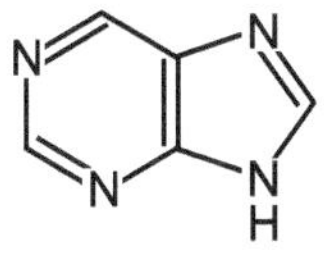	Caffeine from Tea	*Thea sinensis* Family: Theaceae	CNS stimulant

Types of alkaloids	Structure	Example	Biological source and Family	Uses
Tropane		Atropine from Datura	*Datura metel* Family: Solanaceae	Depressant
Quinazolin		Vasicine from Vasaka	*Adhatoda vasica* Family: Acanthaceae	Antitussive
Norlupinane		Lupanine from Lupine	*Lupinus albus* Family: Fabaceae	Carminative, Diuretic

Non-heterocyclic alkaloids:

Types of alkaloids, structure, example, biological sources, family and uses of non-heterocyclic alkaloids are as shown in Table 4.2.

Table 4.2

Types of alkaloids	Structure	Example	Biological source and Family	Uses
Phenyl ethyl amine		Ephedrine from Ephedra	*Ephedra sinica* Family: Ephedraceae	Use for Asthma, stimulant
Steroidal		Connesine from Kurchi	*Holarrhena antidysenterica* Family: Apocyanaceae	Antidysentric
Tropolone		Colchicine from Colchicum	*Colchicum autumnale* Family: Colchicaceae	Gout

Based on Nature/Basicity: They are classified as:

- Primary amines ($R\text{-}NH_2$; Example: Norephedrine),
- Secondary amines ($R_2\text{-}NH$; Example: Ephedrine),
- Tertiary amines ($R_3\text{-}N$; Example: Atropine)
- Quaternary ammonium salt ($R_4\text{-}N$; Example: d-Tubocurarine).

Basicity of alkaloids is as follows: R_2-NH > R-NH_2 > R_3-N. The basicity of alkaloids due to presence of lone pair of electron on nitrogen. The basicity increases if the adjacent group is electron releasing like alkali whereas the basicity decreases if the adjacent group is electron withdrawing like carbonyl and amide group. Hence as per basicity, alkaloids are classified as Weak bases (Example: Caffeine), Strong bases (Example: Atropine), Amphoteric (Examples: Morphine, Narceine) and Neutral alkaloid (Example: Colchicine).

Based on Hegnauer's Classification:

- **True Alkaloids:** They are the alkaloids that derived directly from amino acid. They contain nitrogen in their heterocyclic ring. They are basic in nature due to presence of lone pair of electron on nitrogen atom and strong toxic in nature. They are also very effective. They give positive test for common tests for alkaloids. They occur in plants either in the free state, as salts form and as N-oxides. The primary precursors are viz. amino acids as *l*-ornithine, *l*-lysine, *l*-phenylalanine/*l*-tyrosine, *l*-tryptophan and l-histidine. Examples: Quinine, Morphine, Atropine etc.

- **Proto alkaloids:** They do not have nitrogen in their heterocyclic ring. They are derived from L-Tryptophan, Phenylalanine and Tyrosine. They give positive test for common tests for alkaloids. Examples: Ephedrine, Hordenine, Mescaline.

- **Pseudo alkaloids:** They are not derived from amino acids but derived from the precursors of amino acid (Non-amino acid precursor). They have nitrogen in a heterocyclic ring (acquire nitrogen through transamination process). The nitrogen atom is inserted into the molecule at a late stage. They do not give positive test for common tests for alkaloids. Examples: Caffeine, Coniine, Capsaicin.

(B) Based on Pharmacological action:

Based on pharmacological activity, alkaloids are classified into various groups (Table 4.3).

Table 4.3

Activity	Plant name	Family	Constituent
Narcotic analgesic	Opium (*Papaver somniferum*)	Papaveraceae	Morphine, Codeine
CNS stimulant	Tea (*Thea sinensis*)	Theaceae	Caffeine
	Nux vomica (*Strychnous nuxvomica*)	Loganaceae	Strychnine
Anticancer	Taxol (*Taxus brevifolia*)	Taxaceae	Paclitaxel
	Vinca (*Catharanthus roseus*)	Apocynaceae	Vincrystine, Vinblastine
Antihypertensive	Rauwolfia (*Rauwolfia serpentina*)	Apocynaceae	Reserpine
Bronchodilator	Ephedra (*Ephedra gerardiana*)	Ephedracea	Ephedrine
	Vasaka (*Adhatoda vasica*)	Acanthaceae	Vasicinone
Smooth muscle relaxant	Belladona (*Atropa belladonna*)	Solanaceae	Atropine
	Opium (*Papaver somniferum*)	Papaveraceae	Papaverine

Activity	Plant name	Family	Constituent
Antitussive	Opium (*Papaver somniferum*)	Papaveraceae	Codeine
Mydriatics	Belladona (*Atropa belladonna*)	Solanaceae	Atropine
Myotics	Pilocarpus (*Pilocarpus jaborandi*)	Rutaceae	Pilocarpine
Antiparasitics	Cinchona (*Cinchona calisaya*)	Rubiaceae	Quinine
	Ipecac (*Cephalis ipecacuanha*)	Rubiaceae	Emetine
Local anesthetic	Coca (*Erythroxylum coca*)	Erythroxylaceae	Cocaine
Antiarrythmic	Cinchona (*Cinchona calisaya*)	Rubiaceae	Quinidine

(C) Based on Biosynthesis pathway: They are classified as follows (Table 4.4):

Table 4.4: Classification of alkaloids based on biosynthesis pathway

Pathway	Group of Alkaloid	Example
Ornithine derived	Pyrrolidine	Nicotine
	Tropane	Atropine, Cocaine
Lysine derived	Piperidine and Pyridine	Coniine, Lobaline
	Quinazolidine	Lupinine
Tyrosine derived	Isoquinoline	Morphine, Codeine, Berberine,
	Amino	Colchicine
Tryptophan derived	Indole	Ergot, Vincristine, Reserpine, Strychnine
	Quinoline	Cinchona, Quinine, Quinidine
Histidine derived	Imidazole	Pilocarpine
Phenylalanine derived	Amino alkaloid	Ephedrine

(D) Based on Taxonomical Origin:

Alkaloids are classified on the basis of the biological source. Examples: Quinine from bark of *Cinchona calisaya*, Rauwolfia from roots of *Rauwolfia serpentina*, Morphine from dried latex of *Papaver somniferum* etc.

Functions:

- They are as end products of the metabolism or waste products.
- They are storage reservoir of nitrogen for protein synthesis.
- They act as protective agent for the plants against attack by predators (parasites or herbivore).
- They act as plants stimulants and regulators in activities such as growth, metabolism and reproduction.
- They act as a detoxification agent, which renders harmless certain substances, accumulation of which might cause damage to the plant.

Chemical Tests:

(A) Precipitation reactions:

- Alkaloid sample reacts with Dragendorff's reagent (Potassium-bismuth-iodide solution) which gives **reddish-brown precipitate**.

Reagent Composition: Bismuth nitrate: 8.00 g, Nitric acid: 21.5 g, Potassium iodide: 27.2 g and water to make 100 ml.

- Alkaloid sample reacts with Mayer reagent (Potassium-mercuric-iodide solution) which gives **cream colour precipitate.**

  Reagent Composition: Mercuric chloride: 1.3 g, Potassium iodide: 5.00 g and water to make 100 ml.

- Alkaloid sample reacts with Wagner reagent (Iodine-potassium-iodide solution) which gives **Brown colour precipitate**.

  Reagent Composition: Iodine: 1.3 g, Potassium iodide: 2.0 g and water to make 100 ml.

- Alkaloid sample reacts with Hager reagent (Saturated solution of picric acid) which gives yellow colour precipitate.

  Reagent Composition: Picric acid: 1.0 g, water to make 100 ml.

- Alkaloids react with Valser's test (Mercuric iodide) which gives white colour precipitate.

- Alkaloid sample reacts with acids and gives **buff colour precipitate.**

- Alkaloids react with picrolonic acid and gives **yellow colour precipitate.**

(B) Important Colour reactions:

- **Vitali Morin Test:** This test is positive for solanaceae family drugs such as Belladona, Datura, Henbane, Mandrake, Tobacco etc.

  Test: Sample alkaloid mixed with fuming nitric acid, evaporated to dryness. Dissolved residue in acetone and added methanolic solution of KOH. It produced violet colour. It indicates the presence of tropane group.

- **Van Urk's Test:** This test is positive for Ergot alkaloid.

  Test: Sample reacts with para-dimethyl amino benzaldehyde and dilute sulphuric acid and gives blue colour. It indicates the presence of indole group especially clavine group of alkaloids.

- **Froehd's Test:** This test is positive for opioid alkaloids. Sample reacts with Froehd's reagent (sodium molybdate in concentrated sulphuric acid) and forms brownish black colour due to presence of Isoquinoline group.

- **Thalloquin Test:** This test is positive for Quinine alkaloid. Cinchona powder reacts with bromine water in presence of strong ammonia and gives emerald green colour due to presence of quinoline group.

- **Rosequin Test:** This test is also known as Erythroquinine test. This test is positive for Quinine.

  Test: Sample solution added with dilute acetic acid and few drop of bromine water. Then added a drop of solution of potassium ferrocyanide and added a drop of strong ammonia solution. The solution turns to red colour. In this solution, few ml of chloroform is added then chloroform layer became red colour.

- **Murexide Test:** This test is positive for purine derivative alkaloids, mainly Caffeine.

  Test: Caffeine sample is taken in China dish and added potassium chlorate and dilute HCl. Evaporated to drynesss. It produces red colour. Further expose the China dish on strong ammonia vapour. The red colour is converted into purple or violet colour. When caffeine reacts with HCl it forms tetramethylalloxanthine which further in presence of ammonia forms ammonium salt of tetramethylpurpuric acid (Murexide).

4.3.2 General Extraction Methods

1. Stas-Otto method:

The method is based on the distribution of alkaloidal bases between acid or aqueous solution and immiscible organic solvent (Fig. 4.6).

Powdered drug is mixed with water and alkali to make paste. Alkali is added because it mixed with acids, tannins and other phenolic substances to make free of alkaloids. Thereafter mixed drug is extracted with chloroform or other organic solvents using Soxhlet apparatus. This step is carried out because freed alkaloids are dissolved together with other substances soluble in solvent. Then further re-extract chloroform layer with dilute sulphuric acid in separating funnel and acid layer is collected. This is because alkaloids are converted into alkaloidal sulphate which is soluble in water. Then in acid layer water is added so that soluble constituents are passes into the aqueous solution. Then the aqueous layer is mixed with ammonia to make media alkaline. Then evaporate to dryness and the precipitate is collected and dried. This step is carried out because ammonia converts alkaloidal sulphate to ammonium sulphate which is soluble in water. The free alkaloids which are insoluble in water, are precipitated.

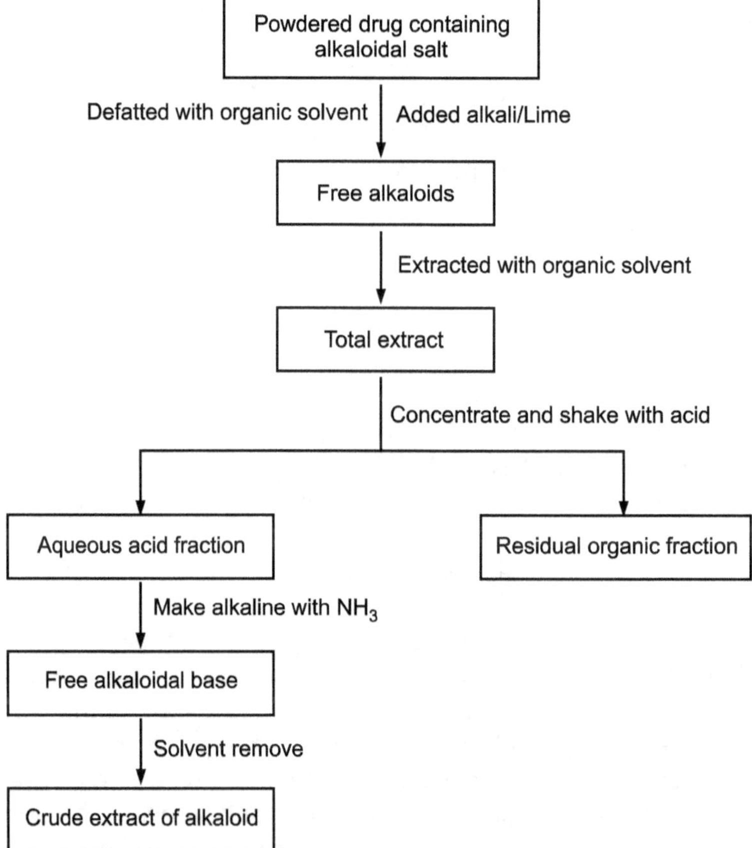

Fig. 4.6: General extraction method of Alkaloid

2. Plant sample extracted with water or alcohol. The aqueous layer further extracted with organic solvent like chloroform to remove pigments or other impurities which are soluble in that solvent. Then shake with acid to form salt of alkaloid in aqueous layer. The aqueous layer is then treated with ammonia to get freed alkaloid which is separated with organic solvents. After evaporation to dryness residue of alkaloidal extract forms (Fig. 4.7).

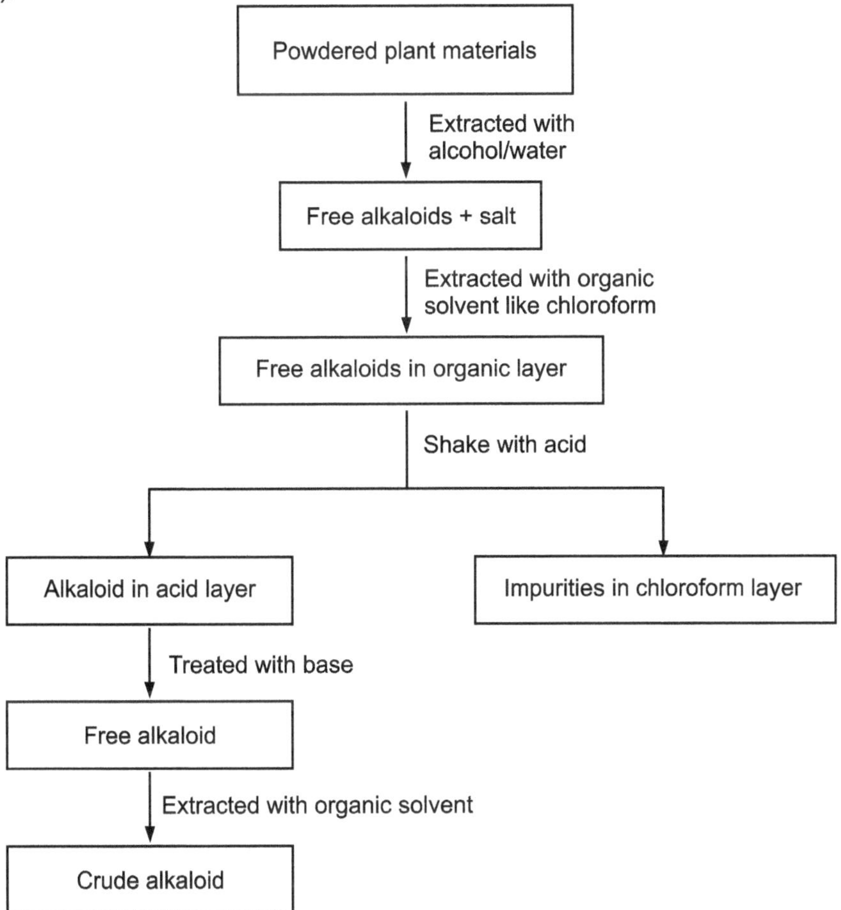

Fig. 4.7: Extraction method of general alkaloids

4.4 GLYCOSIDES

Glycoside is an organic compound contains C, H, and O in their structure. They are natural carbohydrate substances. They are obtained from maximum higher plants but in less quantity. They are also known as internal acetate. They have two parts viz. Sugar part and non-sugar part. Sugar part is known as glycone part whereas non-sugar part is known as aglycone part or genin part. Due to presence of aglycone part, glycosides give therapeutic activities. Sugar and non-sugar parts are linked with glycosidic bridge, known as glycosidic linkage. This linkage is breaks by acid or enzyme hydrolysis and both glycone and genin parts are separated. Glycone part is water soluble but insoluble in organic solvents whereas aglycone parts are vice-versa. They are formed by biochemical reaction which makes water insoluble compound more polar than water soluble molecule. Hence, they are removed from an organic system. Human forms them in liver as part of the process of detoxification and they are excreted through urine. Mammalian glycosides are simple compound whereas plant originated glycosides are much larger and chemically complex. Among the glucose found in nature, D-glucose is available more. They are having two types of stereochemistry namely alpha and beta-glycosides. Example: Methyl D-glucosides.

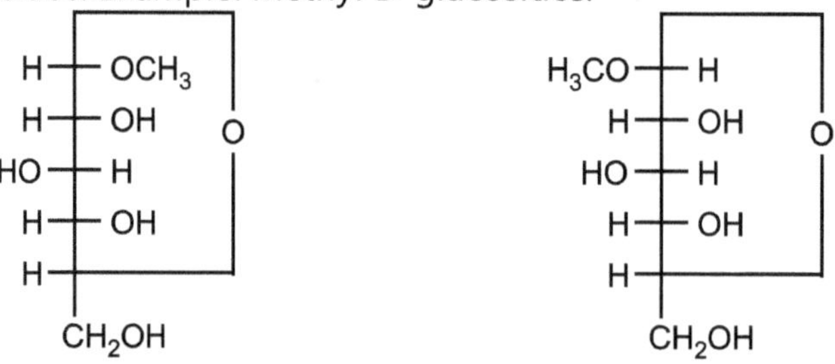

Methyl-Alpha-D-Glucoside   **Methyl-Beta-D-Glucoside**

Separation of Glycosides Parts:

Separation is mainly done in separating funnel. Alcohol and acetone are not used as solvents for aglycone separation because they are water miscible. The best solvent is ethyl acetate to extract aglycone part because the solvent immiscible in water and in separating funnel the solvent present in the upper layer (Fig. 4.8).

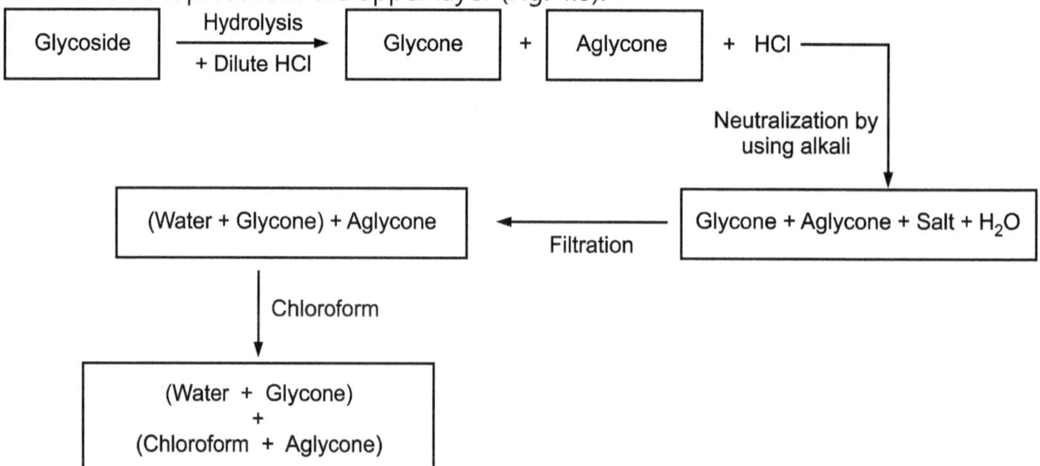

Fig. 4.8: Separation technique of Glycoside

Physical Properties:

- Glycosides are solid and amorphous powder.
- They are colourless but some are coloured (Except: Anthraquinone is red or orange, Flavoniods are yellow).
- They are water soluble but insoluble in organic solvents.
- They are mostly bitter in taste (Except: Glycyrrhizin, Stevioside, Populin).
- They are odourless (Except: Saponin glycoside).
- They are non-volatile in nature.
- Many sugar containing glycosides are insoluble in water but soluble in alcohol.
- They are hydrolysed by mineral acids or enzymes to form glycone and aglycone part.
- Glycone part is water soluble whereas aglycone part is alcohol soluble.
- After hydrolysis they react with Molish's reagent and Fehling's test.

Chemical Properties:
- With acid hydrolysis glycoside separated into sugar and non-sugar parts. The acetal linkage is more readily cleaved than the linkage between the individual sugars of the sugar chain. But C-glycosides are resistant to acid hydrolysis.
- With strong and mild alkali, they are hydrolyses the ester group. They open lactone rings. Example: Cardiac glycosides.
- With enzymatic hydrolysis sugars are splits stepwise from the terminal sugars. Enzymes are specific for some types of glycosides to split. Like Emulsin hydrolyses beta-glycosides, Invertase hydrolyses alpha-glycosides, Myrosin hydrolyses sulphur-glycosides etc.

4.4.1 Classification

Glycosides are the larger group of natural secondary metabolites obtained from many higher plants. They are broadly classified into several groups. They are as follows:

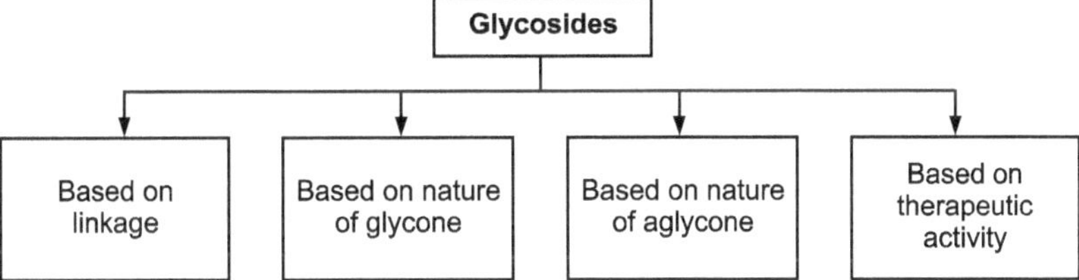

Fig. 4.9: Classification of glycosides

1. Based on Linkage:

Glycosides are classified based on linkage between glycone and aglycone part where OH groups reacting with any of the medicates like, OH, CN, SH, NH product in aglycone part and as per that they are of four types.

(a) C-glycoside:

$$\text{Glycone-OH} + \text{HC –aglycone} \longrightarrow \text{Glycone-C-aglycone} + H_2O$$

Some of the anthraquinone glycosides like cascaroside in cascara, aloin in aloes shows the particular linkage. C-glycosides are called aloin type glycoside present in aloes. They do not hydrolysed by heating with dilute acid or alkalis but occur by oxidative hydrolysis with $FeCl_3$.

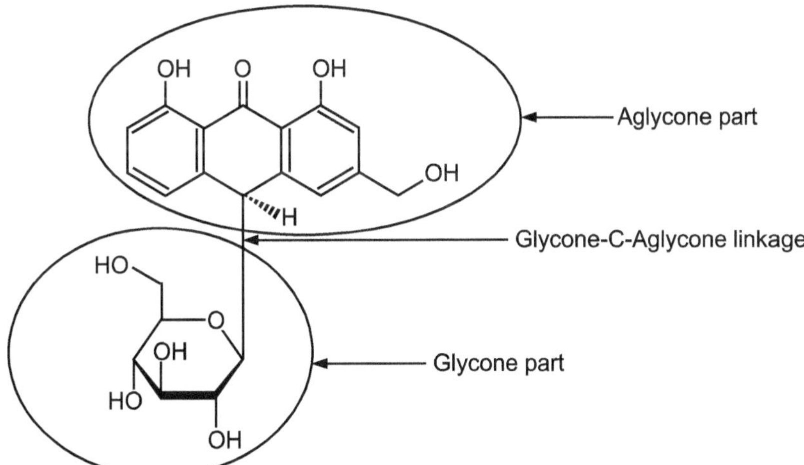

Fig. 4.10: C-Linkage of Aloin in Aloes

Another example is Carminic acid which is obtained from Cochineal insect (Fig. 4.11).

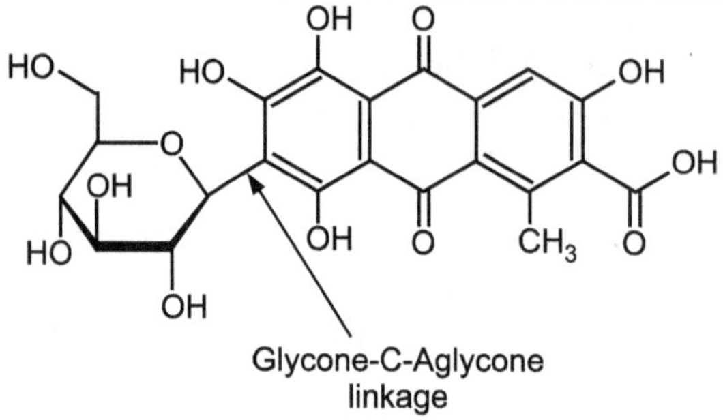

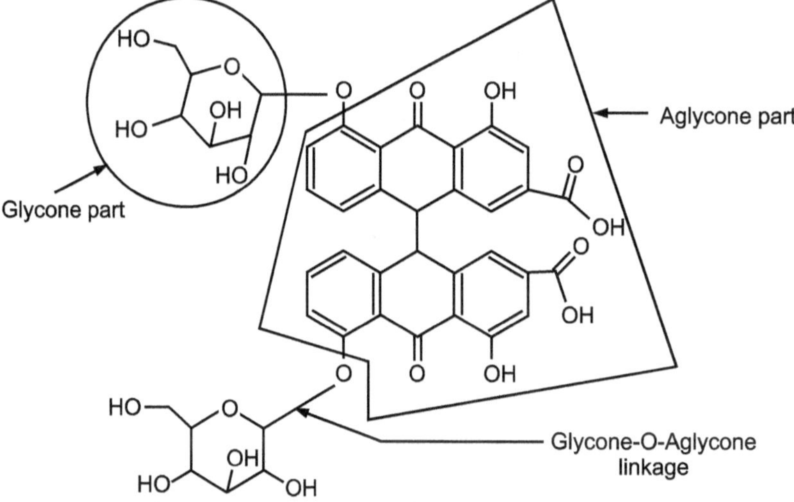

Fig. 4.11: C-Linkage of Carminic acid in Cochineal

(b) O-glycoside:

$$\text{Glycone-OH + HO-aglycone} \longrightarrow \text{Glycone-O-aglycone} + H_2O$$

They are common in higher in plants. Example: Senna, Rhubarb (Fig. 4.12). They are hydrolysed by treatment with acid or alkali into glycone and aglycone portion.

Fig. 4.12: O-Linkage of Sennoside in Senna

(c) S-glycoside:

$$\text{Glycone-OH + HS-aglycone} \longrightarrow \text{Glycone-S-aglycone} + H_2O$$

They occurrence of this glycoside is in isothiacyanate glycoside like sinigirin in black mustard formed by the condensation of sulphohydryl group aglycone to OH group of glycone (Fig. 4.13).

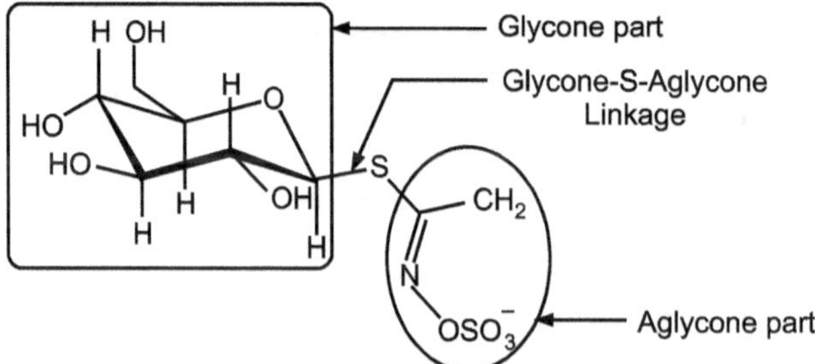

Fig. 4.13: S-Linkage of Sinigrin in Black Mustard

(d) N-glycoside:

$$\text{Glycone-OH + HN–aglycone} \longrightarrow \text{Glycone-N-aglycone + H}_2\text{O}$$

They are mostly present in the nucleoside where the amino group reacts with OH group of ribose or deoxyribose resulting into N-glycoside (Fig. 4.14).

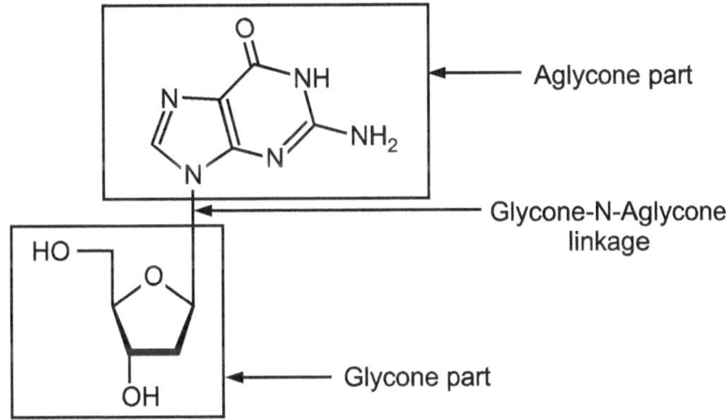

Fig. 4.14: N-Linkage of Nucleoside

(e) C and O-Glycosides:

This is one more type of glycosidic linkage where glucose molecule attached with aglycone part by both C and O linkages. Example: Cascarosides from Cascara (Fig. 4.15). Some flavonols glycosides are also contain this type of linkage.

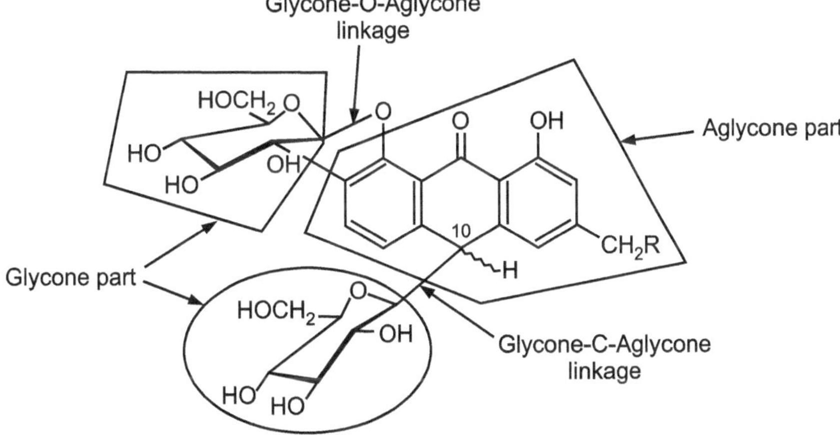

Fig. 4.15: C and O linkage in Cascaroside of Cascara

2. Based on the Chemical Nature of Non-sugar Moiety:

Type of glycoside	Aglycone part	Structure	Examples	Constituents
Anthraquinone	Anthraquinone		Senna	Sennosides

Type of glycoside	Aglycone part	Structure	Examples	Constituents
Sterol or cardiac	Digitoxigenin	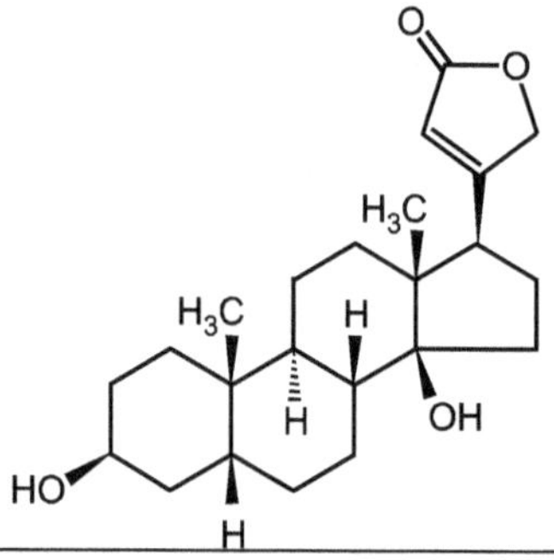	Digitalis	Digitoxin
Saponin	Glycyrrhetinic acid	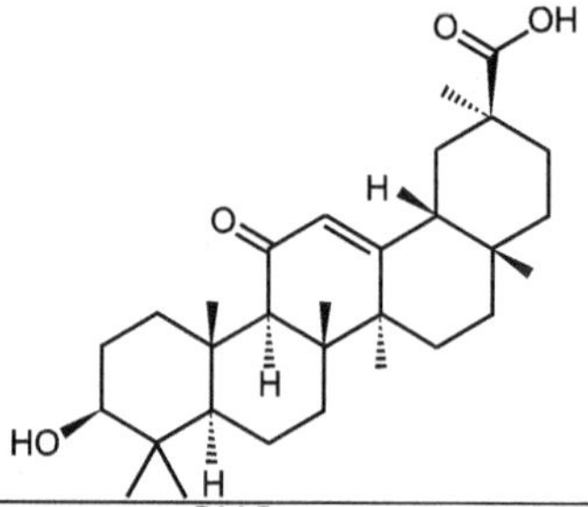	Liquorice	Glycyrrhizin
Cyanogentic	Benzaldehyde and Hydrocyanic acid	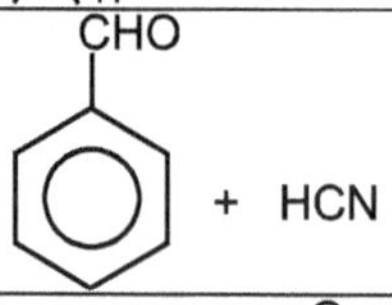	Bitter Almond	Amygdalin
Bitter	Mesogentiogenin	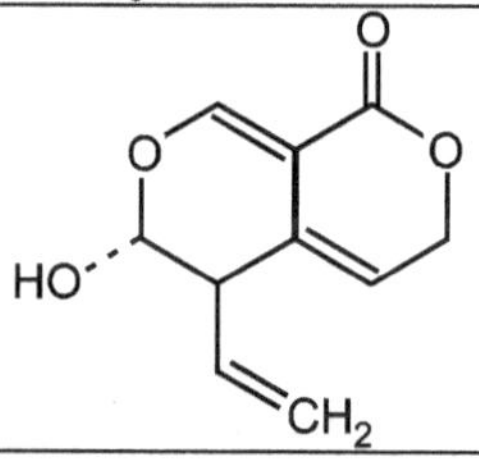	Gentian	Gentiopicrin
Isothiocynate	Allylisothiocyanate	CH_2-CH-CH_2-N=C=S	Black Mustard	Sinigrin
Flavonoid	Quercetin	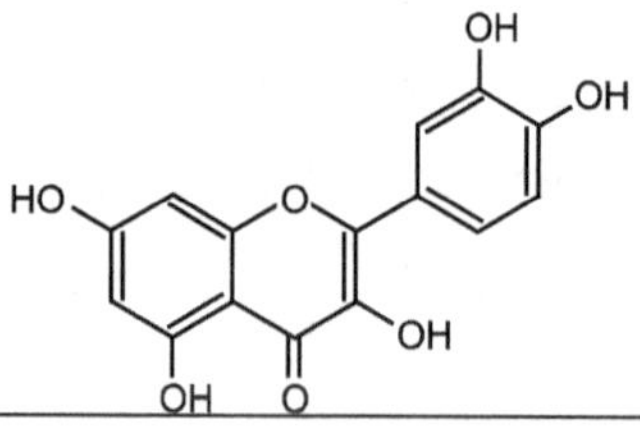	Ruta	Rutin
Coumarin glycoside or furano coumarine	Apigenin	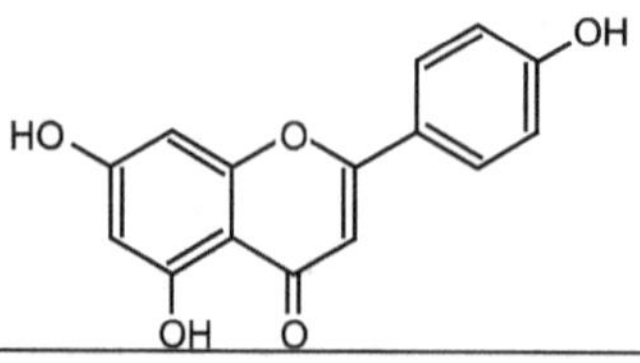	Celery	Apiin

Type of glycoside	Aglycone part	Structure	Examples	Constituents
Aldehyde	Vanillic acid		Vanilla	Vanillic acid
Phenol	Hydroquinone		Uva Ursi	Arbutin
Alcohol	Saligenin		Salix	Salicin
Antibiotic	Streptodine		Micro-organism	Streptomycin

3. **Based on the Nature of Sugar Moiety:**
   (a) **Glucoside:** Sugar portion is glucose.
   (b) **Rhamnoside:** Sugar portion is rhamnose.
   (c) Pentoside sugar portion is pentose.
   (d) Fructoside sugar portion is fructose.
   (e) Arabinoside sugar portion is arabinose.
4. **Based on Therapeutic Nature of Glycoside:**
   • Cardiac glycoside: Examples: Digitalis, Squill.
   • Laxative glycoside: Examples: Senna, Aloe.
   • Anti-ulcer glycoside: Examples: Liquorice.
   • Bitter glycoside: Examples: Chirata, Quassia wood.
   • Local irritant: Examples: Black and white mustard.
   • Analgesic and antipyretic: Example: Salix bark.

General Extraction:

Stas-otto method:

The drug containing glycoside is finely powdered and subjected to successive extraction in a Soxhlet apparatus with alcohol or suitable solvent. After extraction, extract is collected and treated with lead acetate to precipitate tannins. Filtered the solution and to the filtrate H_2S gas is passed. Precipitate of lead sulphide form which is removed by filtration. The filtrate is subjected to fractional crystallization, distillation or chromatography gives pure glycoside. Further the molecular structure is determined by the Spectrophotometer, Ultra Red assays, Infra-red, NMR and Mass spectroscopy etc.

General Chemical Tests:

1. Test for General Glycoside:

Test–A: Treated few mg of powdered drug with sulphuric acid and then 5% NaOH solution is added for neutralization. Finally Fehling's solution A and B are added to the above mixture. The solution produces red colour.

Test-B: Dissolved few mg of powdered drug with sufficient amount of water to make a solution. This solution is tested with Fehling's solution A and B. Red colour is produced. This indicates reducing sugar is present in the drug.

Both the red colours in separate test tubes are compared. If the colour of test A is more intense than test B then presence of glycoside is confirmed.

2. Test for Anthraquinone Glycoside:

(a) Brontrager's Test: This test is performed for the O-glycosides. Senna gives positive test. Powdered drug is dissolved in few ml dilute sulphuric acid and mixture is boiled. Filtered the solution, filtrate is then extracted with organic solvent like chloroform. Chloroform layer is separated and to that ammonia is added. The ammonia layer gives rose pink colour. This indicates the presence of O-glycosides.

(b) Modified Brontrager's Test: This test is performed for the presence of C-glycosides. This test is positive for Aloes. Powdered drug is mixed with dilute hydrochloric acid and $FeCl_3$. This solution converts C-glycoside to O-glycoside. Filtered the solution, filtrate is then extracted with organic solvent like chloroform. Chloroform layer is separated and to that ammonia is added. The ammonia layer gives rose pink colour. This indicates the presence of C-glycosides.

Tests for Cardiac Glycoside:

(a) Kedde's Test: Chloroform extract of drug mixed with 90% alcohol and 2% 3, 5-dinitrobenzoic acid. Further 7% NaOH is added. The solution turns to blue or violet colour. This confirms the presence of cardenolide aglycone.

(b) Antimony Trichloride Test: To a powdered drug added solution of antimony trichloride and trichloroacetic acid then heated the mixture. The solution appears blue or violet colour. This indicates the presence of Cardenolides and Bufadienolides.

(c) Keller–Killiani Test: Powdered drug is extracted with chloroform. Then few ml of acetic acid and $FeCl_3$ is added. After that concentrated sulphuric acid is added to the side tube slowly. The acid layer shows reddish purple ring. This indicates the presence of deoxy sugar, digitoxose.

(d) Raymond's Test: Small quantity of powdered drug dissolved in ethanol. In this solution, 1% solution of m-dinitrobenzene, methanol and few drops of sodium hydroxide are added. Violet colour confirms the presence of cardiac glycosides. After standing, the violet colour slowly changes to blue colour. This indicates presence of methylene group at C-21 position in the lactone ring.

(e) Legal's Test: This test is performed by using pyridine and alkaline sodium nitroprusside. The solution produces red colour. This indicates the presence of cardiac glycoside.

(f) Baljet Test: In the powdered drug sample, picric acid and sodium picrate is added. The solution becomes orange colour. This indicated the presence of cardiac glycoside.

3. **Test for Cyanogenetic Glycoside:**

    (a) Sodium Picrate Test: Drug is mixed with dilute sulphuric acid. After the addition of sodium picrate red colour is produced. This indicates presence of cyanogenetic glycoside.

    (b) Mercuric Acetate Test: Drug solution is mixed with mercuric acetate and forms drug acetate and mercury is separated out. This confirms the presence of cyanogenetic glycoside.

4. **Test for Flavonoids:**

    (a) Shinoda Test: Powdered extract mixed with few ml of 95% ethanol, few drops of conc. HCl and 0.5 g magnesium turnings. Pink colour observed. It indicates the presence of flavonoid.

    (b) To the extract few ml of lead acetate solution is added. Yellow coloured precipitate is formed. Addition of increasing amount of sodium hydroxide to the residue show yellow colour but becomes colourless after addition of acid.

5. **Test for Triterpenoid:**

    Few mg of dried extract dissolved in acetic anhydride, heated to cool. Then few ml of concentrated sulphuric acid is added along the side tube. Formation of pink colour indicates presence of triterpenoid.

    Salkowski Test: The extract is treated with few drops of concentrated sulphuric acid, red colour at lower layer indicates presence of steroids and formation of yellow coloured lower layer indicates presence of triterpenoids.

6. **Test for Saponins:**

    (a) Froth Formation Test (Foam): The solution of drug placed in water in a test tube, shake well, stable froth (foam) is formed.

    (b) Haemolysis Test: Solution of saponin (prepared in 1% normal saline) sample is added to few ml of blood in normal saline and mix well. Centrifuged and note the red supernatant formed which compare with control tube containing few ml of 10% blood in normal saline diluted with normal saline.

4.4.2 Functions of Glycoside

In Plants:

- They convert toxic materials into non-toxic form.
- They transfer water insoluble substances by using monosaccharide.
- They are the sources of energy by storage of sugar.
- They store harmful plant products such as phenol.
- They regulate growth.
- Some glycosides have antibacterial activity so they protect the plant from bacterial and other diseases.

In Animals:
- Glycosides have wide groups of chemical natures due to that they are used as many therapeutic activities. Such as laxative, cardioprotective, analgesic, local irritants etc.
- Sugar part in glycoside helps in the solubilisation of non-sugar parts for increasing the bioavailability of the drugs.
- Phenolic glycosides are used as urinary antiseptic effect.
- Alcohol glycosides are used as analgesic, antipyretic, anti-inflammatory action.
- Cardiac glycosides are used for heart disease.
- Bitter substances have antimicrobial as well as antibiotic actions.
- Thiol glycosides are used as pain killer.
- Anthraquinone glycosides are used as laxative action.

4.5 FLAVONOIDS

Flavonoids are polyphenolic compound and vastly available in maximum plant species. They are generally yellow coloured pigments. They are larger group of glycoside. They are 2-phenylbenzopyrones derivatives and produce a large number of physiological activities. Flavonoids are the largest group of naturally occurring phenols and occur in free states in the plants as glycosides. They may be described as a series of C_6-C_3-C_6 compounds (Fig. 4.16). They are largely found in Polygonaceae, Rutaceae, Fabaceae and Rosaceae families.

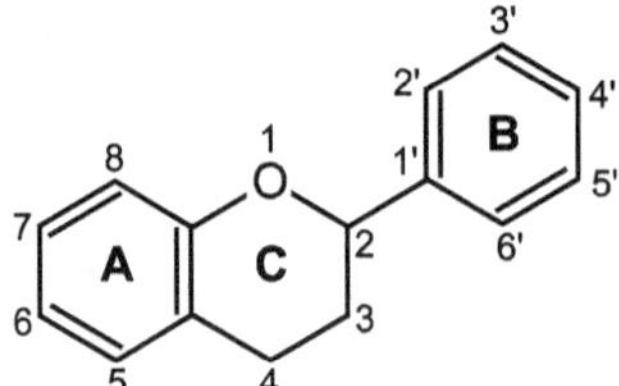

Fig. 4.16: General structure of Flavonoid

Physical Properties:
- They are crystalline substances with certain melting point.
- Catechins, Flavanes, Isoflavanes, Flavanones, Flavanonoles are colourless crystals whereas Flavones, Flavonols, Chalcones are yellow coloured crystals. Anthocyanidins are red in acidic media and blue in alkaline media.
- Anthocyanes are sap pigments. The actual colour of the plant organ is determined by the pH of the sap. Example: Blue colour of the cornflower and red colour of roses are due to these glycosides.
- Flavonoid glycosides are generally soluble in water and alcohol but insoluble in organic solvents.
- Aglycone parts of flavonoids are soluble in diethylether, acetone, alcohols etc.
- Flavanols are optically active.
- Flavanones and flavonones are unstable compounds.
- Flavonoid O-glycosides are undergoes hydrolysis when treated with acid, alkali.
- Rutin is yellow crystalline powder, soluble in alkali but slightly soluble in water.
- Rutin on hydrolysis gives quercetin, rhamnose and glucose whereas hesperidin yields hesperitin, rhamnose and glucose.
- Under the UV light flavonoids shows fluorescence of different colours (yellow, orange, brown, red).

Chemical Properties:

- Chemically flavonoids are based upon a fifteen-carbon skeleton (C15) consisting of two benzene rings (A and B) linked via a heterocyclic pyrane ring (C).
- They occur as aglycones, glycosides, and methylated derivatives.
- Six-member ring condensed with the benzene ring is either a α-pyrone (flavonols and flavanones) or its dihydroderivative (flavonols and flavanones).
- The position of the benzenoid substituent divides the flavonoid class into flavonoids (2-position) and isoflavonoids (3-position).
- Flavonols differ from flavanones by hydroxyl group at the 3-position and a C2–C3 double bond.
- Flavonoids are often hydroxylated at positions 3, 5, 7, 2, 3', 4', and 5'. Methyl ethers and acetyl esters of the alcohol group are known to occur in nature.
- The glycosidic linkage is normally located in flavonoid at positions 3 or 7.

4.5.1 Classification

Broadly flavonoids are classified into two classes namely based on groups and based on place of B-ring location (Fig. 4.17).

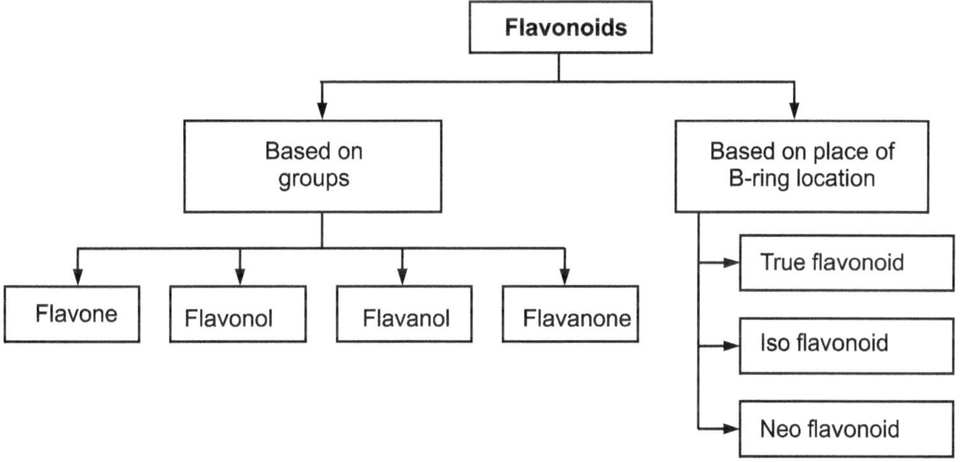

Fig. 4.17: Classification of flavonoids

1. Based on Groups:

Flavonoids are classified into flavones (e.g. apigenin, and luteolin), flavonols (e.g. quercetin, kaempferol, myricetin, and fisetin), flavanones (e.g. flavanone, hesperetin, and naringenin), Flavanol (Example: Catechin) (Table 4.5).

Table 4.5: Classification of Flavonoids as per group

Group	Example	Biological source	Structure
Flavone	Apigenin	*Apium petroselinum* (Apiin)	

Group	Example	Biological source	Structure
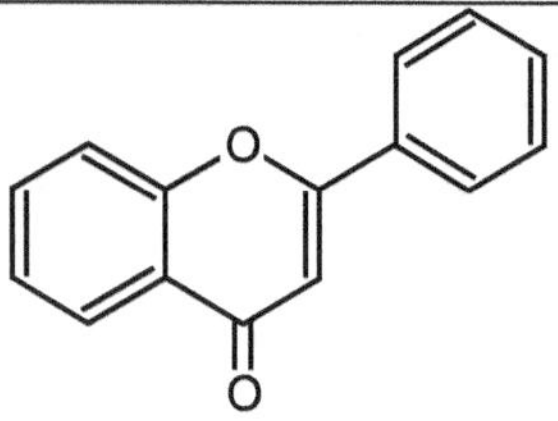	Luteolin	*Salvia tomentosa* (Salvia)	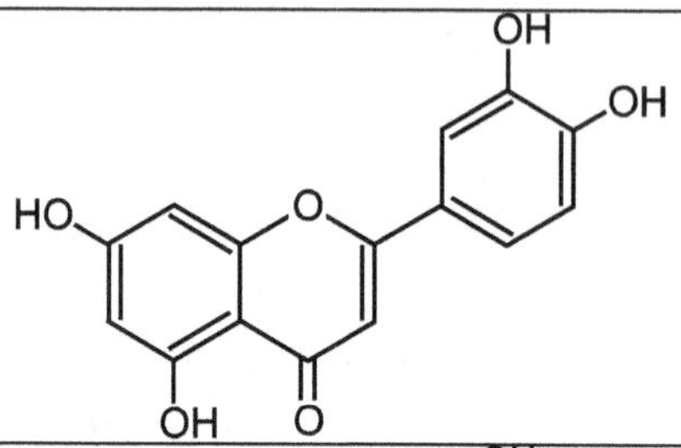
Flavonol 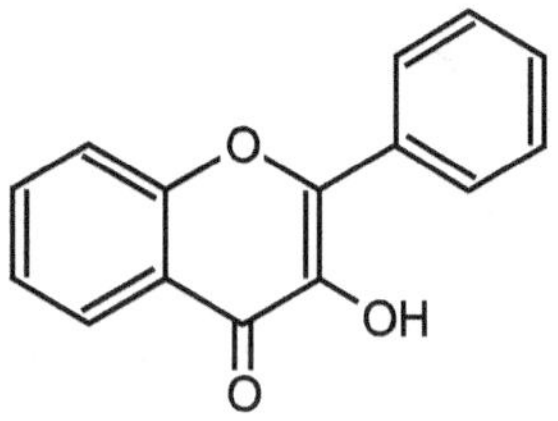	Quercetin	*Quercus alba* (Oak)	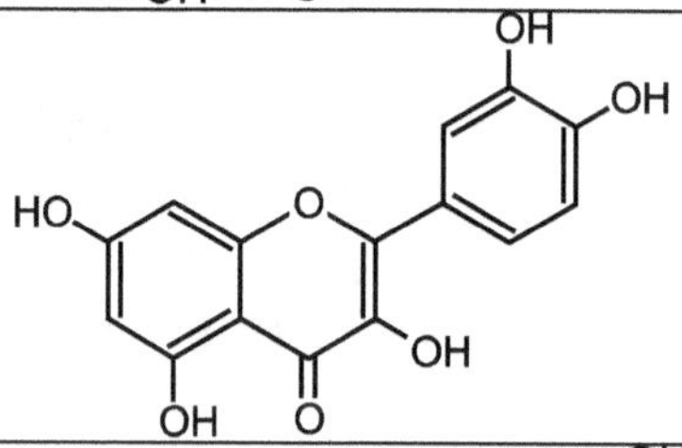
	Kaempferol	*Pinus sylvestris,* (Pine) *Aloe vera* (Aloe)	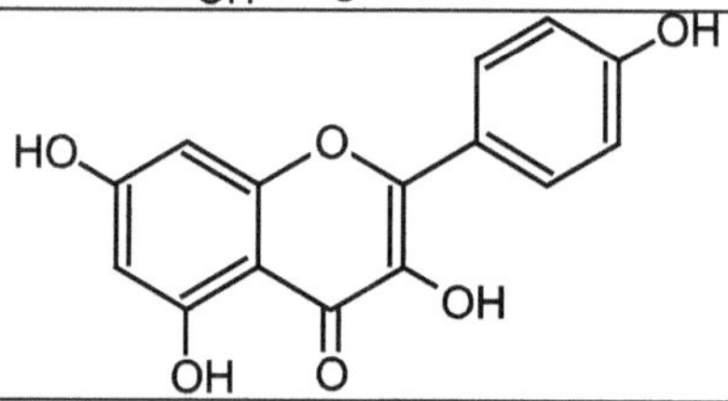
	Myricetin	*Rosa damascene* (Rose)	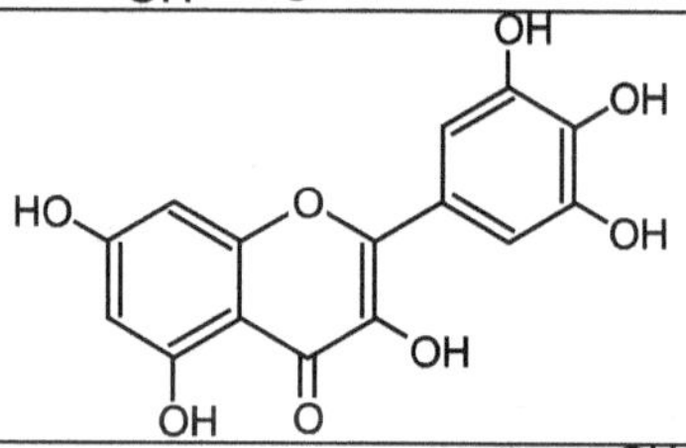
	Fisetin	*Fragaria ananassa* (Strawberry)	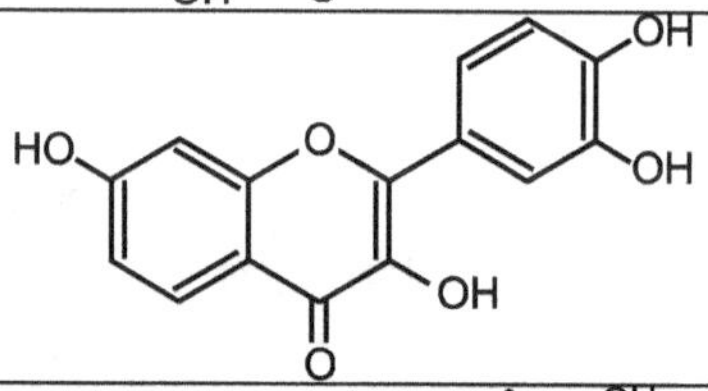
Flavanol 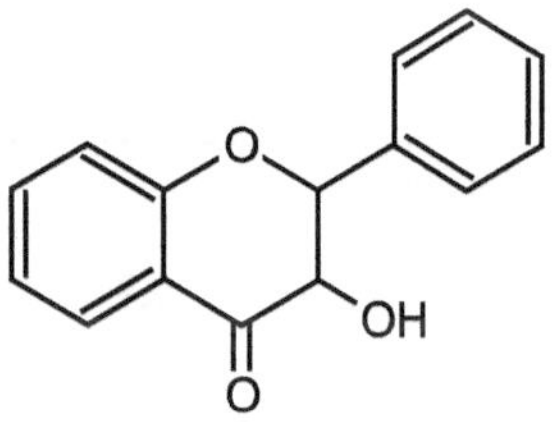	Catechin	*Camellia sinensis* (Green Tea)	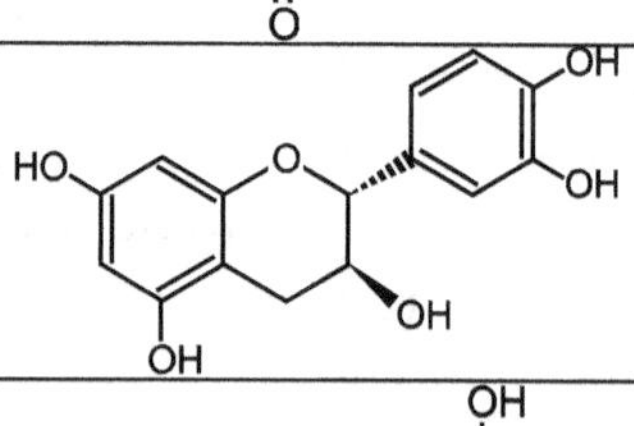
	Epigallo catechin	*Camellia sinensis* (Green Tea)	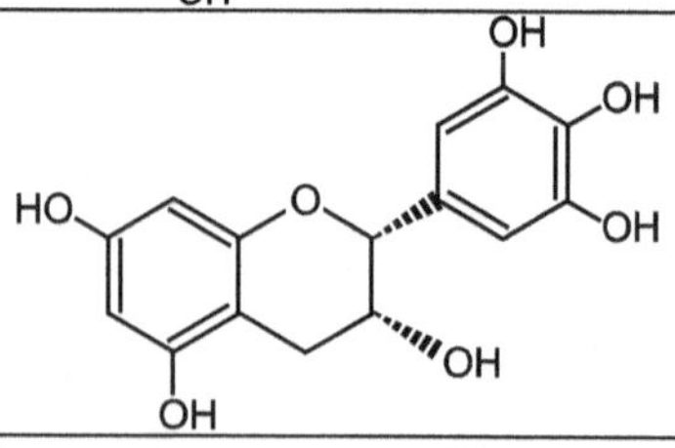

Group	Example	Biological source	Structure
Flavanone 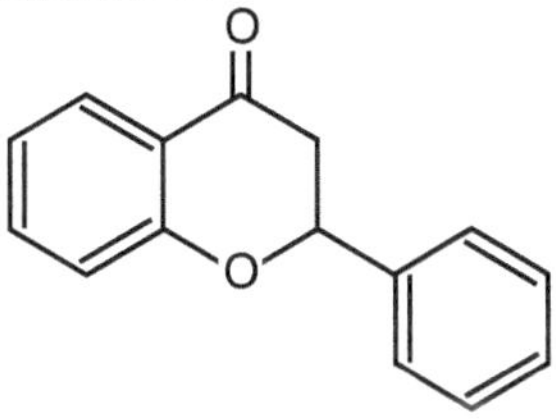	Hesperetin	*Citrus sinensis* (Orange)	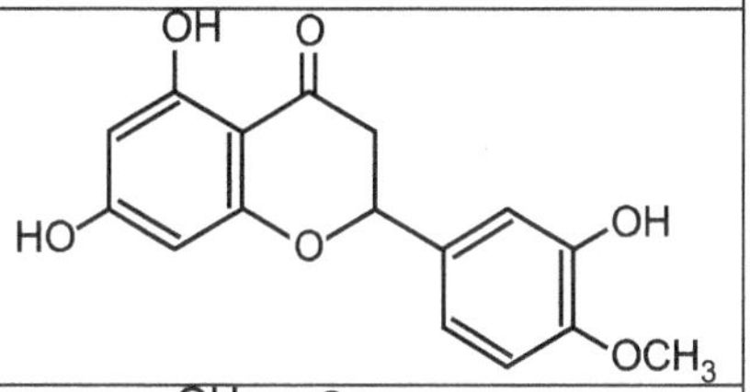 OH, O, HO, OH, OCH₃
	Naringenin	*Citrus paradise* (Grape fruit)	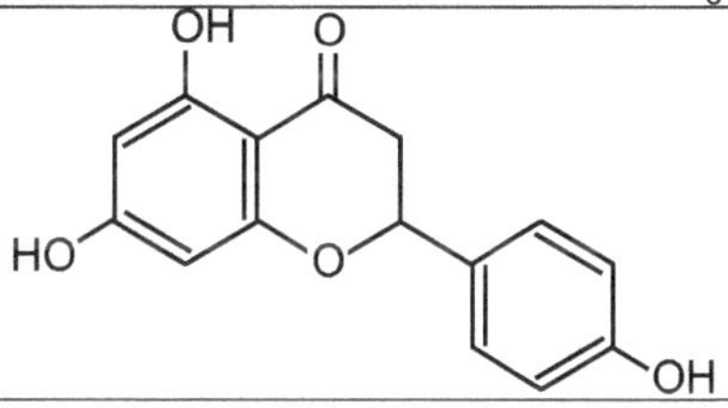 OH, O, HO, OH

2. As per the Place of B-ring location:

As per the location of the B-ring, they are three types like true flavonoids, isoflavonoid and neoflavonoid. True Flavonoids are derived from 2-phenylchromen-4-one (2-phenyl-l, 4-benzopyrone) structure. Isoflavonoids are derived from 3-phenylchromen- 4-one (3-phenyl-1,4-benzopyrone) structure and Neo-flavonoids are derived from 4-phenyl-coumarine (4-phenyl-1,2-benzopyrone) structure. True Flavonoids are also known as bioflavonoid due to origin from plants. Bioflavonoids are anthoxanthin i.e. mixture of flavones and flavonols (Table 4.6).

Table 4.6: Classification of flavonoids based on position of B-ring

Group	Example	Biological source	Structure
True Flavonoid 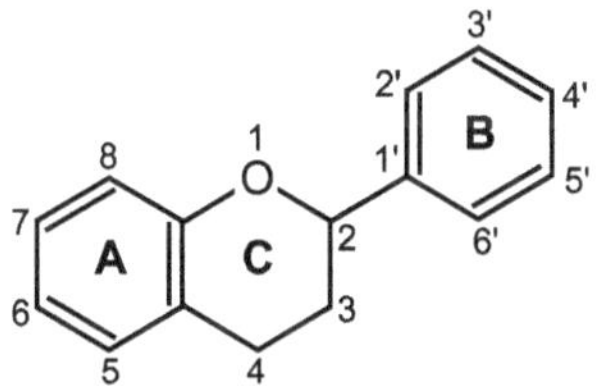	Apigenin	*Apium petroselinum* (Apiin)	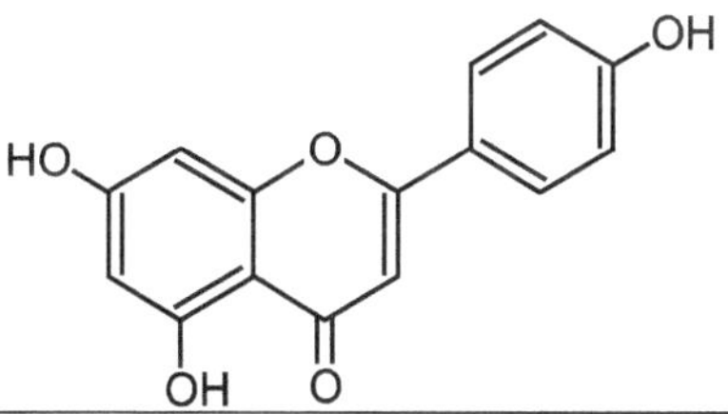 OH, HO, O, OH, O
	Luteolin	*Salvia tomentosa* (Salvia)	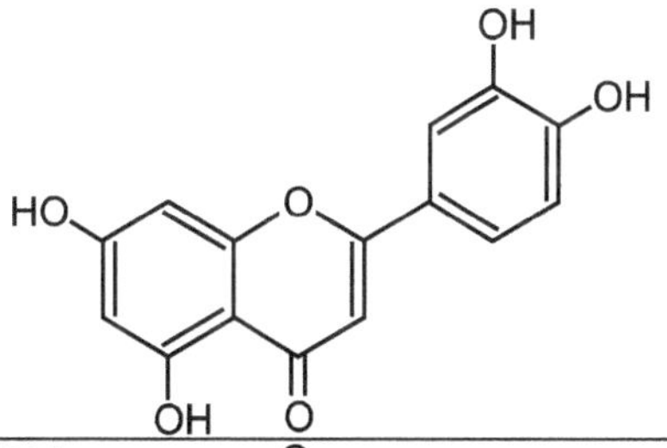 OH, OH, HO, O, OH, O
Isoflavonoid	Genistein	*Glycine max* (Soya bean)	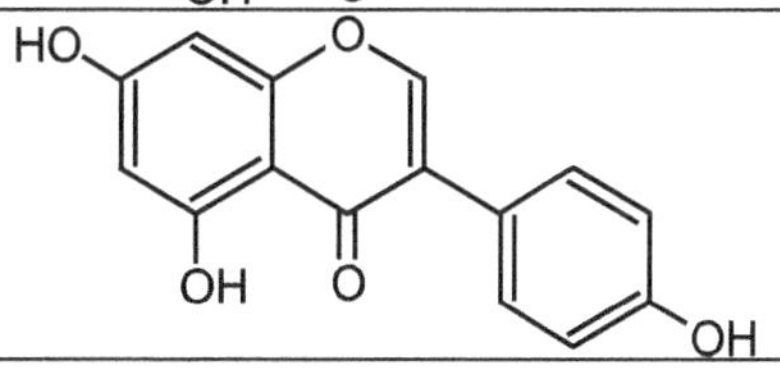 HO, O, OH, O, OH

Group	Example	Biological source	Structure
	Diadzein	*Glycine max* (Soya bean)	
	Glycitein	*Glycine max* (Soya bean)	
Neoflavonoid	Calophyllolide	*Calophyllum inophyllum* (Indian Doomba oil tree, Laurelwood)	
	Dalbergichromene	*Dalbergia sissoo* (North Indian Rosewood)	
	Nivetin	*Echinops niveus* (Globe thistles)	

General Extraction:

Dried plant materials are powdered and extracted with various solvents based on the type of flavonoids such as less polar flavonoids (like Isoflavones, flavanones, flavonols) are extracted with chloroform, diethyl ether or ethyl acetate whereas more polar flavonoid glycosides are extracted with alcohol or mixed solvent of alcohol and water. Soxhlet method is used for the extraction. N-Hexane solvent is used for defatted the plant materials followed by ethyl acetate solvent is used for the extraction of flavonoids.

Generally, successive solvent extraction method is used for the extraction. First, dichloromethane is used for extraction of flavonoid aglycone and other less polar constituents. Then alcohol is used for extraction of glycone part of flavonoid and other polar constituents. The crude extract is purified by using shaking with sodium carbonate or sodium bicarbonate (for strong acidic OH group) or by column chromatography using polyamide column, Sephadex LH-20 column. Sephadex LH-20 column is suitable for separation of proanthocyanidins where alcohol is used as an eluent and acetone is used for separation of high molecular weight polyphenols.

Easy method for common flavonoids extraction is described in Fig. 4.18.

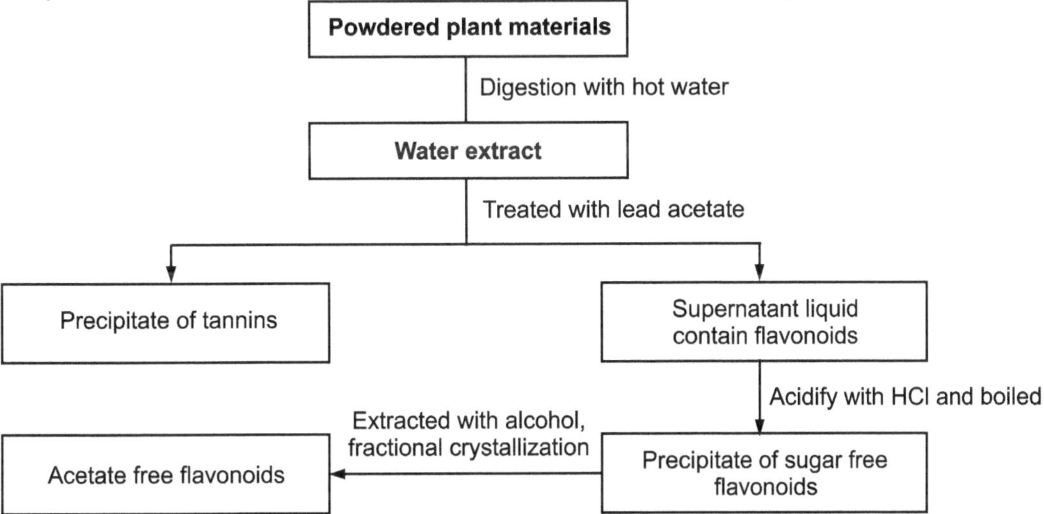

Fig. 4.18: General extraction method of flavonoids

Chemical Tests for Flavonoid:

1. **Shinoda Test:** The alcoholic solution of flavone or flavonol when treated with metallic magnesium (or Zinc) and hydrochloric acid gives an orange, red or violet colour. This test is also known as cyanidin reaction.

2. **Lead Subacetate Test:** To small quantity of residue, add lead subacetate solution. Yellow coloured precipitate is formed. Addition of increasing amount of sodium hydroxide to the residue shows yellow colouration, which decolouration after addition of acid.

3. **Wilson's Reaction:** Flavonoids form complexes with boric acid which is not destroyed by addition of citric acid alcoholic solution (or oxalic acid).

4. **Antimony Pentachloride Test:** Alcoholic solution of sample when reacts with antimony pentachloride the solution produces red or violet colour.

Functions:

- They act as powerful antioxidant like Quercetin, Xanthohumol, Isoxanthohumol etc.
- They control the plant growth.
- They inhibit and activate plant enzymes.
- They having a role in the biochemistry of reproduction.
- They have fungicidal properties.

- They protect the plant from parasites attack.
- They are the pigments of flowers that attract insects for pollination.
- They are having significant therapeutic efficacy such as antiviral, antiallergic, antiplatlets, anti-inflammatory, antitumor etc.

4.6 TANNINS

They are naturally occurring non-nitrogenous compound. They are belongs to water soluble polyphenols with high molecular weight, ranging from 500 to 3000 (Gallic acid esters) upto 20,000 (Proanthocyanidins). First time the term tannin is coined by Seguin in 1796. They have number of hydroxyls and carboxyl groups to form strong complexes with various macromolecules. The tannins enter into the class of semiochemicals which act as messengers within or between species. Based on that, semiochemicals are divided into two classes viz. pheromones and allelochemicals. Pheromones are involved in the communication between the same species while allelochemicals interact with different species. They are widely distributed in many higher plant species such as Aceraceae, Actinidiaceae, Bixaceae, Burseraceae, Combretaceae, Ericaceae, Myricaceae (Dicot plants) and Najadaceae, Typhaceae (Monocot plants) families. They are mainly located in the vacuoles or surface wax of plants. They occur normally in the roots, wood, bark, leaves, and fruits of many plants. They also occur in galls as pathological growths prevent insect attacks.

Physical Properties:
- Tannins are dark brown or reddish brown.
- They are amorphous, non-crystalline in nature.
- They are available in the form of powder, flakes or spongy mass.
- They are water, alkali, alcohol soluble but sparingly soluble in chloroform and other organic solvents.
- They form colloidal solution with water.
- They form protective coating in place of wound injury.
- They have astringent taste.
- They combine with skin and hide to form leather. They react with gelatine to form an insoluble compound.

Chemical Properties:
- Tannins form precipitation with proteins, gelatine, alkaloids etc.
- They have antioxidant properties due to presence of polyhydroxy phenolic compounds.
- They have astringent properties due to formation of precipitation with proteins.
- They yield purple, violet or black precipitate with iron compounds.
  Examples: Hydrolysable tannins reacts with ferric salt to form blue black precipitation whereas condensed tannins form brownish green precipitation with the same.
- They react with potassium ferricyanide in presence of ammonia to form deep red colour solution.
- They are precipitated by metallic salts like potassium dichromate, and lead acetate and sub-acetate.
- They are used in the clarification of wine and beer.
- As a constituent it reduces viscosity of drilling mug for oil wells.

4.6.1 Classification

Based on identity of phenolic nuclei and the linkage, tannins are classified into two main categories (Fig. 4.19).

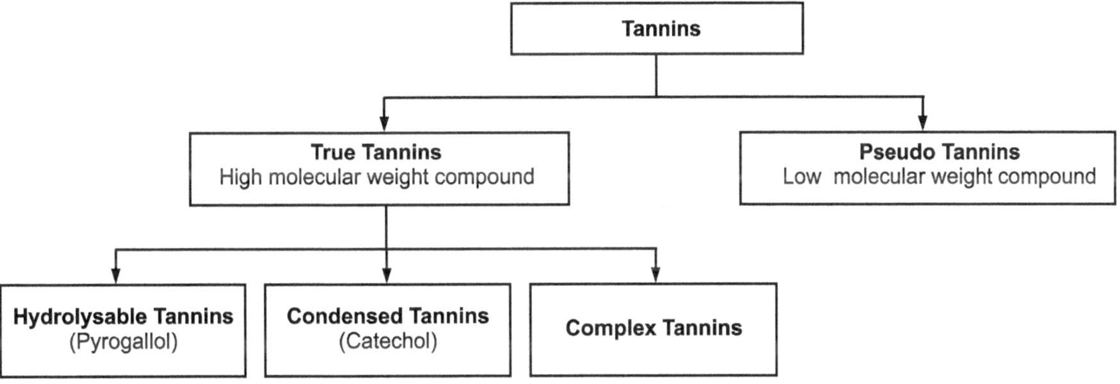

Fig. 4.19: Classification of tannins

(a) Hydrolysable Tannins:

These tannins are basically esters of sugar mainly glucose with one or more trihydroxybenzene carboxylic acid. These tannins are hydrolyzed by acids, or enzyme (Tannase). Their structures composed with several polyphenolic acid molecules such as gallic acid and ellagic acid which are bound through ester linkage to a central glucose molecule. Based on the phenolic acid produced, hydrolysable tannins are classified into gallotannins and Ellagitannins.

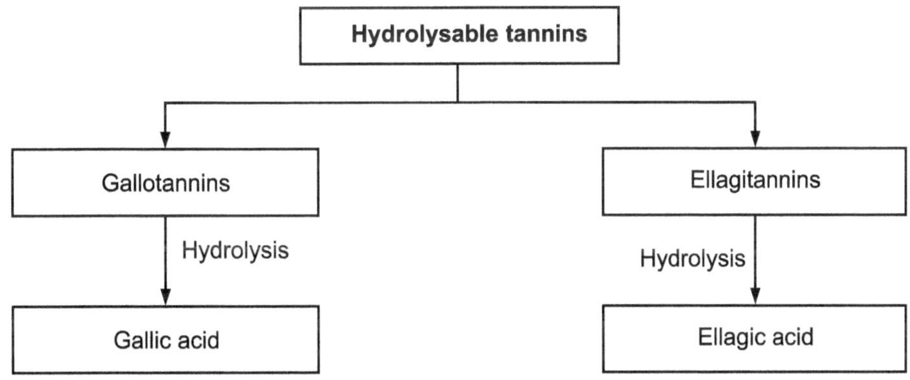

Fig. 4.20

Therefore, gallic acid is hydrolysable product of gallitannins and ellagic acid is hydrolysable product of ellagitannins. The gallic acid is found in rhubarb, clove whereas ellagic acid is found in eucalyptus leave and myrobalans and pomegranate bark. These tannins treated with ferric chloride to produced blue or black colour. Gallitannins are rapidly soluble in water whereas ellagitannins are slowly soluble in water.

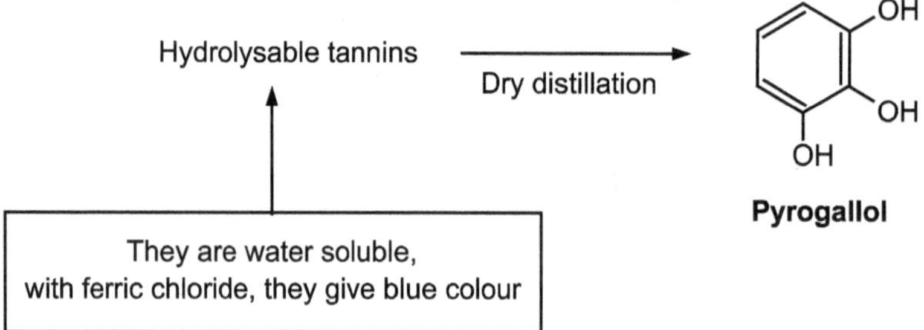

Ellagic acid   **Gallic acid**

Gallotannins are mainly extracted from Tara (*Caesalpinia spinosa*), sumac (*Rhus coriaria*) and gallnuts (*Quercus infectoria* and *Rhus semialata*). The ellagitannins, made from ellagic acid glycosides, are one of the components of oak wood (*Quercus robur, Quercus petraea* and *Quercus alba*), chestnut wood (*Castanea sativa*) and myrobalan (*Terminalia chebula*).

Hydrolysable tannins are also known as pyrogallol tannins as the component of phenolic acid on dry distillation converts pyrogallols and phenolic compounds.

Hydrolysable tannins ⟶ Dry distillation **Pyrogallol**

They are water soluble,
with ferric chloride, they give blue colour

Hydrolysable tannins: Examples: Myrobalan, Bahera, Amla, Arjuna.

(b) Condensed Tannins:

These tannins are resistant to hydrolysis (do not contain sugar moiety) and they derived from the flavonols, catechins and flavan-3, 4-diols. Catechin occurs with tannins and flavan-3, 4-diols are intermediates in the biosynthesis of polymeric molecules. On treatment with acids or enzymes they are decomposed into phlobaphenes (Red insoluble compound). On dry distillation they produce catechol hence they are also known as catechol tannins. These tannins are found in cinchona bark, male fern, wild cherry bark, Black catechu, Pale catechu, Ashoka, Pterocarpus etc. They produce brownish green colour with ferric chlorides. They are further divided into two main categories namely proanthocyanidin and profisetinidin. Proanthocyanidins are oligomeric flavonoids and naturally present in grapes (*Vitis vinifera*) consisting of various flavonoids which release anthocyanins and other insoluble molecules when they are treated under acid hydrolysis. They are mainly diffused in the skins and seeds of grapes, and therefore you can find them in red wines. Cocoa beans contain the highest concentrations of Proanthocyanidins. Profisetinidins are formed from leuco-fisetinidin, the leucoanthocyanidin form of fisetinidin. They extracted from the quebracho wood (*Schinopsis lorentzii*).

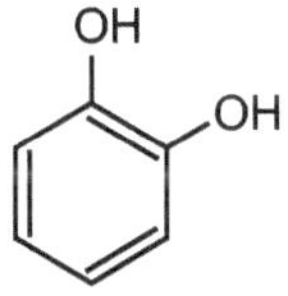

Catechol

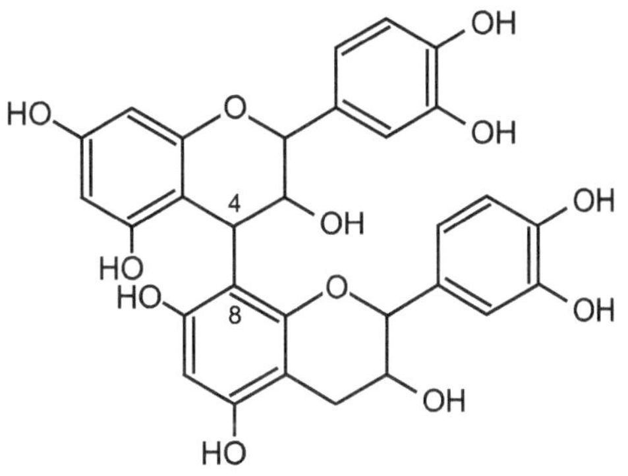

Proanthocyanidin

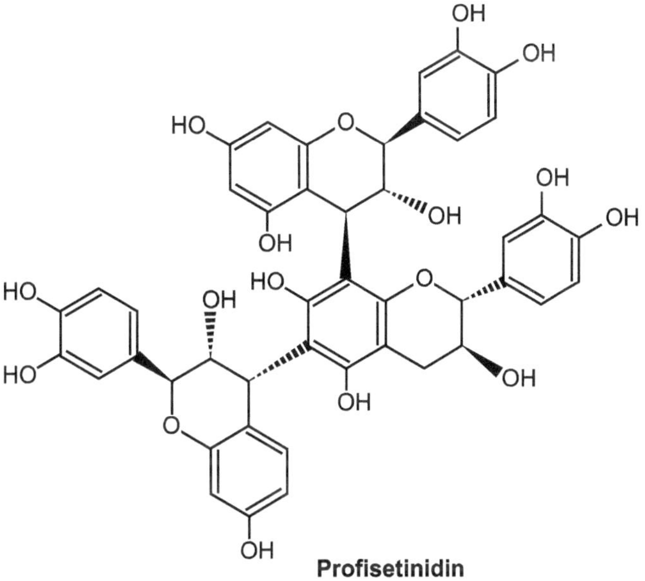

Profisetinidin

(c) Complex Tannins:

They are the group of tannins that biosynthesized from both hydrolysable tannin (C-glucoside ellagitannin) and condensed tannin (Flavono-ellagitannin). Example: Acutissimin. It is prepared by reacting a substance called vescalagin, extracted from oak wood, with a flavanoid from grapes called catechin. Some other examples like tea (*Thea sinensis*), Oak (*Quercus infectoria*), hamamelis (*Hamamelis virginiana*) leaves and bark, chestnuts (*Castanea sativa*) contain both hydrolysable and condense tannins.

(d) Pseudo Tannins:

They are sub-group of tannins because they do not response Gold beaters skin test. They have low molecular weight compound. They are simple phenolic compounds. They are found mainly dead tissues and dying cells of plants. In concentrated solution, they form precipitate with gelatin. They are found in catechu and nux-vomica, etc. Examples: Chlorogenic acid in coffee and Nux vomica, ipecacuanhic acid in Ipecac, catechins in cocoa. Chlorogenic acid is identified by extracting the drug with water followed by oxidation, produces green colour.

(e) Phloro Tannins:

Recently, a third class of tannins has been identified, the phloro tannins, present in many species of dark brown algae such as kelps and rockweeds or sargassacean. It is also available in some red algae. These compounds are oligomers of phloroglucinol (polyphloroglucinols) and based on arrangement of the phloroglucinol monomers they are further classified. They are known as tannins because they form precipitate by reaction of proteins. They are distributed in six main sub-groups namely fucols, phlorethols, fucophloretols, fuhalols and eckols, which are only found in Alariaceae family. As per the linkage, they are classified into four subclasses viz. phlorotannins with an ether linkage (fuhalols and phlorethols, fuhalols are constructed of phloroglucinol units that are connected with para- and ortho-arranged), with a phenyl linkage (fucols), with an ether and a phenyl linkage (fucophlorethols) and with a dibenzodioxin linkage in eckols and carmalols (derivatives of phlorethols containing a dibenzodioxin moiety).

Phloro tannin

Difference between Hydrolysable and Condense Tannins:

Hydrolysable tannins	Condense tannins (Non-hydrolysable)
1. They are known as pyrogallol tannins.	1. They are known as catechol tannins.
2. They became hydrolysed with the help of acid or enzyme.	2. They are resistance to hydrolysis because glucose moiety is absent.
3. With 5% $FeCl_3$ solution, it gives bluish black colour.	3. With 5% $FeCl_3$ solution, it gives brownish green colour.
4. With bromine water it do not form precipitate.	4. With bromine water it forms buff coloured precipitate.
5. Examples: Arjuna, Tannic acid, Amla, Myrobalan.	5. Examples: Ashoka, Black and Pale catechu.

Difference between Gallotannins and Ellagitannins:

Gallotannins	Ellagitannins
1. Upon hydrolysis it gives gallic acid.	1. Upon hydrolysis it gives ellagic acid.
2. It is rapidly soluble in water.	2. It is slowly soluble in water.
3. Free gallic acid in plant is converted to gluco-gallotannins.	3. Present in plant in open and ring forms as hexa hydroxyl diphenic acid.
4. Galloyl groups are linked through depside (polyphenolic compound having linked with ester bond) bonds.	4. Galloyl group are linked through C-C bonds.
5. More available in Clove, Rhubarb, Hamamelis.	5. More available in Eucalyptus, Promegranate.

Chemical Tests:

1. **Gelatin Test:** To a solution of tannin, aqueous solution of gelatin and sodium chloride are added. A white buff coloured precipitate is formed.
2. **Goldbeater's Skin Test:** A small piece of goldbeater skin (membrane prepared from the intestine of an ox) is soaked in 20% hydrochloric acid, rinsed with distilled water and placed in a solution of tannin for 5 minutes. The skin piece is washed with distilled water and kept in a solution of ferrous sulphate. A brown or black colour is produced on the skin due presence of tannins.
3. **Phenazone Test:** A mixture of aqueous extract of a drug and sodium acid phosphate is heated then cooled and filtered. A solution of phenazone is added to the filtrate. A bulky coloured precipitate is formed.
4. **Match Stick Test:** A match stick is dipped in aqueous plant extract, dried near burner and moistened with concentrated hydrochloric acid. On warming near flame, the matchstick wood turns pink or red due to formation of phloroglucinol. This test is also known as Catechin test.
5. **Chlorogenic Acid Test:** An extract of chlorogenic acid containing drug is treated with aqueous ammonia. A green colour is formed on exposure to air.
6. **Vanillin-hydrochloric Acid Test:** Sample solution and added vanillin-hydrochloric acid reagent (Vanillin 1 gm, alcohol 10 ml, concentrated hydrochloric acid 10 ml) a pink or red colour is formed due to formation of phloroglucinol.

General Extraction:

Both hydrolysable and condense tannins are water and alcohol soluble but insoluble in organic solvents. Hence, tannin containing compound (Gallic acid, ellagic acid, other tannins) are extracted with using water or alcohol as solvent. Chloroform containing drugs are removed through ether extraction. Collected aqueous layer and concentrated to get crude extract of tannins.

Functions:

- Medicinally they used as antidotes, antiseptics, astringent properties.
- They used in ink manufacturing industries.
- They used as preservatives.
- They used for vegetable tanning.
- They used to inhibit lipid peroxidation and plasmin.
- They used for lipolysis in fat cells.
- They are used to treat tonsillitis, pharyngitis, hemorrhoids, and skin eruptions.

4.7 VOLATILE OIL

Plants that contain aromatic liquids (derived from shrubs, flowers, trees, roots, bushes, herbs, and seeds) are known as essential oils. These oils provide protection to the plants from insects, harsh environmental conditions, and disease. They are concentrated hydrophobic liquid contain volatile aroma and they are also known as **volatile oils, ethereal oils, aetherolea**, or simply as the **oil of the plant.** Due to presence of essence, they are commonly known as essential oils.

Essential oils are usually hydrophobic and lipophilic compounds. They are not miscible with water but diluted in solvents like pure ethanol and polyethylene glycol.

Terpenes and Terpenoids:

The abundant distributed compounds that present in essential oils are the terpenes and sesquiterpenes and also their oxygenated compounds. The term "terpene" is hydro-carbons which has basic simple isoprene (C_5H_8) molecule. Further "Terpenoids" are a compound having features same like the terpene structure. The terms terpene and terpenoids usually refer not only to the hydrocarbons but also to their oxygenated compounds. The most characteristic group present in essential oils is the monoterpenes and their oxygenated compounds with the empirical formulae $C_{10}H_{16}$; $C_{10}H_{16}O$; $C_{10}H_{18}O$. Isoprene is a precursor in biogenesis of terpenic compounds. In essential oils, Terpenes occur as acyclic, monocyclic, bicyclic, and tricyclic. A saturated acyclic hydrocarbon with 10 carbon atoms has the formula $C_{10}H_{22}$; a compound $C_{10}H_{16}$ may be acyclic with three double bonds, or monocyclic with two double bonds, or bicyclic (one double bond), or tricyclic (no double bonds). They also occur in many redox stages therefore, compounds with more or fewer hydrogens are also found. The oxygenated derivatives contain maximum functional groups such as hydroxyl, methoxyl, carbonyl, carhoxyl, etc. Example: Acyclic terpenes $C_{10}H_{16}$ with three double bonds (below structure):

Terpenes: They are diverse group of organic hydrocarbons produced by a wide variety of plants. They are important building block for certain odours, hormones, vitamins, pigments, steroids, resins, essential oils etc. They are naturally released from plants when temperature is higher, helps to seed clouds which then cool the plants. They synergistically interact with each other for different smells and effects.

Examples:

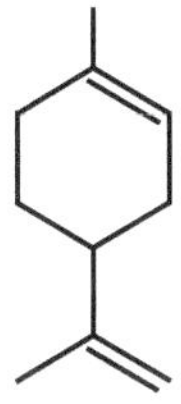

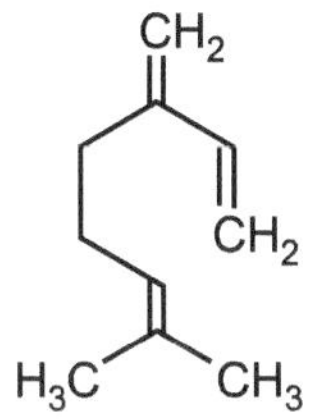

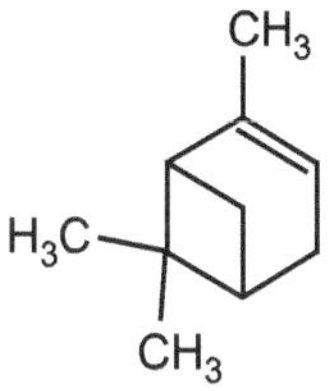

Limonene	**Myrcene**	**Pinene**

Terpenoids: The **terpenoids** are also known as **isoprenoids**. They are large and diverse class of naturally occurring organic chemicals similar to terpenes. They derived from five-carbon isoprene units assembled and modified in various ways. Terpenoids are likely to be as modified terpenes, wherein methyl groups are removed and oxygen atoms added. Hence, they are oxygenated hydrocarbon compounds. They are classified according to the number of isoprene units (Fig. 4.23) as well as classified according to the number of cyclic structures present in the structure. Meroterpenes are also natural products, having a partial terpenoid structure.

Table 4.7: Classification of Terpenoids

Isoprene units	Carbon Atoms	Classification	Example
1	5	Hemiterpene	Isoprene, Prenol
2	10	Monoterpene	Geraniol, Limonene, Pinene, myrcene
3	15	Sesquterpene	Farnesol
4	20	Diterpene	Retinol
5	25	Sesterterpene	Rare compound
6	30	Triterpene	Squalene
8	40	Tetraterpene	Lycopene, Beta Carotene
>8	>40	Polyterpene	Rubber, Polyisoprene

Properties:

- Most of terpenoids are colourless or pale yellow liquids. They are lighter than water and boiled between 150 and 180°C.
- They are insoluble in water but soluble in organic solvents. Many of the essential oils are optically active.
- They undergo polymerization and dehydrogenation in the ring.
- They are very easily oxidized by all the oxidizing agents due to presence of olefin bonds.
- They readily isomerize in the presence of acids into more stable forms.
- On thermal decomposition, they yield isoprene as one of the products.
- They are unsaturated compounds (open-chain or cyclic with one or more carbon atom rings) having one or more double bonds.
- They also form characteristic addition products with NO, NOCl and NOBr. These addition products are useful in the identification of terpenoids.

Some Useful Extraction Methods:

- **Expression Method:** In this method, the plant material is crushed and the juice is centrifuged in a high-speed centrifugal machine when nearly half of the essential oil is extracted. The other half of the oil is generally not extracted and such residue is used for the isolation of inferior quality of oil by distillation. Examples: Citrus, lemon and grass oils are extracted by this method.

- **Steam Distillation:** This method is widely used in the laboratory. In this method, the plant material is macerated and then steam distilled, when the essential oils go into distillate by the use of pure organic volatile solvents, like light petroleum. In this method, some essential oils are decomposed during distillation and some (ester) are hydrolyzed to none or less fragrant compounds so the method should be used carefully.
- **Extraction by Mean of Volatile Solvent:** In this method, heat sensitive essential oils are extracted. The plant material is directly treated with light petrol at 50°C, and the solvent is removed by distillation under reduce pressure.
- **Adsorption in Purified Fats:** This method is also known as **Effleurage**. The fat is spreaded in glass plates and warmed to about 50°C, then its surface is covered with the flower petals and it is allowed to keep for several days until the fat is saturated with the essential oils for which the old petals are replaced by the fresh ones. The petals are then removed and fat is digested with ethyl alcohol when the essential oils present in the fat are dissolved in ethyl alcohol and if some fat is also dissolve during digestion it is removed by cooling to about 20°C. The extract having ethyl alcohol and essential oils is distilled under reduced pressure to remove the solvent.

Application of Essential Oil:

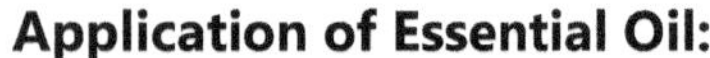

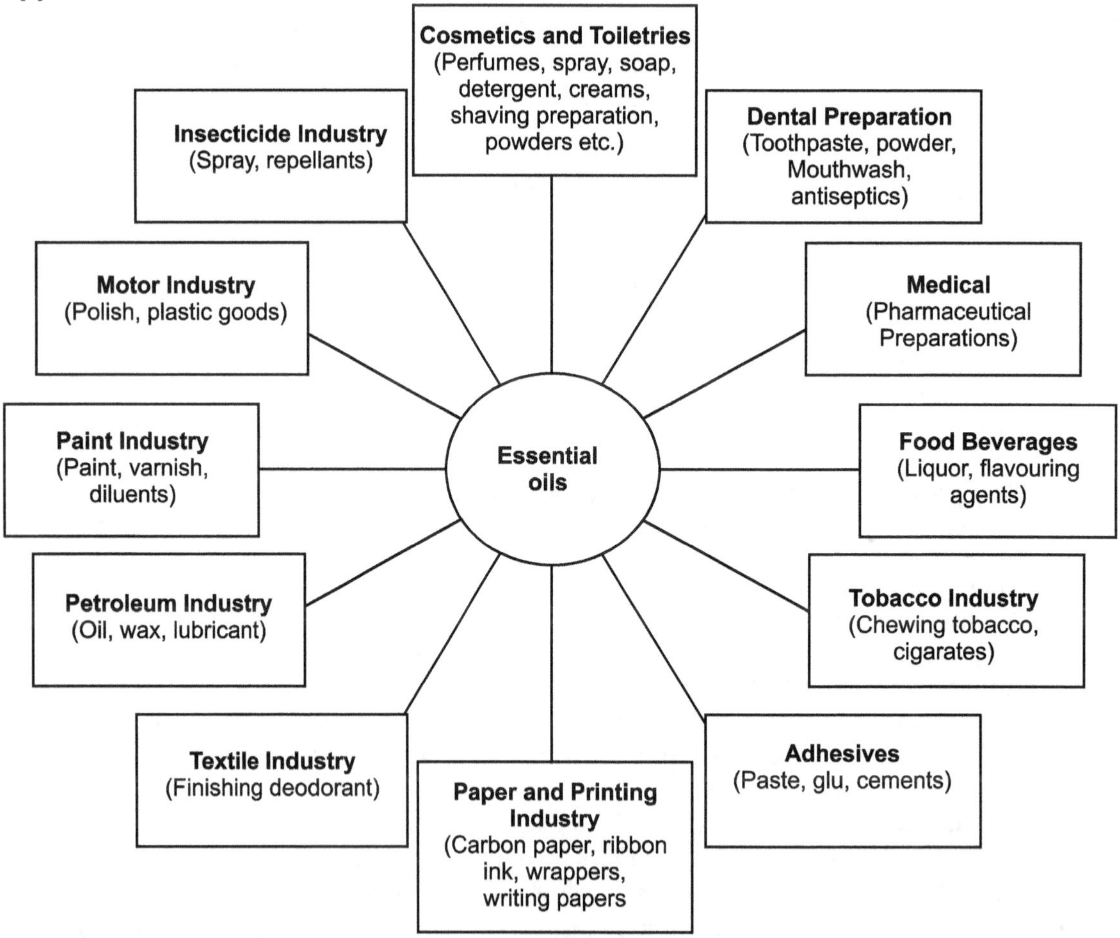

Fig. 4.21

General Chemical Test:

Test	Observation	Inference
To the section of the drug, add alcoholic solution of sudan III.	Red colour obtained by globules.	Presence of volatile oil.
To the thin section of the drug, add a drop of tincture alkaline.	Red colour is obtained.	Presence of volatile oil.

4.8 RESINS

Resins are the amorphous products of complex chemical nature. They are simply extractions of plant material, are taken either from the whole plant or from specific parts of the plant (bark of trees, flowers of herbs, and buds of shrubs) depending on the availability and desired effect. They are produced in special resin cells known as schizogenous cells in the plants or at the site of injury of the plants and oozes out through the bark and hardens on exposure to air. Commercial resins are collected from fossil material. Resinous substances may occur alone or in combination with essential oils or gums. They consist primarily of secondary metabolites or compounds that apparently play no role in the primary physiology of a plant. Resin production is widespread in nature, but only a few families are of commercial importance viz. Anacardiaceae, Burseraceae, Dipterocarpaceae, Guttiferae, Hammamelidaceae, Leguminosae, Liliaceae, Pinaceae, Styracaceae and Umbelliferae. Resin is dark brown in colour and it has different levels of hardness and opacity, based on the clarity. Resins are collected from the wood or the bark of the plants that secrete it or ooze out, and they are often collected from plants when the tissues are leached by alcohol. Raw resins are distilled to take away the terpene elements to make products.

Properties:

1. Resins are transparent or translucent solids, semisolids or liquid substances.
2. They are brittle solid in nature.
3. They are fusible and flammable organic substances.
4. They are not soluble in water but heavier than water.
5. They are soluble in volatile oils, ether and alcohol.
6. They become harden when exposed to air.
7. They are generally produced by woody plants.
8. They do not play a role in the fundamental processes of the plant.
9. When heated, they form smoky flame.

Chemistry:

- Resins are mixture of essential oils.
- They are oxygenated products of terpene and carboxylic acid.
- Chemically they contain esters, acids and alcohols.
- Some resins are chemically inert, known as resenes.
- Resins generally form soap when boiled with alkali.

- With heat they become soft, clear and form adhesive fluids.
- Resins are also combined with glycosidal manner with sugar.
- They are non-nitrogenous compound.
- The common terpenes in resin are the bicyclic terpenes alpha and beta pinene and sabinene, the monocyclic terpenes limonene and terpinolene and smaller amounts of the tricyclic sesquiterpenes.
- They are associated with volatile oils (oleoresins), with gum (gum resins) or with oil and gum (oleo-gum resins).
- Electrically they are non-conductive masses.
- Specific gravity is 0.90-1.25.

Sources of Resins: They are mainly three types that are given in Fig. 4.22.

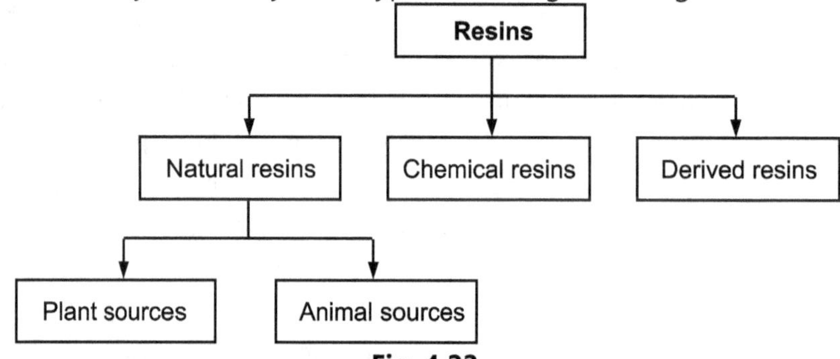

Fig. 4.22

(a) **Natural Sources:** The resins that are obtained from the plant and animal sources are known as natural sources resins. They are obtained in different parts of plants and by various methods depending on the nature of the resins. They are found inside plants or are exuded by plants, such as sap, latex or mucilage forms. Some examples of plant source resins are Asafoetida, Myrrh, Balsam, Benzoin, Ginger, Colophony, Jalap, Podophyllum etc. Some examples of animal source resins are Shellac or Lac. Sometimes animals and plants resins are obtained from fossils, they are known as fossilized resin. Example: *Amber* which is fossilized tree resin, often known as Copal.

(b) **Chemical resins:** They are synthetic resins and are useful in various preparations like nail polish. It is made up of organic compounds. They are generally liquid monomers of thermosetting plastics. Typical examples of synthetic resins are *epoxy resin, acrylic phenolic resin, urea formaldehyde resin* etc.

(c) **Derived Resins:** They are transparent or translucent mass, derivatives of the resins that are not produced directly from plants or animals, e.g., rosin. It is prepared by solidified resin from which the volatile terpene components have been removed by distillation. It has vitreous fracture and a faintly yellow or brown colour, non-odorous or having only a slight turpentine odor and taste. It is insoluble in water but soluble in alcohol and other organic solvents like ether. It melts under the influence of heat and burns with a bright smoky flame.

Preparation of Resin:

As per the method of preparation, resins are classified as follows:

(a) Natural Resins: They occur as exudates from plants, are produced normally or as result of pathogenic conditions. It may happen by artificial punctures e.g., mastic or deep cuts in the wood of the plant e.g., turpentine or by hammering and scorching like balsam of Peru.

(b) Prepared Resins: The resins are powdered and extracted with alcohol till exhaustion. The concentrated alcoholic extract is either evaporated or poured into water and the precipitated resin is collected, washed and dried. Depending on the solvent used in the extraction they are further classified as Oleoresins and gum resins. Ether or acetone is used for the extraction of oleoresins whereas alcohol is used for the extraction of gum resins.

Occurrence in Plants: Based on the sources, resins are collected from different parts of plants namely, resin cells (Ginger), Schizogenous cells (Pine) and glandular hairs (Cannabis).

4.8.1 Classification of Resins

Resins are classified into three types which is tabulated in below Fig. 4.23.

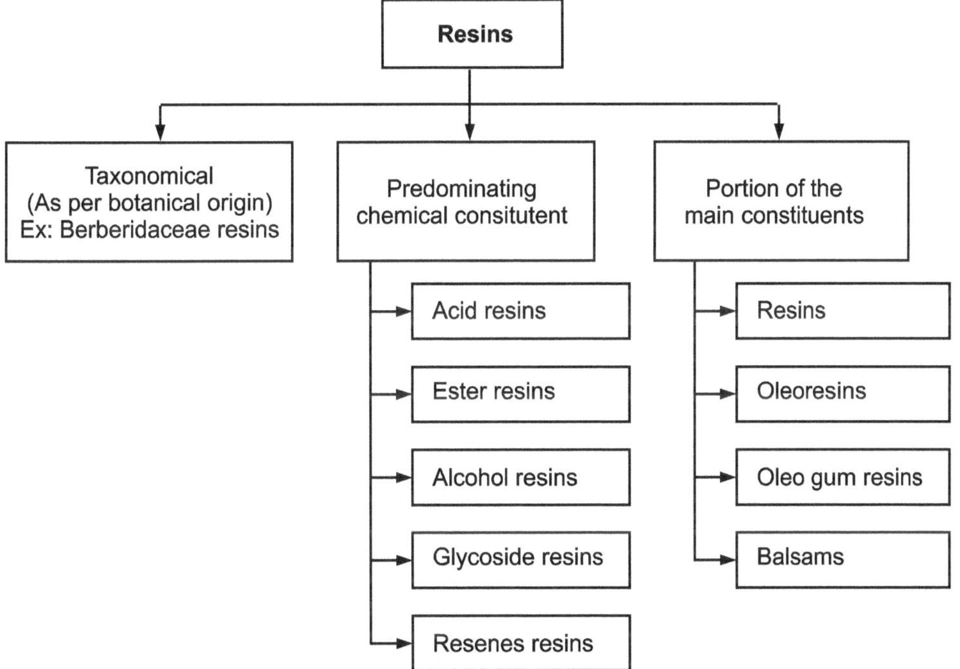

Fig. 4.23: Classification of Resin

Taxonomical Classification: As per the botanical origin, the resins are classified, as Coniferous resins: Colophony, Berberidaceae resins: Podophyllum etc.

Chemical Classification: These types of resins are classified as per the predominating chemical constituents present in the resin structure:

Acid Resins: They are mixtures of carboxylic acids, found in tree. They have the basic skeleton of three fused ring fused with the empirical formula $C_{19}H_{29}COOH$. Resin acids are tacky, yellowish gums that are water-insoluble. They are used to produce soaps.

Examples: Abietic acid from Colophony, Commiphoric acid from Myrrh, Alleuritic acid from Shellac etc.

Ester Resins: Ester groups are present in the basic structure of the resins.

Examples: Benzyl benzoate in Benzoin, Cinnamyl cinnamate in Storax etc.

Alcohol Resins: High molecular weight alcoholic group and present in the structure of resins. They sometimes form complex and are found either in free state or as ester form.

Examples: Peruresinotannol from Balsam of Peru, Guaicresinol from Guaiam, Gurjuresinol from Gurjan etc.

Resin alcohols are of two types, namely resinotannols and resinols. Resinotannols are the alcohol that gives specific tannin reaction with iron salts. They are of various types like *Aloe resinotannoil* (e.g: Aloes), *Ammo resinotannol* (eg: Ammoniacum), *Galba resinotannol* (e.g.: Galbanum), *Peru resinotannol* (e.g.: Balsam of Peru), *Sia resinotannol* (e.g.: Benzoin) and *Tolu resinotannol* (e.g.: Balsam of Tolu).

Resinols: They are the resins that gives sowing negetive specific tannin reaction with iron salts. They are of different types like *Benzo resinol* (e.g.: Benzoin), *Sto resinol* (e.g.: Storax), *Gurju resinol* (e.g.: Gurjun balsam) and *Guaia resinol* (e.g.: Guaiacum resin).

Glycoresins: They are the combination of resin and sugar.

Examples: Jalap resin from jalap, Podophylloresin from dried roots and rhizome from *Podophyllum hexandrum* etc.

Resenes Resins: They are chemically inert substances and have no chemical properties. They do not undergo hydrolysis or any salt formation.

Examples: Dracoresens from Dragon's blood, Fluavil from Gutta percha, Mastic from *Pistacia lentiscus* etc

Classification Based on Constituents of Resin: They are classified as per the major constituents present in the resins or in resin combinations. They are further sub-classified as:

Resins: They are unorganized hydrocarbon compounds present in the plants. They are produced in resin ducts and are excreted through canals or glands.

Examples: Colophony, Cannabis.

Oleoresins: They are concentrated liquid form of the spice. Oleoresins can be defined as the true essence of the spices and can replace whole/ground spices without impairing any flavor and aroma characteristic.

A naturally occurring mixture of essential oils and a resin, extracted from various plants. They obtained by extraction with a non-aqueous solvent followed by removal of the solvent by evaporation and by super critical fluid extraction.

Examples: Copaiba, Ginger, Pine, Balsam.

Advantages of Oleoresins:

- Easy to store and transport.
- More stable when heated.
- More economical to use.
- Easier to control quality and cleaner than the equivalent ground spices.
- Free from contamination.

- Concentrated form reduces storage space and bulk handling and transport requirements.

- Concentrated and moisture-free form ensures longer shelf life due to minimal oxidative degradation or loss of flavour.

Oleo Gum Resins: It is a solid plant exudation consisting of a mixture of volatile oil, gum and resin. It is a combination of oleo gum and resin. Therefore, an oleo-gum- resin has a nature that is partly soluble in water and alcohol and looks oily.

Examples: Asafoetida, Myrrh, Turmeric.

Balsams: They are also known as turpentine. They are the resinous exudate or sap from certain kinds of trees and shrubs. They mainly contain cinnamic and benzoic acid or their esters in the structures. They are oily and odorous substances. Among the true balsams are the Balm of Gilead, or Mecca, which is cultivated in Arab, Egypt and Syria and they are extremely costly. The Copaiva balsam, Balsam of Peru and Tolu are found chiefly in South America.

Examples: Balsam of Tolu, Balsam of Peru, Balsam of Mecca (Liquid balsam obtained from the tree *Commiphora gileadensis*).

Uses of Resins: Broadly resins are used for paints, varnishes, perfumery preparations and various pharmaceutical aids. Therapeutic graded resins are used for expectorants, antiseptics, flavoring agents, carminatives, stomachic etc.

Chemical Tests:

Test	Observation	Inference
To the extract add 5 ml of distilled water.	Turbidity is formed.	Presence of resins.
Alcoholic solution of colophony.	It turns blue litmus to red.	Presence of diterpenic acid.
Alcoholic solution of balsam of tolu.	Gives green colour with $FeCl_3$.	Presence of toluresino tannols.
To a petroleum ether solution of benzene, add 2-3 drops of H_2SO_4 in a china dish.	Sumatra benzoin: reddish brown colour Slam benzoin: purple red colour.	Presence of resins.
0.1 g in 10 ml $(CH_3CO)_2O$ with aid of gentle heat, cool and add 0.05 ml of H_2SO_4.	A light purplish red colour to violet.	Presence of resins, Colophony.
0.1 g powder in 10 ml of $(CH_3CO)_2O$ in a test tube and add a drop of concentrated H_2SO_4.	Purple colour.	Presence of resins, Colophony.

EXERCISE

Long Essays:

1. Explain Ayurveda and Siddha systems of medicines.
2. Explain Allopathy and Homeopathy Systems of medicines.
3. Explain Unani and Chinese systems of medicines.
4. Explain Alkaloids.
5. Explain Glycosides.
6. Explain Tannins.
7. Explain Volatile oils.
8. Explain Flavonoids.
9. Explain Resins.

Short Essays:

1. Explain role of Pharmacognosy in Ayurveda and Chinese medicines.
2. Explain role of Pharmacognosy in Homeopathy and Unani medicines.
3. Explain principle involved in Ayurveda and Siddha systems of medicines.
4. Explain principle involved in Unani and Homeopathy systems of medicines.
5. Explain principle involved in Chinese system of medicines.
6. Explain classification and biological role of alkaloids.
7. Explain classification and biological role of Glycosides.
8. Explain classification and biological role of Tannins.
9. Explain classification and biological role of Resins.
10. Explain classification and biological role of Flavonoids.
11. Explain classification and biological role of Volatile oil.
12. Explain general chemical tests of Alkaloids and glycosides.
13. Explain general chemical tests of Tannins and Resins.
14. Explain general chemical tests of Flavonoids and Volatile oil.
15. Explain difference between Ayurveda and Homeopathy.
16. Explain difference between Allopathy and Homeopathy.
17. Explain difference between Ayurveda and Allopathy.
18. Explain general physical and chemical properties of glycosides and alkaloids.
19. Explain general physical and chemical properties of Tannins and Flavonoids.
20. Explain general physical and chemical properties of Volatile oil and Resins.

Multiple Choice Questions (MCQs):

1. The plant which is directly used in Allopathic medicine system is ......
   - (a) Aconite
   - (b) Digitalis
   - (c) Senna
   - (d) Kurchi
2. Traditional Knowledge Digital Library has set up in the year ......
   - (a) 1971
   - (b) 1990
   - (c) 2001
   - (d) 2004

3. "Veda" stands for ……
   (a) Life   (b) Knowledge
   (c) Soul   (d) Mind
4. "Pitta" is belongs to ……
   (a) Panchabhuta   (b) Kapha
   (c) Dshas   (d) Vedas
5. As per Ayurveda one of the components is not belongs to Pachabhuta ……
   (a) Air   (b) Earth
   (c) Ether   (d) Metal
6. "Vata" composed of ……
   (a) Air and water   (b) Ether and earth
   (c) Air and fire   (d) Air and ether
7. "Kapha" composed of ……
   (a) Water and earth   (b) Fire and water
   (c) Air and water   (d) Air and earth
8. "Basti" indicates ……
   (a) Toxic element   (b) Purgation
   (c) Enema   (d) Vomiting
9. Siddha medicine system originated from ……
   (a) Karnataka   (b) Kerala
   (c) Tamil Nadu   (d) Andhra Pradesh
10. "Kabam" means ……
   (a) Old age   (b) Childhood
   (c) Adult   (d) None of these
11. "Muscle" in Siddha system termed as ……
   (a) Ooner   (b) Ischeneer
   (c) Oon   (d) Elumbu
12. The term "Elumbu" stands for ……
   (a) Fatty tissue   (b) Bone
   (c) Bone marrow   (d) Blood
13. "Vaadham" stand for ……
   (a) Air   (b) Fire
   (c) Earth   (d) Water
14. Metals that are used in Siddha system ……
   (a) Mercury and Gold   (b) Mercury and Sulfur
   (c) Sulfur and Gold   (d) Gold and copper
15. One of the four humours is ……
   (a) Phlegm   (b) White bile
   (c) Hawa   (d) Water
16. Which one is not belongs to Unani treatment ……
   (a) Naum-o-Yaqzah   (b) Hawa
   (c) Harkat-o-sakoon nafsaniah   (d) Harkat-wo-Mashroob

17. "Dau Sadaf" is known as ......
    (a) Psoriasis   (b) Vatiligo
    (c) Fever   (d) Hepatitis
18. As per Homeopathy medicine system, potency indicates with the symbol ......
    (a) C   (b) P
    (c) X   (d) M
19. "Like with Like" is the principle of ......
    (a) Homeopathy   (b) Ayruveda
    (c) Unani   (d) Siddha
20. "Yin and Yang" theory is based on the ......
    (a) Principle of Chu   (b) Principle of Yin
    (c) Principle of Chi   (d) Principle of Xing
21. As per Chinese medicine system, one of the vital five organs is ......
    (a) Eye   (b) Lungs
    (c) Tongue   (d) Skin
22. As per Chinese medicine system, five elements are known as ......
    (a) Yin and Yang   (b) Yin and Yu
    (c) Xing Wu   (d) Wu Xing
23. "Yin and Yang" stand for ......
    (a) Fire and wind   (b) Heat and cold
    (c) Cold and heat   (d) Pulse and Headache
24. Amorphous solid alkaloid is ......
    (a) Datura   (b) Emetine
    (c) Ephedra   (d) Caffeine
25. Example of dextrorotatory alkaloid is ......
    (a) Caffeine   (b) Papaverine
    (c) Coniine   (d) Morphine
26. Optically inactive alkaloid is ......
    (a) Quinine   (b) Papaverine
    (c) Coniine   (d) Nicotine
27. Orange colour alkaloid is ......
    (a) Colchicine   (b) Betanin
    (c) Nicotine   (d) Betanidine
28. Volatile liquid alkaloid is ......
    (a) Colchicine   (b) Betanin
    (c) Nicotine   (d) Quinine
29. Non-volatile liquid alkaloid is ......
    (a) Colchicine   (b) Betanin
    (c) Nicotine   (d) Pilocarpine
30. Secondary amino alkaloid is ......
    (a) Norephedrine   (b) Ephedrine
    (c) Atropine   (d) Caffeine

31. Pyrrolidine derivative alkaloid is ......
    (a) Lobeline
    (b) Nicotine
    (c) Hygrine
    (d) Piperine
32. Pilocarpine belongs to derivatives of alkaloid is ......
    (a) Pyrrolidine
    (b) Piperidine
    (c) Imidazole
    (d) Indole
33. Vasicine belongs to derivatives of alkaloids is ......
    (a) Norlupinane
    (b) Purine
    (c) Quinazolin
    (d) Pyridine
34. Tropolone derivative alkaloid is ......
    (a) Atropine
    (b) Connesine
    (c) Ergometrine
    (d) Colchicine
35. Example of Proto alkaloid is ......
    (a) Quinine
    (b) Mescaline
    (c) Capsaicin
    (d) Atropine
36. Pseudo alkaloid is ......
    (a) Atropine
    (b) Ephedrine
    (c) Ipecac
    (d) Coniine
37. Indole alkaloid is derived from ......
    (a) Tryptophan
    (b) Tyrosine
    (c) Ornithine
    (d) Histidine
38. Imidazole alkaloid is derived from ......
    (a) Tryptophan
    (b) Tyrosine
    (c) Ornithine
    (d) Histidine
39. Source of Quinine is ......
    (a) Root
    (b) Bark
    (c) Leaves
    (d) Stem
40. Composition of Mayer's reagent is ......
    (a) Pot-bismuth iodide
    (b) Iodine pot Iodide
    (c) Pot-mercuric iodide
    (d) Mercuric iodide
41. Alkaloid forms white colour precipitate when reacts with ......
    (a) Picrolonic acid
    (b) Sulphuric acid
    (c) Mercuric iodide
    (d) Hager's reagent
42. One of the reagents used in Vitali Morin test is ......
    (a) Sulphuric acid
    (b) Chloroform
    (c) Amino benzaldehyde
    (d) KOH
43. Sodium molybdate in concentrated Sulphuric acid is known as ......
    (a) Rosequin reagent
    (b) Van Urk's reagent
    (c) Froehd's test
    (d) None
44. Solvent that is not use for separation of aglycone ......
    (a) Chloroform
    (b) Acetone
    (c) Ether
    (d) Pet. ether

45. Populin is what type of secondary metabolite?
    (a) Alkaloid   (b) Glycoside
    (c) Tannin   (d) Resin
46. Beta-glycosides are hydrolysed by ......
    (a) Myrosin   (b) Invertase
    (c) Glucosidase   (d) Emulsin
47. Sulfur glycosides are hydrolysed by ......
    (a) Myrosin   (b) Glucosidase
    (c) Invertase   (d) Emulsin
48. Example of O-linkage glycoside is ......
    (a) Aloe   (b) Cochineal
    (c) Rhubarb   (d) Gentian
49. Aglycone part of rutin is ......
    (a) Apigenin   (b) Coumarin
    (c) Vanilic acid   (d) Quercetin
50. Arbutin is a constituent of ......
    (a) Vanilla   (b) Salix
    (c) Celery   (d) Uva Ursi
51. Analgesic and Antipyretic glycosidic drug is ......
    (a) Quassia   (b) Salix
    (c) Wild Cherry bark   (d) Celery
52. Presence of Cardinolides and Bufadinolides are identified by ......
    (a) Keddy Test   (b) Raymond test
    (c) Antimony trichloride test   (d) Keller Killiani Test
53. Cyanogenetic glycosides react with sodium picrate and sulphuric acid to form ......
    (a) Red   (b) Yellow
    (c) Orange   (d) Blue
54. Shinoda test is perform to confirm ......
    (a) Alkaloid   (b) Cardiac glycoside
    (c) Tannin   (d) Flavonoid
55. Flavonoids are ......
    (a) 2-Phenylbenzoic acid   (b) 2-Phenyl benzopyrone
    (c) 2-Benzopyrone   (d) 2-Phenyl hippuric acid
56. Structural formula of flavonoid is ......
    (a) C_3-C-C_3 (b) C_3-C-C_6
    (c) C_6-C_3-C_6 (d) C_6-C_3
57. Glycosidic linkage in Flavonoids occurs at ......
    (a) Position 3 or 5   (b) Position 3 or 7
    (c) Position 5 or 7   (d) Position 10 or 9
58. Hesperetin belongs to what type of flavonoid?
    (a) Flavone   (b) Flavanone
    (c) Flavocrystallin   (d) Flavonol

59. Example of flavones glycoside ……
    (a) Luteolin   (b) Catechin
    (c) Querrcetin   (d) Naringenin
60. Isoflavonoids are derivatives of ……
    (a) 2-phenylchromen-4-one (2-phenyl-1 ,4-benzopyrone) structure
    (b) 3-phenylchromen-4-one (3-phenyl-1,4-benzopyrone) structure
    (c) 4-phenylcoumarine (4-phenyl 1,2-benzopyrone) structure
    (d) 2-phenylchromen-4-one (3-phenyl-2, 2-benzopyrone) structure
61. Plant sample reacts with potassium ferricyanide and ammonia to form red colour solution indicates presence of ……
    (a) Glycoside   (b) Tannin
    (c) Flavonoid   (d) Volatile oil
62. Gallic acid is found in ……
    (a) Eucalyptus   (b) Rhubarb
    (c) Myrobalan   (d) None of these
63. Ellagitannins are present in ……
    (a) Sumac   (b) Chestnut
    (c) Gallnut   (d) Tara
64. Proanthocyanidins are ……
    (a) Monomeric flavonoid   (b) Isomeric
    (c) Oligomeric   (d) None of these
65. Complex tannins are found in ……
    (a) Oak   (b) Hamamelis
    (c) Grape   (d) (a) and (b) both
66. Phloro tannins are found in ……
    (a) Blue algae   (b) Kelp
    (c) Brown algae   (d) (b) and (c)
67. Phenazone test is for ……
    (a) Tannin   (b) Volatile oil
    (c) Resin   (d) None of these
68. Squaline belongs to ……
    (a) Tetraterpene   (b) Triterpene
    (c) Diterpene   (d) None of these
69. Volatile oil extracted from rose petal through ……
    (a) Stem distillation   (b) Fractional distillation
    (c) Enflurage   (d) None of these
70. Resins are ……
    (a) Heavier than water   (b) Lighter than water
    (c) Missible in water   (d) None of these

71. Chemically resins are ......
    (a) Methylated product of terpene
    (b) Oxygenated product of terpene
    (c) Carbonated product of terpene
    (d) None of these
72. Amber resin is ......
    (a) Natural
    (b) Chemical
    (c) Derived
    (d) None of these
73. Resin is example of ......
    (a) Natural
    (b) Chemical
    (c) Derived
    (d) None of these
74. Pine is ......
    (a) Oleo gum
    (b) Oleo resin
    (c) Resenes
    (d) None of these
75. Sumatra benzoin reacts with petroleum ether, few drops of H_2SO_4 and forms ......
    (a) Reddish brown
    (b) Reddish black
    (c) Black
    (d) Greenish brown

ANSWERS

1. (b)	2. (c)	3. (b)	4. (c)	5. (d)	6. (d)	7. (a)	8. (c)	9. (c)
10. (a)	11. (c)	12. (b)	13. (a)	14. (b)	15. (a)	16. (d)	17. (a)	18. (c)
19. (a)	20. (c)	21. (b)	22. (d)	23. (c)	24. (b)	25. (c)	26. (b)	27. (d)
28. (c)	29. (d)	30. (b)	31. (b)	32. (c)	33. (c)	34.(d)	35. (b)	36. (d)
37. (a)	38. (d)	39. (b)	40. (c)	41. (c)	42. (d)	43. (c)	44. (b)	45. (b)
46. (d)	47. (a)	48. (c)	49. (d)	50. (d)	51. (b)	52. (c)	53. (a)	54. (d)
55. (b)	56. (c)	57. (b)	58. (b)	59. (a)	60. (b)	61. (b)	62. (b)	63. (b)
64. (c)	65. (d)	66. (d)	67. (a)	68. (b)	69. (c)	70. (a)	71. (b)	72. (a)
73. (c)	74. (b)	75. (a)						

STUDY OF PRIMARY METABOLITES, PLANT AND MARINE SOURCES NATURAL DRUGS

♦ LEARNING OBJECTIVES ♦

After completing this unit, reader should be able to understand:

❖ Plant products that are originated from plant sources.
❖ Marine sources of natural drugs for novel medicinal uses.
❖ Detail study about primary metabolites.
❖ Some drugs that are sources of carbohydrates.
❖ Detail study about proteins and enzymes and some crude drugs that are procured from the same.
❖ Lipid and some lipid containing drugs.

5.1 PLANT PRODUCTS

5.1.1 Fibres

Fibres are natural or synthetic strings. They are used as a component of composite materials. In alternate, fibres are threads or filaments from which a vegetable tissue, mineral substance or textile is formed. By textile word, fibres are defined as unit of matter characterized by flexibility, fineness and a high ratio of length to thickness. Depending on the sources, fibres are classified broadly in two categories (Fig. 5.1).

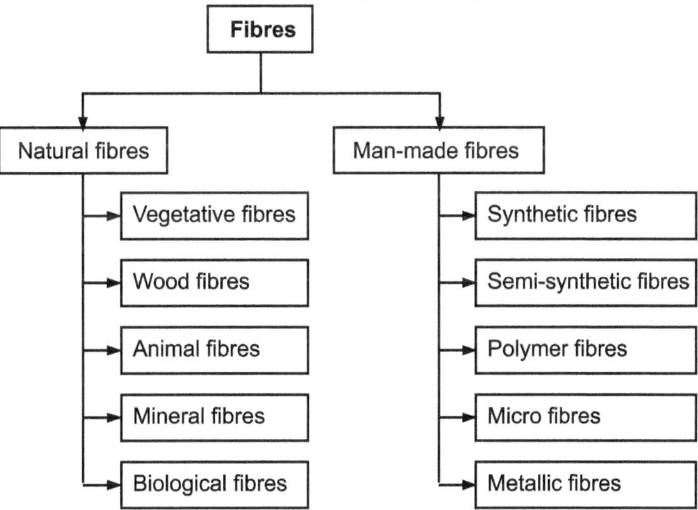

Fig. 5.1: Classification of fibres

Vegetable Fibres or Bast Fibres: They are also known as skin fibres. They are collected from the phloem (the "inner bark" or the skin) or bast surrounding the stem of certain plant i.e., mainly dicotyledonous plants. They support the conductive cells of the phloem and provide strength to the stem. They are separated from the xylem by retting method by treating with microorganisms either on land or in water or by chemicals or by pectinolytic enzymes. They are generally based on arrangements of cellulose, often with lignin. They have higher tensile strength. Examples include cotton, hemp, jute, flax, banana, sisal etc. They are employed in the manufacture of various ropes, yarn, in paper and textile industries. Dietary fibres are important for human nutrition as they are used as laxatives (Fig. 5.2).

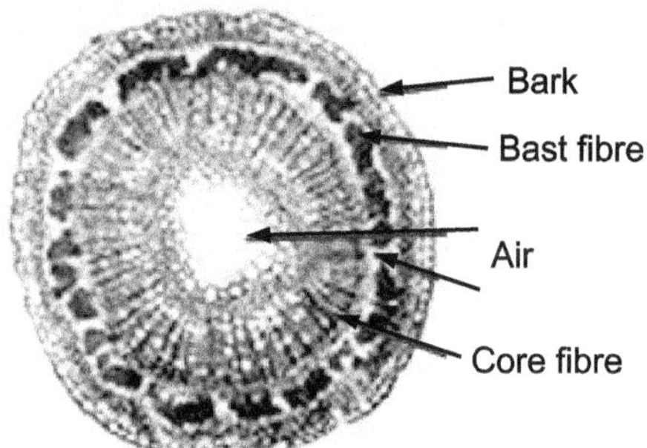

Fig. 5.2: Location of Bast Fibre

Bast fibres from stem: Examples: Flax, Hemp, Jute etc.

Bast fibres from leaf: Examples: Ananas, Agave, Palm etc.

Bast fibres from seed: Examples: Cotton, Soya, Coir etc.

Bast fibres from fruit: Examples: Luffa, Coir etc.

Bast fibres from grass: Examples: Bamboo, Totora etc.

Bast fibres from wood: Examples: Hard wood, Soft wood etc.

Wood fibres: They are usually cellulose elements that are extracted from trees and are used to make materials including paper. There are different forms of wood fibres including ground wood, thermomechanical pulp and bleached or unbleached sulfite pulps. Sulfite pulp is obtained by pulping process that is used to remove the lignin bonding the original wood structure.

Animal fibres: They are obtained from different parts of animals and consist largely of particular proteins. **Examples:** Silkworm silk, catgut, wool; Hair such as cashmere wool, mohair and angora; Fur such as sheepskin, rabbit, mink etc.

Mineral fibres: They include the asbestos group and are long fibres. Six minerals have been classified as "asbestos" including chrysotile, amosite, crocidolite, tremolite, anthophyllite and actinolite. Short mineral fibres are wollastonite, palygorskite etc.

Biological fibres: They are also known as fibrous proteins. They consist of biologically important proteins, mutations etc. Examples: Collagen, actin.

Synthetic fibres: They are man-made fibres derived from the natural fibres, mainly cellulose, e.g., nylon and terylene. Nylons are polymers of adipic acid and hexamethyl diamine, whereas terylene is a polymer of ethylene glycol and terephthalic acid.

Semi synthetic fibres: Semi-synthetic fibres are made from raw materials with natural long-chain polymer structure and are only modified and partially degraded by chemical processes. Generally they are regenerated cellulose derivatives. Examples: Rayon, bamboo fibres etc.

Polymer fibres: They are based on synthetic chemicals and made from polyamide nylon, polyester, polyvinyl chloride etc.

Micro fibres: They are ultra-fine fibres often used in filtration. In textiles micro fibres are referred as sub-denier fibres.

Metallic fibres: These fibres are prepared from the metals such as copper, gold or silver and extruded or deposited from more brittle ones such as nickel, aluminum or iron.

Differences between Natural Fibres and Synthetic Fibres:

- Natural fibres are derived from plants and animals, whereas synthetic fibres are almost entirely man made.
- Fabrics made of natural fibres are generally more comfortable than synthetic ones.
- Natural fibres are expensive compared to synthetic fibres.
- In synthetic fibres, spinnerets are used to produce the filaments; whereas, in natural fibres, it is made naturally.
- Natural fibres have limited usage when compared to synthetic fibres.
- Natural fibres are biodegradable, hence environmental friendly, whereas synthetic fibres are not.

Differences between Plant and Animal Fibres:

1. On ignition, animal fibres give bad smell; whereas plant fibres do not give smell.
2. Plant fibres are soluble in cuoxam solution (ammoniacal copper oxide), whereas animal fibres are 50% soluble in alkaline hydroxide solution.
3. Plant fibres form blue colour when reacted with iodine in the presence of dilute sulphuric acid; whereas animal fibres form permanent yellow stain when reacted with picric acid.
4. Plant fibres react with Molish's reagent to form violet colour; whereas with Millon's reagent, animal fibres give red stain.

COTTON

Biological source: Cotton is a natural source of fibres consisting of the hairs of the seeds of Gossypium species like *Gossypium hirsutum* L., *G. barbadense* L and *G. herbaceum*.

Family: Malvaceae.

Distribution: The plant is a shrub native to tropical and subtropical regions around the world, including the America, Africa, Australia and India. *Gossypium hirsutum* is native to Central America, the Caribbean and southern Florida, *G. barbadense* is native to tropical South America, *G. arboreum* is native to India and Pakistan. In India, the major production of the plant is in Maharashtra, Gujarat, Punjab, Andhra Pradesh and Madhya Pradesh.

Description of plant: The plant is a perennial and annual and about 6 to 12 feet tall. Underground, the cotton plant develops a strong taproot with many lateral branches, penetrating as deeply as 8 to 10 feet. The leaves are heart-shaped with pointed lobes. There are three to five lobes at the ends of each leaf blade, which measures up to 7 inches long and across. Leaves are fuzzy and are arranged in an alternating pattern on the stems and branches. The flowers are five-petaled and a creamy white or yellow in colour. After pollination, the three- to four-chambered ovary inside ripens to form a green capsule or "boll." This long, spherical capsule contains a few oil glands as well as many dark brown seeds that are encased in lint and fuzz. Capsule contains numerous seeds (Fig. 5.3).

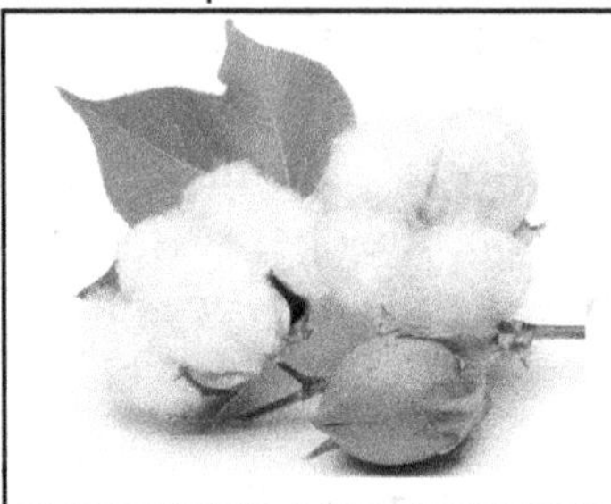

Fig. 5.3: Cotton with cotton boll

Preparation of Cotton: A fertilized flower takes about 20-45 days to become an open boll. After the plant flowers, the cotton fibres (lint) develop on the seed in the boll in three stages. In the "elongation" stage (0 to 27 days), the fibre cell develops a thin, expandable primary wall surrounding a large vacuole. During the "thickening" stage (15 to 55 days), the living protoplast shrinks, while a secondary wall composed almost entirely of cellulose is deposited inside the primary wall. By the "maturation" stage, the secondary wall fills most of the fibre cell volume, leaving a small central cavity (the lumen) containing the cytoplasm and the vacuole. As the boll opens, the fibre cells rapidly desiccate, collapse and die. As the tubular cells collapse, they assume a flat, ribbon-like form with twists, called "convolutions." The fibre removed from the plant also contains the cotton seeds and is referred to as "seed cotton." The harvested seed cotton is transported to the gin. Ginning is the process of separating cotton fibres from the seeds. Seed cottons are then cleaned with dilute soda solution under pressure for several hours to remove the impurities like wax, fatty matters and finally treated with suitable bleaching agent and then packed for transportation.

Three broad types of cotton are generally recognized on the basis of the length, strength and structure of fibre.

(i) Long Staple Cotton: It has the longest fibre whose length varies from 24 to 27 mm. The fibre is long, fine and shiny. It is used for making fine and superior quality cloth. It is largely grown in Punjab, Haryana, Maharashtra, Tamil Nadu, Madhya Pradesh, Gujarat and Andhra Pradesh.

(ii) Medium Staple Cotton: The length of its fibre is between 20 mm and 24 mm. About 44% of the total cotton production in India is of medium staple. Rajasthan, Punjab, Tamil Nadu, Madhya Pradesh, Uttar Pradesh, Karnataka and Maharashtra are its main producers.

(iii) Short Staple Cotton: This is inferior cotton with fibre less than 20 mm long. It is used for manufacturing inferior cloth. It is grown in U.P., Andhra Pradesh, Rajasthan, Haryana and Punjab.

Physical Properties:

Colour	:	White, creamy white
Odour	:	Odourless
Taste	:	Tasteless
Tensile strength	:	It is a strong fibre. It has a tenacity of 3-5 g/den. The wet strength is 20%.
Elongation at break	:	5-10%
Elastic recovery	:	Inelastic and rigid fibre. At 2% extension it has elastic recovery of 74%.
Specific gravity	:	1.54
Moisture regain	:	8.5%
Effect of heat	:	It turns yellow at 120°C, and is decomposed at 150°C. It burns in air. It is damaged after few minutes at 240°C.
Effect of sunlight	:	Cotton is exposed to sunlight and turns yellow. The degradation of cotton by oxidation is done by heat.
Dielectric constant	:	3.9 - 7.5
Micronaire	:	2.0 - 6.5
Denier	:	0.7 - 2.3 (Upland cotton)
Length	:	0.9 - 1.2 inches
Diameter	:	9.77 - 27.26 Å

Chemical Properties:

Effect of acids	:	It disintegrates with hot dilute acid or cold concentrated acid.
Effect of alkali	:	It swells in sodium hydroxide, but is not damaged.
Effect of organic solvent	:	It is dissolved by copper complexes, like cuprammonium hydroxide, cupriethylene diamine and 70% sulphuric acid.
Effect of bleach	:	It is resistant to bleach, hydrogen peroxide, calcium chlorohypochloride.

Chemical Constituents: Cotton mainly contains cellulose, moisture, protein, ash, pectin, oil, fat and some pigments. The whole cotton fibre contains 88 to 96.5% of cellulose (Fig. 5.4), the rest are non-cellulosic polysaccharides constituting up to 10% of the total fibre weight.

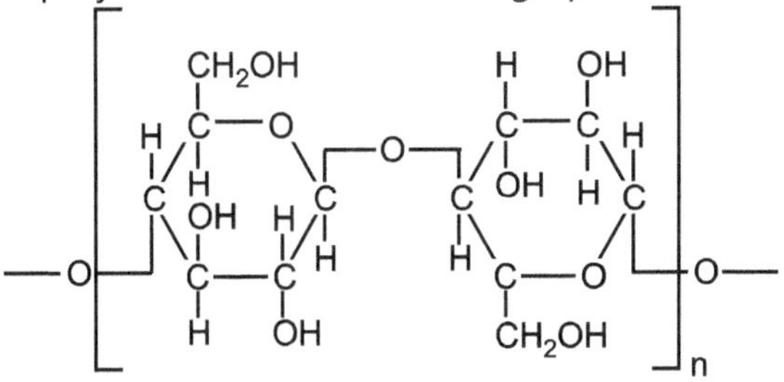

Fig. 5.4: Cellulose

Non-cellulosic constituents consist of pectins, fats and waxes, proteins and natural colorants. The secondary wall contains about 92-95% cellulose and 8-9% moisture.

Chemical Tests:

1. Cotton fibres are soaked in iodine water and then 80% sulphuric acid is added. The trichomes become bluish-green in colour.
2. Raw cotton fibres dissolve in cuoxam solution and form balloon-like structure, whereas absorbent cotton dissolves completely and swells in the same solution.

Uses: The long cotton fibres are used to make cloth and the short fibres are used in the paper industry. Further in pharmaceutical field, cotton is used as filtering media and various surgical dressings. It is also used as an insulating material.

Storage: Cotton in wrapped condition, is stored in cool place with dust proof cupboard.

JUTE

Biological Source: The jute fibre is collected from the stem bark of the white jute plant and to a lesser extent tossa jute belongs to species Corchorus i.e. *C. capsularis* and *C. olitorius*.

Family: Tiliaceae or Malvaceae.

Distribution: Jute is cultivated in Bangladesh, Nepal, Myanmar, India, Thailand, China, Pakistan, Japan, UK, France, Egypt and Spain. In India, the major production of jute is in West Bengal, Assam and Bihar.

Description of Plant: The plants are annual herbs with 2-4 m height. They are unbranched or with a few side branches. The leaves are alternate, simple and lanceolate in shape (Fig. 5.5). They are 5-15 cm long, with an acuminate tip and a finely serrated or lobed margin. The flowers are 2-3 cm in diameter and are yellow in colour.

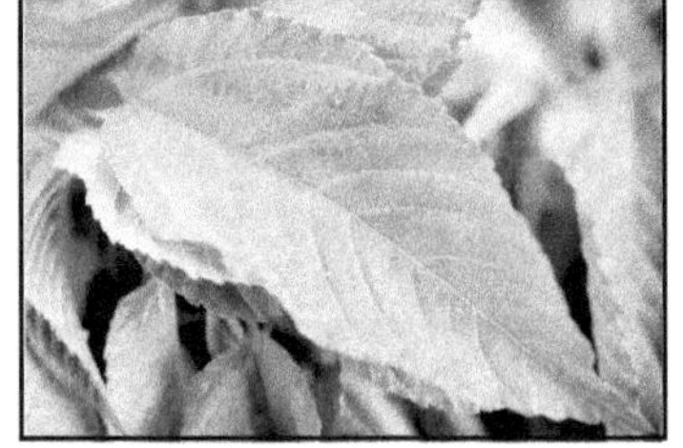

Fig. 5.5: Jute leaves

Production of Fibre: The unbranched stems of the jute plant are cut and formed a bundle. This should carry out before flowering stage. The jute fibre comes from the stem and ribbon (outer skin) of the jute plant. The fibres are first extracted by retting method either in pond or any water logged condition. Retting is a microbial process by which the jute plant is immersed in water and the fibre is loosened from the woody core of the jute plant. This process softens the tissues and breaks the hard pectin bond between the bast and jute hurd (inner woody fibre stick) and the process permits the fibres to be separated. It has been found that jute stems ret most rapidly at 34°C. At this temperature it takes generally 8-12 days for complete retting. The retting process consists of bundling jute stems together and immersing them in slow running water. After the retting process, stripping begins. In the stripping process, non-fibrous matter is scraped off, leaving the fibres to be pulled out from within the stem and washed in clear, running water. Then they are hung up or spread on thatched roofs to dry. After 2-3 days of drying, the fibres are tied into bundles. The jute fibres are graded according to colour, length and smoothness of the fibres (Fig. 5.6).

Physical Properties:

Colour	:	Golden yellow
Odour	:	Characteristic
Taste	:	None
Size	:	Average length is 1 to 4 m and diameter from 17 to 20 microns
Appearance	:	Jute is long, soft and shiny
Specific gravity	:	1.5 g/mm^3
Moisture regain	:	13.75% Strength
Elongation	:	1.7% at the break

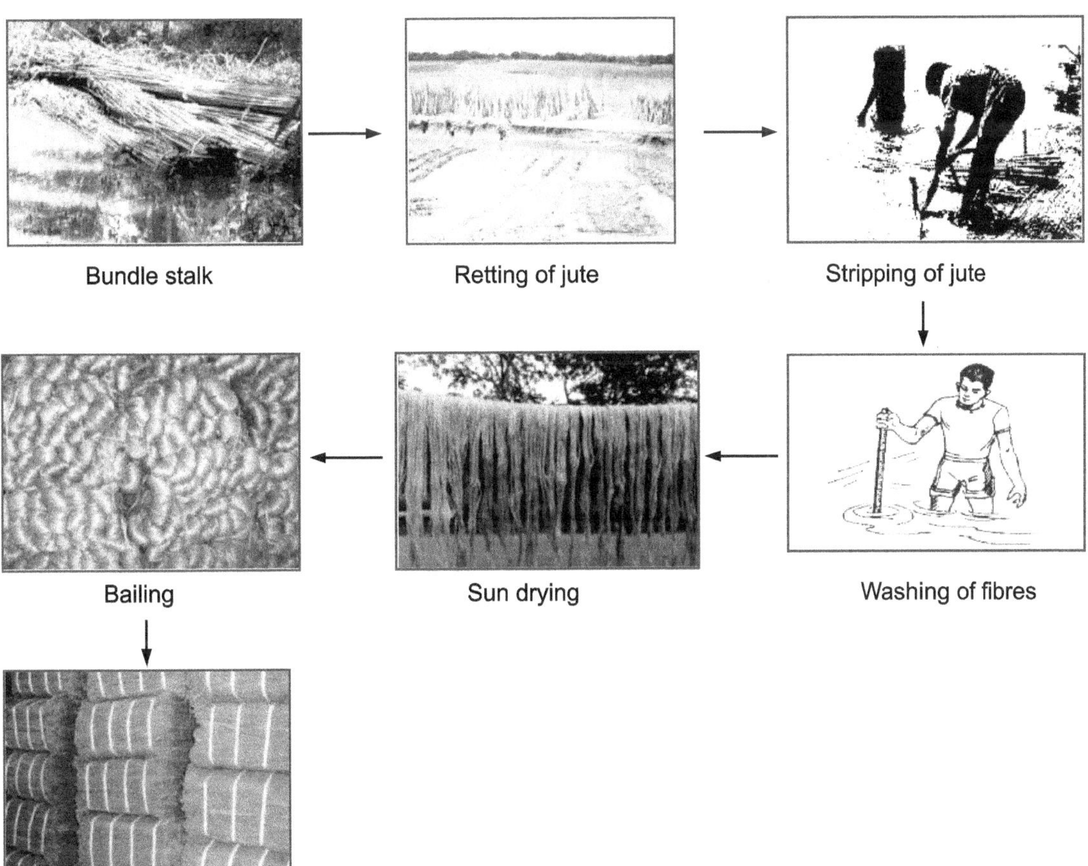

Fig. 5.6: Production of jute fibres

Chemical Properties:

Effect on acids	:	Easily damaged by hot dilute acid or cold concentrated acid
Effect on alkali	:	Fibres are damaged by strong alkali, on heating with sodium hydroxide, fibres losses weight
Effect of light	:	Due to presence of lignin, fibres change the colour slightly.
Effect of dyes	:	Basic dyes are used to colour the fibres
Effect of bleaches	:	No effect with H_2O_2, $KMnO_4$.

Chemical Constituents: Jute fibres contain mainly cellulose (60%) and hemicellulose (24%). Apart from that Lignin, fats and wax are also present.

Uses: Jute is the second most important vegetable fibre after cotton. Jute is used chiefly to make cloth for wrapping bales of raw cotton, and to make sacks and coarse cloth. The fibres are also woven into curtains, chair, coverings and carpets. The fibres are used alone or blended with other types of fibres to make twine and rope.

Substitutes: Fibres of *Hibiscus cannabinus* are used as substitutes for jute fibres.

HEMP

Biological Source: The pericyclic fibre is obtained from the plant of *Cannabis sativa*.

Family: Cannabinaceae.

Distribution: The hemp is originated from central Asia, mainly from China. It is cultivated in India, Romania, Hungary, Poland and Turkey. In India, MP, Himachal Pradesh and Jharkhand are cultivating hemp for industrial use.

Description of Plant: The plant grows up to 5 m in height. The slender stalks are hollow except at the tip and base. The leaves are compound with palmate shape. The flowers are small and greenish yellow (Fig. 5.7).

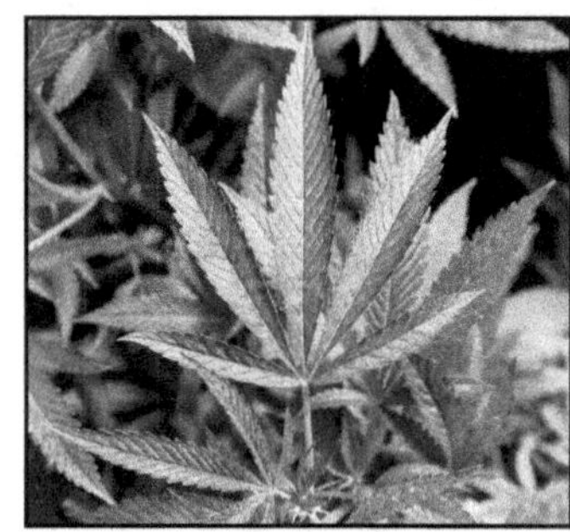

Fig. 5.7: Hemp Leaves

Preparation of Fibres: Fibres are obtained by subjecting the stalks to retting, drying and crushing. Finally a shaking process completes separation from the woody portion, and releases the long, fairly straight fibre, or line. Recently new technologies such as ultrasound and steam explosion have been developed for separation of the fibres from the stalk. There are two principal types of fibres in hemp viz. bast or long fibres and hurds or inner short fibre. Bast fibres are of two types namely, primary bast fibres and secondary bast fibres. The primary bast fibres are made up of approximately 70% of the fibres and are long. They contain high cellulose and low lignin. Primary bast fibres are the most valuable part of the stalk, and are generally considered to be among the strongest plant fibres known. Secondary bast fibres are made up of the remaining 30% of the bast fibres and are medium in length and higher in lignin.

Physical Properties:

Colour	:	Yellowish, greenish, or a dark brown or gray
Odour	:	Odourless
Taste	:	Tasteless
Appearance	:	Made of individual cylindrical cells with an irregular surface, they are longer and less flexible than flax.
Size	:	Strand is about 5.8 feet (1.8 metre) long and blunt rounded ends and the diameter ranges from 16-50 micron. Elongation at break: Stress easily
Moisture regain	:	12%

Effect of heat   :   Resistant to heat, but temperature between 160°C and 260°C results in softening of lignin

Tensile strength   :   Depends on the diameter of the fibres, but an average is 900 MPa (Mega Pascal)

Specific gravity   :   1.5 g/ mm^3

Modulus of elasticity : 34 GPa (Giga Pascal)

Chemical Properties:

Effect of acids   :   Hemp fibres disintegrate with hot dilute acids or cold concentrated acid

Effect of alkalis   :   Good resistance to alkalis

Effect of organic solvents : No effect

Ability to dye   :   Not suitable

Chemical Constituents: Hemp fibres mainly contain 77% cellulose and 10% hemicellulose. Apart from that lignin, fat, wax and pectin are also present.

Uses: Natural fibres from the hemp stalk are extremely durable and can be used in the production of textiles, clothing, canvas, rope, cordage, archival grade paper, paper, and construction materials. Long hemp fibres are used in clothing, home furnishing textiles and floor coverings, whereas short fibres are used in making insulation products, fibreboard and erosion control mats.

HALLUCINOGENS

Hallucinogens are psychoactive agents. They cause hallucinations, perceptual anomalies and other substantial subjective changes in thoughts, emotion, and consciousness. All hallucinogens contain nitrogen and are classified as alkaloids. They are found in the various parts of the plant such as roots, leaves, seeds, bark and/or flowers parts like many hallucinogens contain chemical structures similar to those of natural neurotransmitters. They affect neural circuits in the brain involving the neurotransmitter serotonin, and dissociative drugs cause their effects by disrupting the actions of the glutamate system of the brain. The regions of the brain that are affected by hallucinogens control mood, sensory perception, sleep, hunger, body temperature, sexual behaviour and muscle control. They are administered in various ways namely smoked or snuffed, swallowed fresh or dried, drunk in decoctions and infusions, absorbed directly through the skin, placed in wounds or administered as enemas. They are mainly of three types: psychedelics, dissociatives and deliriants.

1. **Psychedelics:** They are class of drugs that trigger psychedelic experiences via serotonin receptor agonism, causes thought and visual or auditory changes and altered state of consciousness.

2. **Dissociatives:** They produce analgesia, amnesia and catalepsy at anaesthetic doses. They achieve their effect through blocking the signals received by the NMDA (*N*-methyl-D-aspartate) receptor set. They also have CNS depressant activity.

3. **Deliriants:** They induce delirium. They are characterized by extreme confusion and an inability to control one's actions. They are unpopular as recreational drugs due to the severe and sometimes unpleasant nature of the hallucinations produced. They block the muscarnic acetylcholine receptors, hence they are known as anticholinergic drugs.

Some of the important herbal plants which are used as significant psychoactive activity and their effects are described in Table 5.1.

Table 5.1: Significant psychoactive plants and their effects

Plant name	Family	Constituents	Effects
Catha edulis (Khat)	Celastraceae	Cathine	Induce manic behaviours and hyperactivity, causes loss of appetite.
Coffea Arabica (Coffee)	Rubiaceae	Caffeine	Stimulant, temporarily warding off drowsiness and restoring alertness.
Cannabis sativa (Marijuana)	Cannabaceae	Tetrahydrocannabinol	Relaxation and increase in appetite.
Datura stramonium (Datura)	Solanaceae	Hyoscine	Acts as deliriant and can produce intense spiritual visions.
Erythroxylum coca (Coca)	Erythroxylaceae	Cocaine	Stimulant, appetite, suppressant.
Papaver somniferum (Opium)	Papaveraceae	Morphine	Analgesia, sedation, euphoria
Lophophora williamsii (Peyote)	Cactaceae	Mescaline	Hallucinogen.
Nicotiana tobacum (Tobacco)	Solanaceae	Nicotine	Stimulant, relaxant.
Salvia divinorum (Salvia)	Lamiaceae	Salvinorin-A	Induce Hallucination.

TERATOGENS

A **teratogen** is an agent, which can cause a birth defect via toxic effect on an embryo. The study of abnormalities of physiological development is known as Teratology. It results growth retardation, delayed mental development or other congenital disorders without any structural malformations. This condition occurs due to drugs used in pregnancy, lack of nutrients such as folic acid, physical restraint such as Potter syndrome, genetic disorders, alcohol consumption during pregnancy etc. There are three different types of possibilities such as: (1) known teratogens in known teratogenic plants, (2) known teratogenic plants with unidentified teratogens, and (3) suspected teratogenic plants. The details of the plants are tabulated in Table 5.2.

Table 5.2: Teratogenic plants

Known Teratogens in known teratogenic plants			
Biological source	**Family**	**Constituents**	**Effects**
Asparagus racemosus (Shatavari)	Liliaceae	Shatavarin	Cause gross malformations in fetus, can increase the rate of re-absorption in fetus and may also cause intrauterine growth.
Conium maculatum (Hemlock)	Apiaceae	Coniine	Acts directly on the central nervous system through inhibitory action on nicotinic acetylcholine receptors.
Leucaena leucocephala (River Tamarind)	Fabaceae	Mimosine	Inhibits DNA synthesis at the level of elongation of nascent chains by altering deoxyribonucleotide metabolism.
Lupinus mutabilis (Lupine)	Fabaceae	Sparteine	Cause gross malformations in fetus.
Ruta graveolens (Ruta)	Rutaceae	Arborinine	Women for contraception or induced abortion.
Veratrum album (Veratrum)	Liliaceae	Veratramine	Act by increasing the permeability of the sodium channels of nerve cells.
Known Teratogenic Plants With Unidentified Teratogens			
Astragalus gummifer (Tragacanth)	Leguminosae	Bassorin	Use in spermicidal jelly.
Malus domestica (orchard apple)	Rosaceae	Amygdalin (from seed)	Large doses can cause adverse reaction.
Nicotiana tabacum (Tobacco)	Solanaceae	Nicotine	Consume during pregnancy, controls birth.
Trachymene species	Apiaceae	Alkaloids	Roots are a traditional Aboriginal bushfood.
Prunus amygdalus (Almond)	Rosaceae	Cyanide	In large dose causes adverse reaction.
Suspected Teratogenic Plants			
Datura stramonium (Datura)	Solanaceae	Atropine	In large dose it causes bradycardia.
Lycopersicon esculentum (Tomato)	Solanaceae	Solanin	It causes nervous disturbances.
Senecio vulgaris (Groundsel)	Asteraceae	Senecionine	It causes irreversible liver damage.
Solanum tuberosum (Potato)	Solanaceae	Solanin	It causes nervous disturbances.
Solanum melongena (Egg plant)	Solanaceae	Solanin	It causes nervous disturbances.
Sorghum arundinaceum (Sorghum)	Poaceae	Prussic acid	In high dose it causes poisoning.

5.1.2 Natural Allergens

Allergens:

Allergens are a type of antigen that produces an abnormally vigorous immune response. They are inciting agents of the allergy. That means they are the substances that are capable of sensitizing the body in such a way that an unusual response occurs, in hypersensitive person. It may be biological, chemical or synthetic origin. The substances such as pollens, danders, dust etc. are as natural allergens. They are protein and glycoprotein in nature. They are mainly of 5 types:

(a) **Inhalants:** They are air borne substances that are chemicals which cause respiratory diseases, inflammation in nose, lungs etc. They are causes by pollen, dust mites, pets and moulds and results Hay fever, Asthma etc. **Symptoms:** Sneezing, lacrimation, coughing, itching eyes, nose etc.

(b) **Ingestants:** These are also known as food allergy. Allergens which are present in food staff and swallowed are termed as ingestants. A food allergy is an immune system that coexists with inhalant allergies. When the foods are digested and the nutrients are absorbed, substances in food stimulate allergic response. Foods induce respiratory symptoms by both reaginic and non-reaginic mechanisms. Most common food allergens ingested by patients are milk, egg, peanut, fish, soy, wheat etc. **Symptoms:** Skin rash, migraine, Bronchial asthma, GIT disturbance etc.

(c) **Injectants:** They are injectable preparations and some insects. They cause allergy in hypersensitive person. **Symptoms:** Itching, peeling of skin, Erythema etc. The natural sources of injectable allergens are produced by the sting of bees, wasps, hornets etc.

(d) **Contactants:** Allergens produce manifestation of hypersensitivity at the site of skin or other mucous. Aeroallergens such as the various pollen grains containing oils trichomes from various leaves, flowers are carried by smoke originating from brush fires, grass fires are also cause for contact allergens. A number of plant products used as additives in cosmetic preparations are irritants and cause skin allergy. Wool fats in cosmetics, soap, soap powder, enzyme detergents, nail polishes, hair dyes are also major cause of contact dermatitis.

(e) **Infectants:** Allergy caused by metabolic products of living microorganism in the human body. The continual presence of certain types of bacteria, molds, protozoas, in the human body being are responsible for chronic infection. Sometimes bacterial metabolic wastes are considered to be infectant allergens.

Photosensitizing Agents:

These are the drugs that are pharmacologically inactive but when exposed to sun light are converted to their active metabolites to produce a beneficial reaction affecting the diseased tissue. They have property to fluorescence. On expose to visible light it absorbs a quantum of energy and the molecules became activated. This energy is transferred to another molecule such as amino acids, histamine, tryptophan, tyrosine which in turn become activated, subsequently decompose for further reaction. As per the reaction they are of three types:

(a) **Photo allergy/reaction:** It is an allergic reaction of the skin to UV light.

(b) Photophobia: It is the strong desire to avoid all light sources based on a painful sensitivity of the eyes to strong light.

(c) Phototoxicity: It is an irritation of the skin after exposure to UV light. Immediate reactions are included as itching, burning, swelling and rashes.

Photosensitizers are broadly classified as photodynamic and photosensitizing agents.

Photodynamic agents require oxygen for their action. This group includes photodynamic dyes, hypericin, Bengal rose, quinine etc. These substances photo-oxidize terpenene, blood serum and causes haemolysis. They are topically inactive, but cause immediate photoreaction with intra dermal injection.

Photosensitizing agents do not require oxygen for their reaction. They include furanocoumarins and their derivatives. These agents neither cause photooxidation of terpenene nor haemolysis. They combine with UV light and cause photoaging, skin cancers, allergic reaction etc.

They are used for treatment of vitiligo in which melanin formation is less.

Photodynamic therapy is based on the discovery that certain chemicals can kill one celled in presence of light. It is a bio-component therapy method. This method is used for treatment of tumor diseases.

Fungal Toxins:

They are also known as mycotoxin. They are chemicals produced by fungi, molds under certain condition. They are essential for fungal growth and reproduction, but harmful for the human. There are more than 250 fungal toxins available. The diseases, that are caused by mycotoxins, are known as mycotoxicosis. The diseases, that are caused by molds, are known as mycosis.

(a) Aflatoxins: They are produced by *Aspergillus flavus*. There are five types of aflatoxins likely B1, B2, G1, G2 and M. Aflatoxins are extremely toxic and their target organ is liver. Aflatoxin B1 is 3 times more potent than G1. They are naturally occurring hepatocarcinogens.

(b) Stearigmatocystins: These are produced by *Aspergillus versicolor*. They are also highly toxic in nature same as aflatoxin B1. It is considered as potent carcinogen, mutagen and teratogen. The toxic effect is located in kidney and liver.

(c) Ergotoxins: They are produced from fungal infection of Rye plant *Claviceps purpurea*. They produce alkaloids which cause ergotism in humans. They cause CNS and peripheral disorders and also cause hallucination. It also causes abortion in pregnant women.

(d) Ochratoxins: They are produced by *Aspergillus ochraceus*. Ochratoxin A has been associated with the disease known as Balkan nephropathy. They can form in cold temperature on cheese and cake. Ochratoxin B is non-toxic. The toxic effect is located in kidney followed by liver.

5.2 PRIMARY METABOLITES

5.2.1 Carbohydrates

They are organic compounds found in the major part of fruits, vegetables, legumes and cereal grains. They carry out many functions in all living organisms. These are large biomolecules, consisting of carbon (C), hydrogen (H) and oxygen (O) in their basic structure.

Chemically, they are simple organic compounds that are aldehydes or ketones with many hydroxyl groups added on each carbon atom which are not part of either of these both functional groups. The basic formula is $C_m(H_2O)_n$ where "m" is different from "n". The hydrogen and oxygen ratio is 2 : 1, hence they are known as hydrates of carbon.

So, carbohydrate is defined as polyhydroxy aldehydes or polyhydroxy ketones which give these on hydrolysis and contains at least one chiral carbon atom. Carbohydrates are produced in green plants by photosynthesis and serve as a major source of energy in animals. They also serve as structural components, such as cellulose in plants and chitin in some animals.

Classification:

Carbohydrates are of three types namely simple sugar, polysaccharides and oligosaccharides (Fig. 5.8). The simplest carbohydrates are the three-carbon sugars, i.e. monosaccharides, and further cannot be hydrolysed to simple sugars.

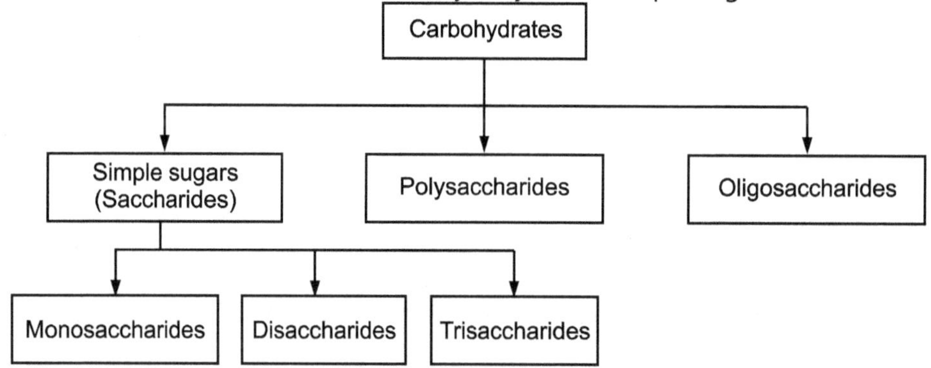

Fig. 5.8: Classification of carbohydrates

Depending on the number of carbon atoms, monosaccharides are further classified into following:

Bioses are two-carbon compounds, but do not occur in free form in the nature.

Trioses are three-carbon compounds. They are in the form of phosphoric esters.

Example: Glyceraldehyde.

Tetroses are four-carbon compounds.

Examples: Erythrose, Threose.

Pentoses are five-carbon compounds and occur in plants. They are the products of polysaccharides such as hemicelluloses, mucilage etc.

Examples: Ribose, Arabinose, Xylose etc.

Hexoses are six-carbon molecules and are abundantly available. On hydrolysis they produce starch and inulin.

Examples: Glucose, Fructose etc.

Monosaccharides are classified according to three different characteristics: the placement of carbonyl group, the number of carbon atoms they contain, and their chiral handedness. If the carbonyl group is an aldehyde, the monosaccharide is an aldose, and if the carbonyl group is a ketone, the monosaccharide is a ketose. Aldose or aldo sugar containing compounds are glucose, galactose, ribose etc., whereas ketose or keto sugar containing compound is fructose. Depending on the chemical nature of the sugar, they are also classified as reducing and non-reducing sugars.

Reducing sugar: Contain a hemiacetal or hemiketal group. Sugars include glucose, galactose, fructose, maltose, lactose.

Non-reducing sugar: Hemiacetal groups are absent. Sucrose and all polysaccharides are present in this group. Heptoses contain seven carbon atoms and so on. Disaccharides are the compounds in which two monosaccharides are joined together and these are the simplest polysaccharides. Examples: Sucrose, lactose etc.

Sucrose = Glucose and Fructose; Lactose = Galactose and Glucose; Maltose = Glucose and Glucose

Trisaccharides are oligosaccharides composed of three monosaccharides with two glycosidic bonds connecting in between them. Examples: Raffinose (Glucose + Fructose + Galactose).

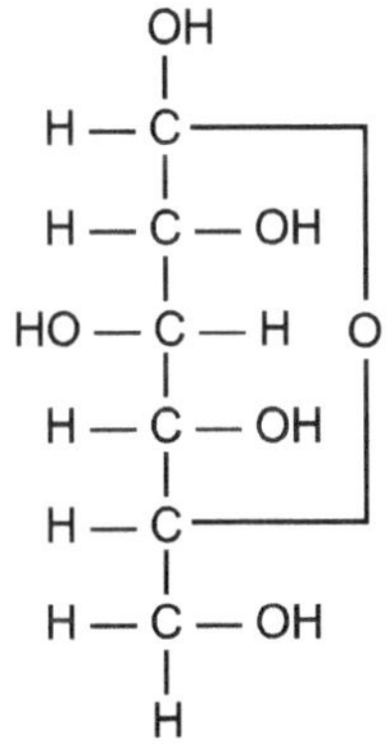

Glucose 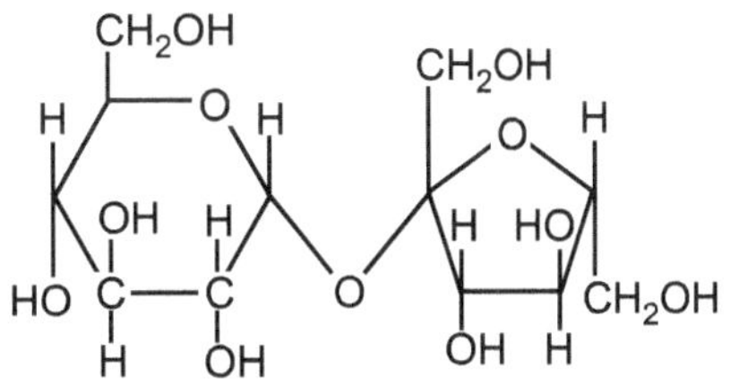   Sucrose

Polysaccharides are polymeric carbohydrates that are composed of long or branched chains of monosaccharide units bounded together by glycosidic bonds. They are of two types viz. Structural polysaccharides and Digestible polysaccharides. Former one are digestible by herbivorous species — cellulose, lignin, dextrans, mannans, inulin, pentosans, pectic acids, algic acids, agar and chitin. Later one is starch.

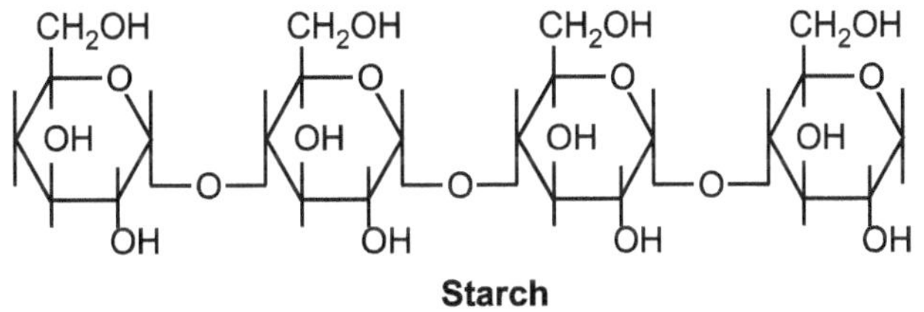

Starch

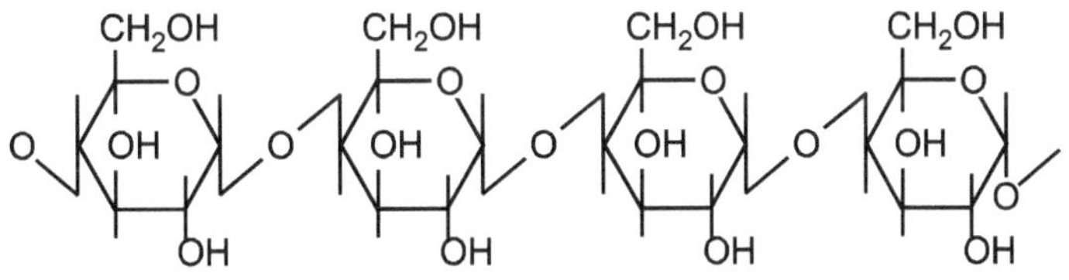

Cellulose

Oligosaccharides are saccharide polymers containing a small number of simple sugars. Some examples are fructo-oligosaccharides (FOS), which are found in many vegetables.

Function:

- They are used for energy storage and production. Starch and glycogen, respectively in plants and animals, are stored as carbohydrates from which glucose can be mobilized for energy production.
- They exert a protein-saving action.
- The presence of carbohydrates is necessary for the normal lipid metabolism.
- Glucose is indispensable for the maintenance of the integrity of nervous tissue and red blood cells.
- Two sugars, ribose and deoxyribose, are part of the bearing structure, respectively of the RNA and DNA and present in the nucleotide structure.
- They take part in detoxifying processes. For example, at hepatic level glucuronic acid, synthesized from glucose, combines with endogenous substances, as hormones, bilirubin etc.
- Carbohydrates are also found linked to many proteins and lipids. Within cells they act as signals that determine the metabolic fate or intracellular localization of the molecules which are bound.
- Two homopolysaccharides, cellulose and chitin, serve as structural elements.
- The cellulose in plants is used to manufacture paper, wood for construction, and fabrics.

Chemical Tests:

Molisch Test: Molisch reagent is mixed with a dilute solution of carbohydrate. The test reagent dehydrates pentoses to form furfural (top reaction) and dehydrates hexoses to form 5-hydroxymethyl furfural (bottom reaction). The furfurals further react with alpha-naphthol present in the test reagent to produce a purple product. Pentoses and hexoses form five-member oxygen containing rings on dehydration. This test is known as Molisch test and is used to detect carbohydrates in several substances.

Fehling's Test: Fehling's solution (containing Cu^{2+}) changes colour from blue to red/brown in the presence of reducing sugars.

Benedict's Test: This test is performed to identify the reducing sugars. Few ml of a sample solution is placed in a test tube. Two ml of Benedict's reagent (a solution of sodium citrate and sodium carbonate mixed with a solution of copper sulfate) is added. The solution is then heated in a boiling water bath for three minutes. A reddish precipitate will form within three minutes.

Barfoed's Test: This test is performed to distinguish between mono and disaccharides. Barfoed's reagent is copper acetate in acetic acid and is not as reactive as Benedict's reagent. A positive reaction may only be a light red precipitate. Monosaccharides produce the red precipitate in 2 to 3 minutes; disaccharides produce the precipitate in 10 minutes.

Iodine Test for Starch and Other Poly-saccharides: Starch is a polysaccharide that can be easily identified by the iodine test. Cellulose do not form colour complex with Iodine solution. Starch reacts with iodine solution and forms blue-violet color. Many glucose in starch trap iodine molecule and form the colour.

Seliwanoff's Test: Seliwanoff's test is used to distinguish aldohexoses from ketohexoses. A ketohexose like fructose will form a deep red colour with Seliwanoff's reagent (a solution of resorcinol in HCl), while an aldohexose will show a light pink colour and takes a longer time to develop the colour.

Bial's Test: This test is used to distinguish pentoses and hexoses. Pentoses give a positive test with Bial's reagent (contains orcinol, HCl and ferric chloride). In the presence of concentrated HCl, pentoses form a five-membered ring, known as furfural. A positive test is the formation of a bluish colour within 5 minutes without the formation of a precipitate. Hexoses generally react to form green, red, or brown products.

5.2.2 Carbohydrate Related Drugs

ACACIA

Biological source: It is a dried gummy exudation obtained from stem and branches of *Acacia arabica, A. senegal.*

Family: Leguminosae.

Distribution: The plant is distributed in West Africa, Central Africa, Europe, Australia, Asia. In India it is collected from Western Ghats, Punjab, Rajasthan, and Gujarat (Fig. 5.9).

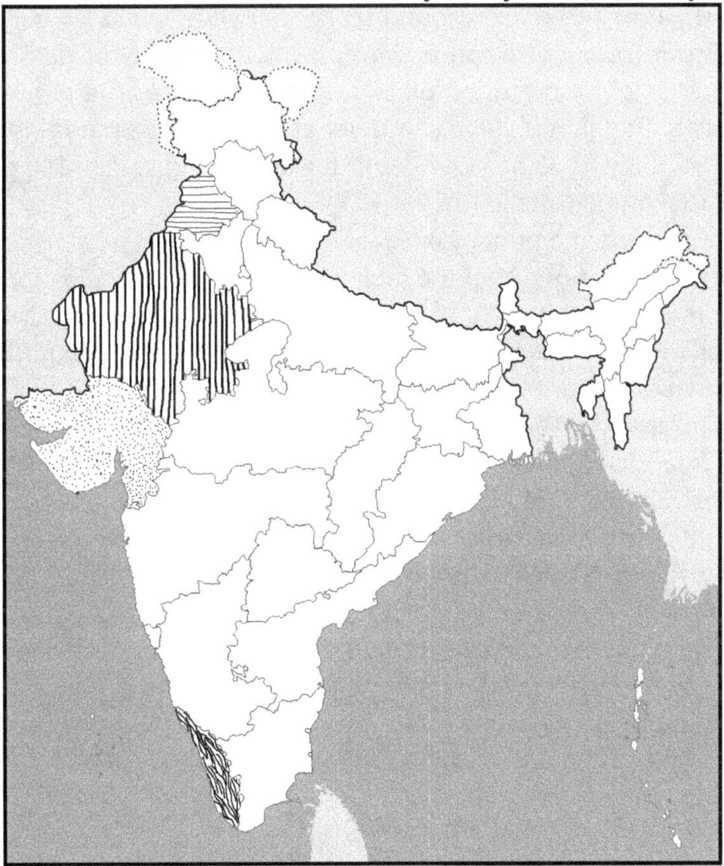

Fig. 5.9: Distribution of Acacia in India

Plant Description: The plants are spiny shrubs or small to large sized trees, but the growth mainly depends on the species. They prefer dry climate and grow to about 10 to 60 feet in height. The branches are purplish to gray with very small glands. The leaves are compound pinnate, but in some species the leaflets are suppressed, vertically flattened.

The bark is light brown in colour with rough surface. The flowers are small with five small petals (Fig. 5.10).

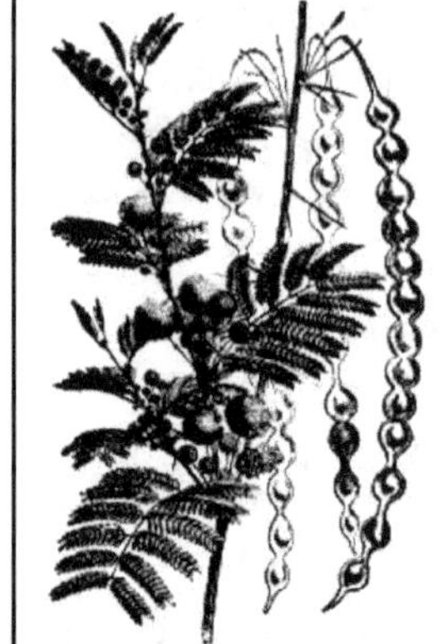

Fig. 5.10: *Acacia arabica* leaves and fruits

Description of Gum: The gum is round tears and white in colour but sometimes light brown or cream brown colour also forms, which is inferior quality of gum. Outer surface of the gum is dull and smooth, but dried gum is brittle in nature. The gum is odourless and mucilaginous in taste. The gum is soluble in water and forms acid, but is insoluble in alcohol. In chemical test, the gum shows negative result for tannin and starch. The gum contains 5% ash and less than 15% of moisture.

Parts Used: Pods, seed and gummy exudation from stem.

Collection and Preparation: After the rainy season, the gum exudes spontaneously from the trunk and principal branches. Since the flow is small in quantity, it is stimulated by incisions in the bark. To facilitate the flow, a thin strip, 2 to 3 feet in length and 1 to 3 inches wide is torn off. In about a fortnight, it thickens and hardens on exposure to the air, in the form of round or oval tears. They are white or red, according to whether the species is a white or red gum tree. Then gum is harvested and marketed as 'Gum Arabica'.

Chemical Constituents: Gum Acacia consists principally of Arabin, a compound of Arabic acid with calcium. It can be obtained as an amorphous precipitate by treating with alcohol an aqueous solution of gum Arabic in the presence of hydrochloric acid. It is soluble in water and insoluble in alcohol. Varying amounts of magnesium and potassium salts of Arabic acid are also present. The gum also contains 12 to 17 per cent of moisture and a trace of sugar. Apart from that it also contains oxidase and peroxidase enzymes. Gum arabic is a complex, slightly acidic polysaccharide.

Arabic Acid

Chemical Tests:

- Aqueous solution of gum + Ruthenium red $\longrightarrow$ No Pink colour.

- Aqueous solution of gum + Hydrogen peroxide + Benzidine in alcohol $\longrightarrow$ Blue colour (Due to presence of oxydase enzyme)
- Aqueous solution of gum + Lead subacetate $\longrightarrow$ Gelatinous form
- Aqueous solution of gum + Ferric chloride $\longrightarrow$ No blackish colouration or blackish precipitate $\longrightarrow$ Tannin absent.
- Aqueous solution of gum + Iodine solution $\longrightarrow$ No blue colour (Starch absent).
- Aqueous solution of gum + dil. HCl $\longrightarrow$ Boil $\longrightarrow$ Add Fehling's A and B $\longrightarrow$ Red colour after heating.

Uses: Acacia gum is used in pharmaceuticals as a demulcent. It is used topically for healing wounds and has been shown to inhibit the growth of periodontic bacteria and the early deposition of plaque. It is used as an emulsifier and a thickening agent in icing, fillings, chewing gum and other confectionery items. It also reduces cholesterol levels and helps to increase weight loss when taken orally. It is also used in diarrhea, irritations, ulcer in the stomach and intestine, bleeding piles, leucorrhoea etc.

Adulterants and Substituents: Gum Senegal is often used as a substituent for Indian gum. It is identified as gum Senegal is yellowish white in colour, tears are ovoid, whereas gum Arabica is whitish in colour, and tears are rounded.

Indian gum is adulterated with gum ghatti obtained from *Anogeissus latifolia.* It is identified as it reacts with lead subacetate, but very less precipitate will form and morphologically, the outer surface of the gum is dull and without fissures. Starch, sterculia gum and dextrins are also used as adulterants for Indian gum.

Storage: In contact with the moisture the gum becomes hardened and darkened in colour and this can affect its quality. Hence, it should be stored in clean, cool and dry place. It does not deteriorate due to long storage under such favourable conditions.

AGAR

Biological Source: It is a dried gelatinous substance obtained from red algae i.e. Gelidium species by aqueous extraction, i.e. *Gelidium amnasi* (Japan species), *Gracilaria confervoides* (Australian species) etc. *Gelidium cartilagenium* collected along the West coast of North America (Mexico) is the common source of bacteriological agar in the U.S.A.

Family: Gelidaceae.

Distribution: It is mainly located in the coastal areas of USA and Pacific coastal areas. Commercially it is produced in Japan, Australia, USA, New Zealand and India. In India it is produced in the coastal areas of Bay of Bengal, mainly in Orissa and Tamil Nadu (Fig. 5.11).

Description of Red Algae: Red algae are red because of the presence of the phycoerythrin. This pigment reflects red light and absorbs blue light. Because blue light penetrates water to a greater depth than light of longer wavelengths, these pigments allow red algae to photosynthesize and live at somewhat greater depths than most other "algae". The most red algae are marine, but few occur in fresh water. Rhodophytes are usually multicellular and grow attached to rocks or other algae, but there are some unicellular or colonial forms. They do not have flagellated cells, and are structurally complex. Many red algae are having pit connections between the cells and their cell walls include a rigid component composed of microfibrils. Agar and carragenin are two red algal mucilages that are widely used for gelling and thickening purposes in the food and pharmaceutical industries.

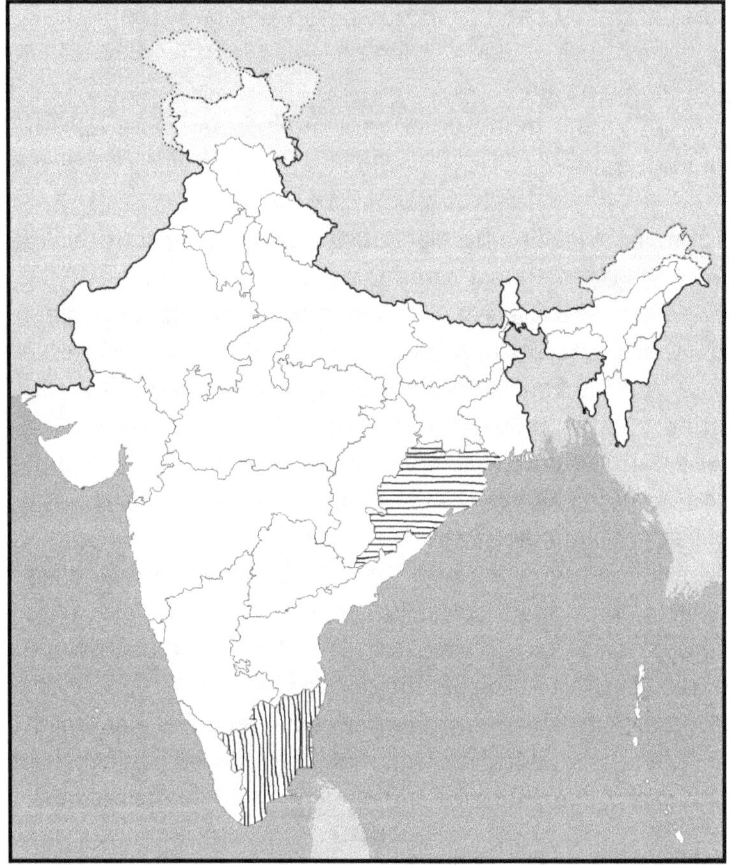

Fig. 5.11: Distribution of Agar in India

Description of Agar: There are two different types of agar, the Gelidium and Gracilaria agars. Bacteriological agar is prepared mostly from Gelidium and Pterocladia. Agar is isolated from the algae as an amorphous and translucent product sold as powder, flakes, or bricks. It is also available in strips which are about 60-65 cm in length and 5 mm in width. It is produced chiefly in Japan, New Zealand, Australia, the United States, and Russia. It is odourless, mucilaginous in taste and is insoluble in cold water. It absorbs as much as 20 times its own weight. It dissolves readily in boiling water; a dilute solution is still liquid at 42°C, but solidifies at 37°C into a firm gel. Agar gels may contain as much as 99.9% water. The stiffness of agarose gels may be due to the aggregation of the double helices forming a network phase which may contain as much as 100 parts of water for each part of agarose. In the natural state, agar occurs as a complex cell wall constituent containing a complex carbohydrate (polysaccharide) with sulfate and calcium, but starch is absent. The aggregate in agarose gels may actually contain 10 to 104 double helices which make agarose very useful in immunology, biotechnology and genetic engineering.

Preparation and Collection: Majority of the agar samples were prepared by Blethen's method from Chilean agar which could have been manufactured from *Gracilaria leanaeformis*, the predominant Gracilaria species of Chile (Fig. 5.12).

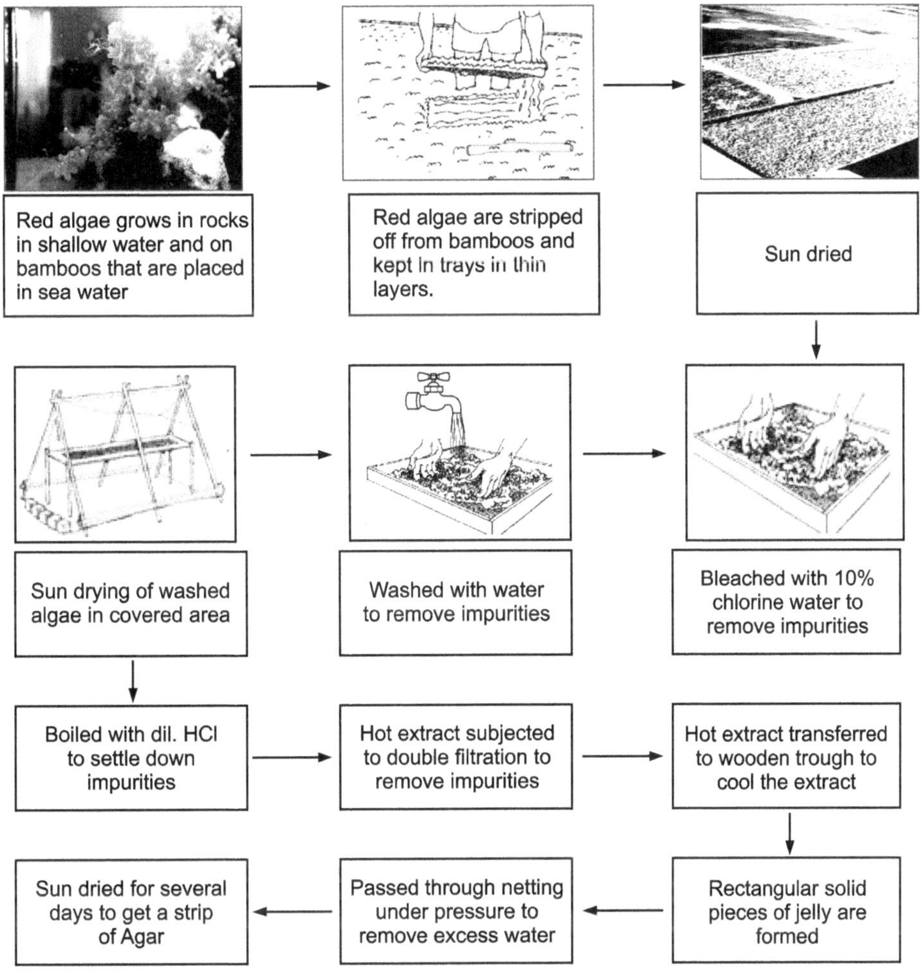

Red algae grows in rocks in shallow water and on bamboos that are placed in sea water
Red algae are stripped off from bamboos and kept in trays in thin layers.
Sun dried
Bleached with 10% chlorine water to remove impurities
Washed with water to remove impurities
Sun drying of washed algae in covered area
Boiled with dil. HCl to settle down impurities
Hot extract subjected to double filtration to remove impurities
Hot extract transferred to wooden trough to cool the extract
Rectangular solid pieces of jelly are formed
Passed through netting under pressure to remove excess water
Sun dried for several days to get a strip of Agar

Fig. 5.12: General production of agar strip

Commercial isolation of agar from red algae (*Gracilaria edulis*) (Fig. 5.13)

Red algae is sun dried and leached in fresh water for 12-18 hours. → It is washed 2-3 times with fresh water in agitator tank. → The algae is softened with dilute HCl for 30 minutes at pH 2-4. → The algae is digested by passing steam in the digester for 2-3 hrs at 50 lb pressure → After 30 minutes agar gel is settled → Agar gel is filtered through filter cloth and collected in aluminium trays. → Agar gel is cooled at room temperature for 1-2 hrs. and then cutted with gel chopper. → It is freezed for 24 hrs. at 0-20°C, then thawed and sun dried → Agar is bleached in 10% chlorine water for 10 min and then cleaned with water 3 times → Then it is dried in sun and finally agar sheets are packed in polythene bags.

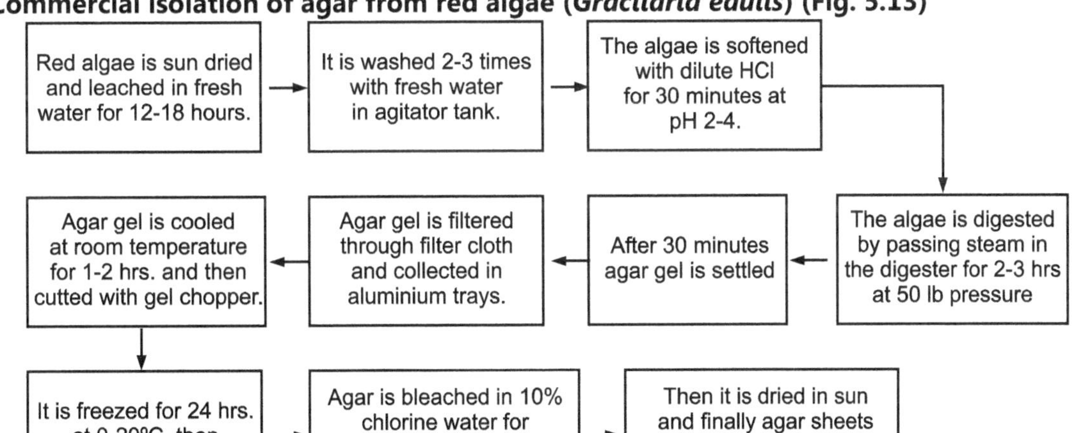

Fig. 5.13: Commercial production of agar from red algae

Chemical Constituents: Agar of *Gelidium amansii* is a mixture of two different polysaccharides, one a neutral agarose which consists of alternating 1,3-linked 3-D-galactopyranose and a 1,4-linked 3,6-anhydro-a-L-galactopyranose and the other a charged agaropectin. About 3-4% cellulose and 6-7% nitrogenous substances are present in agar. It also contains pyruvic acid and D-galactose. The gel strength of agar decreases with an increase in sulfate and a decrease in 3,6-anhydro-α-L-galactose concentration. The gelling temperature increases with an increase in methoxyl content of the agarose. A 1.5% solution of agar-agar forms a gel on cooling to about 32° to 45°C that does not melt below 85°C. Agar normally maintains ash content between 2.5-4%.

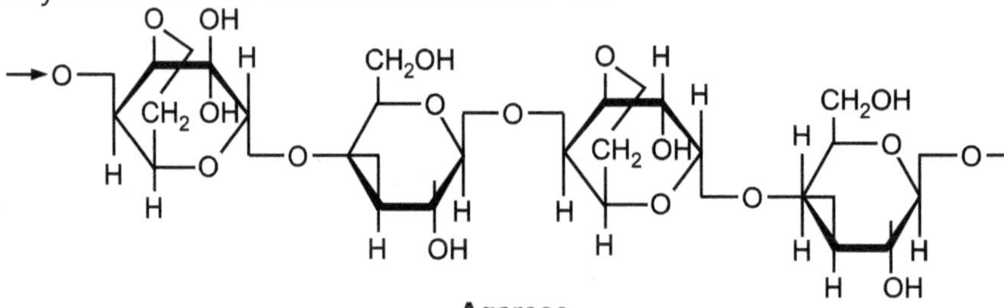

Agarose

Chemical Tests:

- Agar sample is mixed with sufficient water and boiled. After cooling the solution, stiff jelly is formed.
- If agar solution is added with ruthenium red and observed under microscope, the red colour is observed.
- 0.2% agar solution in water when mixed with Tannic acid but no white precipitated.
- Sample solution mixed with soda lime but no ammonium smell.
- Aqueous solution of agar is mixed with dil. HCl and then boiled. After that the solution is divided into two parts. In one part 10% NaOH and Fehling's solution is added that gives red colour due to presence of galactose. In another part barium chloride is added which gives white precipitate due to formation of barium sulphate.

Uses: Agar acts as a solidifying component of bacteriological culture media. It is used in canning meat, fish, and poultry; in cosmetics, medicines, and dentistry. It is used as thickening agent in ice cream, pastries, desserts, salad dressings, and as a wire-drawing lubricant. It functions as food stabilizers. It is also an emulsifying agent and a bulk laxative.

TRAGACANTH

Biological Source: The economical part of the plant is gum which is a dried gummy exudation and obtained from *Astragalus gummifer* or other species of *Astragalus*.

Family: Leguminoseae.

Distribution: The thorny shrubs of tragacanth normally grow at an altitude of 1000-3000 meter and the primary source is the desert highlands of northern and western part of Iran. Apart from Iran it is naturally found in various countries, *viz.*, Iraq, Armenia, Syria, Greece and Turkey. Very few species of *Astragalous* are located in India, *viz.*, Kumaon, Garhwal and Punjab.

Collection of Gum: Collection of gum is described in Fig. 5.14.

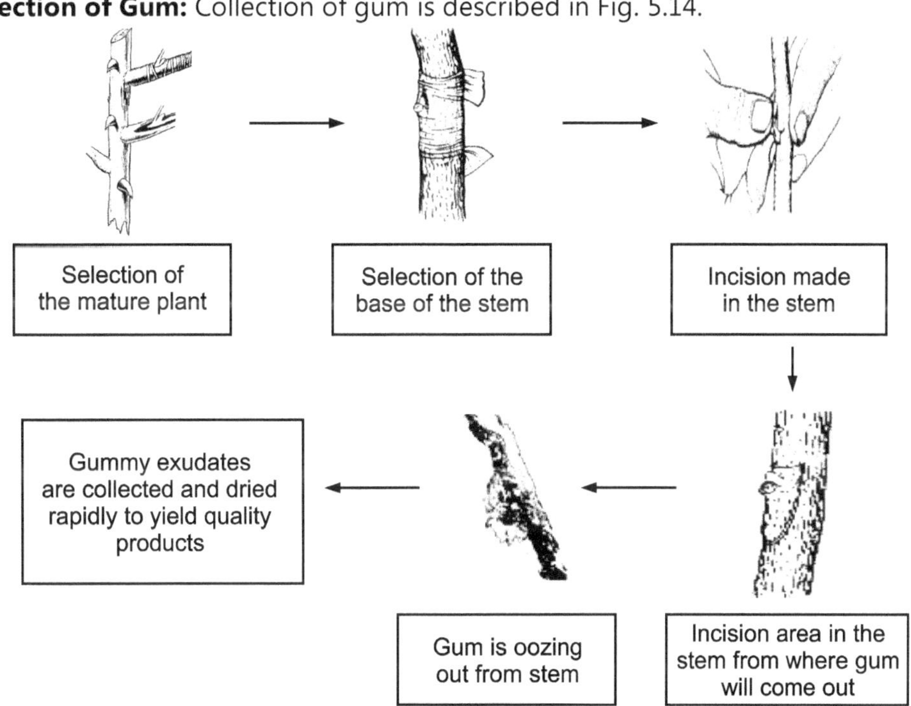

Fig. 5.14: Production and Collection of Tragacanth gum

It takes about a week to collect the gum exudates and this process continues periodically.

Properties of Gum:

- The gum is translucent and the powder is white or pale yellow in colour, odourless and tasteless.
- Gum looks like curved or twisted ribbon, like flakes marked with concentric ridges.
- Fracture of gum is normally short and horny.
- Gum tragacanth is a viscous and water-soluble mixture of polysaccharides.
- It absorbs water to become a gel, which can be stirred into a paste.
- Tragacanthin partially dissolves and partially swells in water yielding a viscous colloid.

Chemical Nature of Gum:

- Tragacanth gum contains linear chains of galacturonic acid in xylose and with varying levels of fructose.
- Tragacanth contains from 20% to 30% of a water-soluble fraction called tragacanthin (composed of tragacanthic acid and arabinogalactan).
- It also contains from 60% to 70% of a water-insoluble fraction called bassorin.
- Tragacanthic acid is composed of D-galacturonic acid, D-xylose, L-fructose, D-galactose, and other sugars.
- Tragacanthin is composed of uronic acid and arabinose and dissolves in water to form a viscous colloidal solution (sol), while bassorin swells to form a thick gel.
- The gum also contains several carbohydrates like L-arabinose, D-galactose, D-Xylose, L-fructose, L-Rhamnose etc.

Chemical Tests:

- Aqueous solution of Tragacanth + Conc. Hydrochloric acid $\longrightarrow$ Boil $\longrightarrow$ No Red colour forms.
- Sample of Tragacanth + Ruthenium red solution $\longrightarrow$ No Pink colour forms
- Aqueous solution of Tragacanth + Drops of Ferric chloride $\longrightarrow$ Deep yellow precipitate froms.
- Sample solution + Lead acetate $\longrightarrow$ Heavy white precipitate forms

Substituents/Adulterants: Gum kondagogu is gummy exudate obtained from the tree bark *Cochlospermum gossypium*. Dextrin, wheat and corn starch etc. are used as substituents for tragacanth gum. Generally, Karaya gum or sterculia gum or Indian tragacanth is used as a substitute for gum tragacanth.

Karaya gum can be identified morphologically, microscopically and by chemical tests. (a) Indian tragacanth is irregular, striated, pale brownish pieces and has acid odour. (b) In Karaya gum powder, sclerenchymatous cells are present, whereas these cells are absent in Tragacanth gum powder. (c) Karaya gum is identified with the ruthenium solution test with formation of red colour, whereas this test is negative for tragacanth.

Citral gum obtained from *Acacia strobiliferus* is used as an adulterant. It can be identified by chemical test. Powdered Tragacanth is mixed with water, guaicol and few drops of hydrogen peroxide. Pure Tragacanth remains colourless, whereas acacia gum forms a brown colour mucilage.

Uses: Tragacanth is used as an emulsifier, binding agent, and demulcent. Orally, tragacanth is used both for diarrhoea and as a laxative. Topically, tragacanth is an ingredient in toothpastes, hand lotions, and vaginal creams and medicinal jellies like spermicidal jelly. It is used as a binding agent for preparations of tablets and pills. In foods, tragacanth is used as stabilizer, thickener and suspending ingredients in salad dressings, foods, and beverages. The mucilage is used as adhesives.

Mechanism of Action: Tragacanth contains ingredients that stimulate the movement of the intestines. It acts as a stabilizer by formation of non-covalent protein–polysaccharide complexes via interactions by the methoxylated galacturonic acid in the soluble part of the gum and by the viscosity increase induced by the insoluble bassorin part.

HONEY

Biological Source: Honey is a saccharine liquid prepared from the nectar of the flower by the honey bees that is deposited in the honey comb. The bees are *Apis mellifera, Apis dorsata* and others.

Family: Apidae.

Geographical Location: Honey is produced in many parts of the world like Africa, Australia, Newzealand, Asia. In India it is abundantly produced in forest area of all the states. Maximum honey production is obtained from Himalayan forest region, Karnataka, West Bengal, Madhya Pradesh and Andhra Pradesh.

Preparation of Honey: It is described in Fig. 5.15.

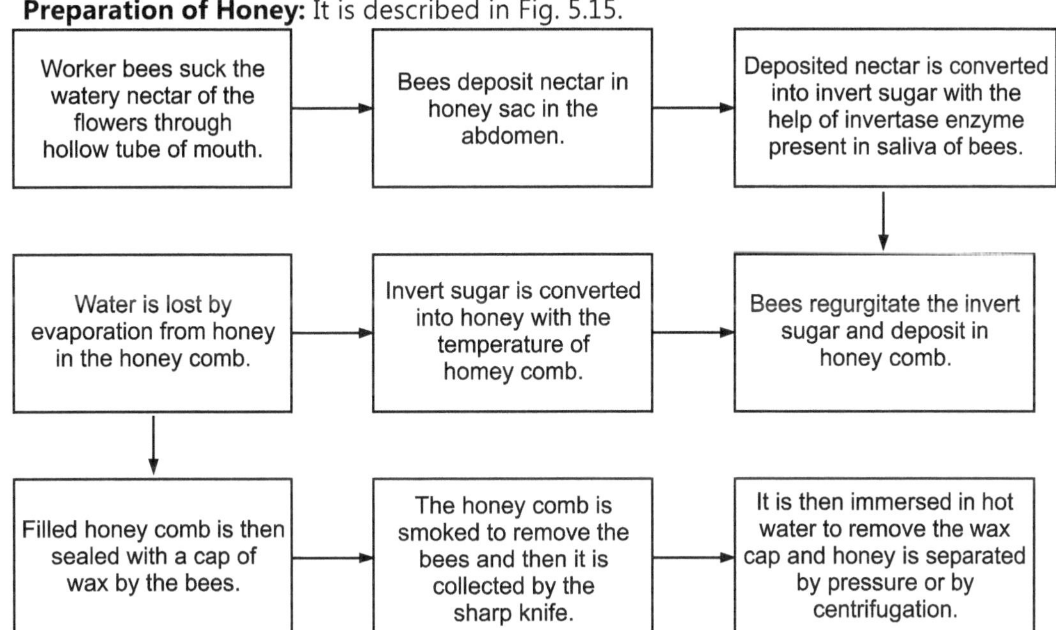

Fig. 5.15: General production of honey

Chemical Constituents: Honey is essentially a concentrated aqueous solution of inverted sugar and contains a highly complex mixture of other carbohydrates, a variety of enzymes, amino acids, organic acids, minerals, vitamins, aromatic substances, pigments, waxes, etc. The main sugars present in honey are fructose (38%) and glucose (31%). The saccharose content varies in accordance with the state of maturity of the honey, and the composition of the oligosaccharide fraction is determined by the plants used in the production process.

Honey contains free amino acids in quantities of around 0.1% of the dry product. Proline is the major amino acid, but other amino acids like arginine, alanine, glutamic acid, aspartic acid, lysine, glycine and leucine are also present. The main acid in honey is gluconic acid and smaller quantities are also found of lactic, citric, succinic, formic, malic, acetic, maleic and oxalic acids.

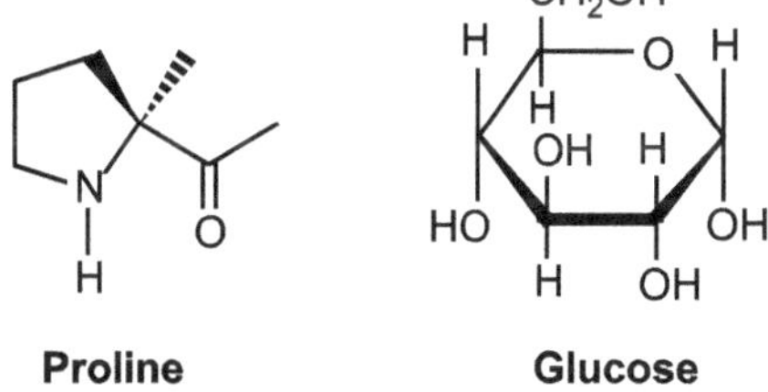

Properties: The physical properties of honey vary, depending on water content, the type of flora used to produce it, temperature, and the proportion of the specific sugars it contains.

1. Honey is translucent, white to pale yellow liquid.
2. Odour is pleasant and characteristic whereas taste is sweet.
3. It is soluble in water but insoluble in alcohol.
4. Fresh honey is a super saturated liquid, containing more sugar than the water.
5. It is hygroscopic in nature.
6. At room temperature, honey is a super cooled liquid, in which the glucose will precipitate into solid granules.
7. The melting point of crystallized honey is between 40 and 50°C.
8. Honey has a glass transition between −42 and −51°C.

9. A honey contains 16% humidity, at 70°C.
10. Honey has more viscosity than water and is around 10,000 cps (counts per second).
11. The refractive index for honey ranges from 1.504 at 13% humidity to 1.474 at 25%.
12. Honey also contains acids, which act as catalysts.
13. The average pH of honey is 3.9, but it can range from 3.4 to 6.1.
14. A product that contains crystallized dextrose is called granulated honey.

Uses: The medicinal uses of honey are as wound dressing material, antimicrobial, anti-inflammatory, antiseptic and reduce tissue damages. In Ayurveda, honey is used for both internal and external applications. It is mainly used for the treatment of eye diseases, cough, thirst, leprosy, diabetes, obesity, worm infestation, vomiting, asthma and diarrhoea.

According to Ayurveda, there are eight different types of honey:

1. **Makshikam:** It is used in the treatment of eye disease, hepatitis, piles, asthma, cough etc.
2. **Bhraamaram:** It is used in the treatment of vomiting with blood.
3. **Kshoudram:** It is used in the treatment of diabetes.
4. **Pauthikam:** It is used in the treatment of diabetes and urinary infection.
5. **Chathram:** It is used in the treatment of worm infestation.
6. **Aardhyam:** It is effective for eye diseases, cough and anaemic condition.
7. **Ouddalakam:** It is used in the treatment of leprosy and poisoning conditions.
8. **Daalam:** It increases digestion and helps in the treatment of cough and vomiting.

Chemical Tests:

1. The amount of hydroxymethyl furfural (HMF) in honey can be determined by Reflectoquant® HMF test by dilute weighed honey sample with distilled water (1 : 4) and by putting the test strip into reflectometer.
2. Sample honey is mixed with ether and then evaporated in room temperature. Then dilute HCl and resorcinol are added to the solution. Acid layer will not form any red or pink colour.

Adulteration: Gas Chromatography (GC), Liquid Chromatography (LC) analysis, Near Infrared Transflectance Spectroscopy (NIR) etc. are suitable for use as a screening technique in the quality control of honey. Generally corn syrup, flour, molasses, glucose, starch, dextrose and other similar products are used as adulterant for honey.

(a) **Honey with Sugar Solution (Sugar + Water):** To detect the adulterant, (a) Pure honey is always in a semi solid state. (b) If adulterated honey is poured in water it will dissolve immediately. If honey is pure, it will not dissolve so soon.

(b) **Honey with Cane Sugar:** Microscopic analysis. Cane sugar exhibited parenchyma cells, single ring vessels and epidermal cells, whereas all these characters are absent in honey.

(c) **Honey with Invert Sugar:** It can be checked with the help of *Fiehe's test*. Sample of honey is mixed with ether and then evaporated in room temperature. Then dilute HCl and resorcinol are added to the solution. Acid layer will not form any red or pink colour.

(d) **Honey with Glucose:** This can be identified by *iodine test*. Sample honey is mixed with same quantity of water and then potassium iodide is added. The solution becomes red or violet. This indicates the presence of glucose. This test is negative for pure honey.

(e) Honey with Commercial Sugar: This can be identified by *Aniline chloride test.* Sample honey + mixture of hydrochloric acid and Aniline (3 : 1) $\longrightarrow$ crimson red colour or the orange colour forms due to formation of aniline chloride by commercial sugar. This test is negative for pure honey.

(f) Honey with Starch or Flour: Starch or flour is added to honey for a simple reason, to increase the weight and whiteness of it. One can add cold water to sample honey and thus be sure whether it is free from flour and starch or not. If they are present in honey then honey falls down to the bottom of the vessel. When they are exposed to heat, they obviously remain in the liquid form, but upon cooling down they turn hard.

5.3 PROTEINS AND ENZYMES

Protein was first described by the Dutch chemist Gerhardus Johannes Mulder and further named by the Swedish chemist Jons Jakob Berzelius in 1838. The term protein, derived from the Greek *proteios*, meaning first, are a class of organic compounds that are present in and vital to every living cell. Proteins are large biochemical compounds (carbon, hydrogen, oxygen, and nitrogen) consisting of one or more polypeptides (amino acid residue) typically folded into a globular or fibrous form in a biologically functional way. A polypeptide is a single linear polymer chain of amino acids bonded together by peptide bonds between the carboxyl and amino groups of adjacent amino acid residues i.e. an amine group (NH_2), a carboxylic acid group (R–C=O–OH) and a side-chain (usually denoted as R) (Fig. 5.16). They required for the structure, function, and regulation of the body's cells, tissues, and organs.

Examples: Hormones, enzymes

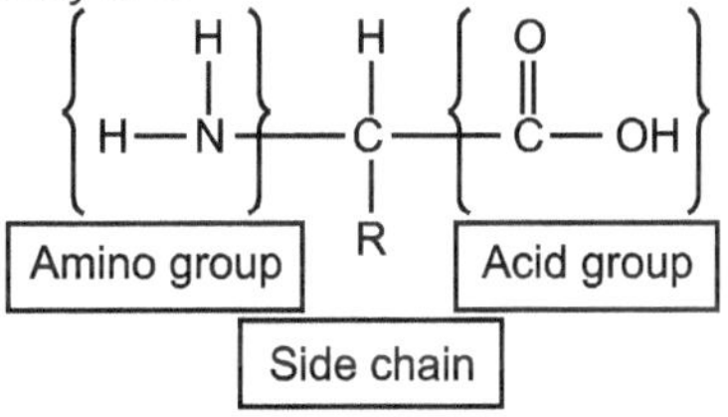

Amino acid structure

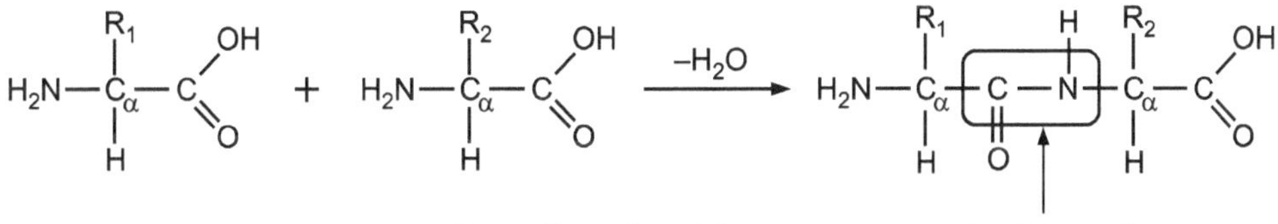

Formation of protein   **Peptide bond**

Fig. 5.16: Building block of protein

They are stored in the form of aleurone grains in plants and can be extracted easily. They are purified from other cellular components using a variety of techniques such as ultracentrifugation, precipitation, electrophoresis, and chromatography techniques.

Chemistry:

- The length of proteins and complexity vary based on the number and type of amino acid chains. There are about 20 different amino acids, each with a different chemical structure and characteristics; for instance, some are polar, others are non-polar. The final protein structure is dependent upon the composition of amino acids.

- They consist of two polypeptide chains, a long chain which is on the left side, consisting of 346 amino acids and a short chain which is on the right side having 99 amino acids. The long chain is also known as heavy chain that contains 5 domains. In that 3 are extracellular domains (N_1, C_1 and C_2) and a transmembrane domain where the polypeptide chain passes through the cell and a cytoplasmic domains (C-terminal) within the cytoplasm of the cell.
- They are hydrolysed with acids or enzymes and break into amino acids.
- They form colloidal solution in water.
- Proteins are amphoteric in nature and get easily denatured due to heat, changes in pH, reaction with organic solvents etc.

Biochemical Importance:

- Proteins are the main structural and functional component of cytoskeleton. They are the main source of replacement of nitrogen in the body.
- Proteins act as biocatalyst. They are enzymes.
- Proteins are immunoglobulins that serve as first line defence against bacteria.
- Structural proteins provide mechanical strength to the body.
- Storage proteins bind with specific substances and are stored in the body. Example, iron is stored in body as ferritin.
- Transport proteins carry out the function of transporting specific substances either across the membrane or in the body fluids.

Classification of Proteins:

Broadly proteins are classified in three types tabulated in Fig. 5.17.

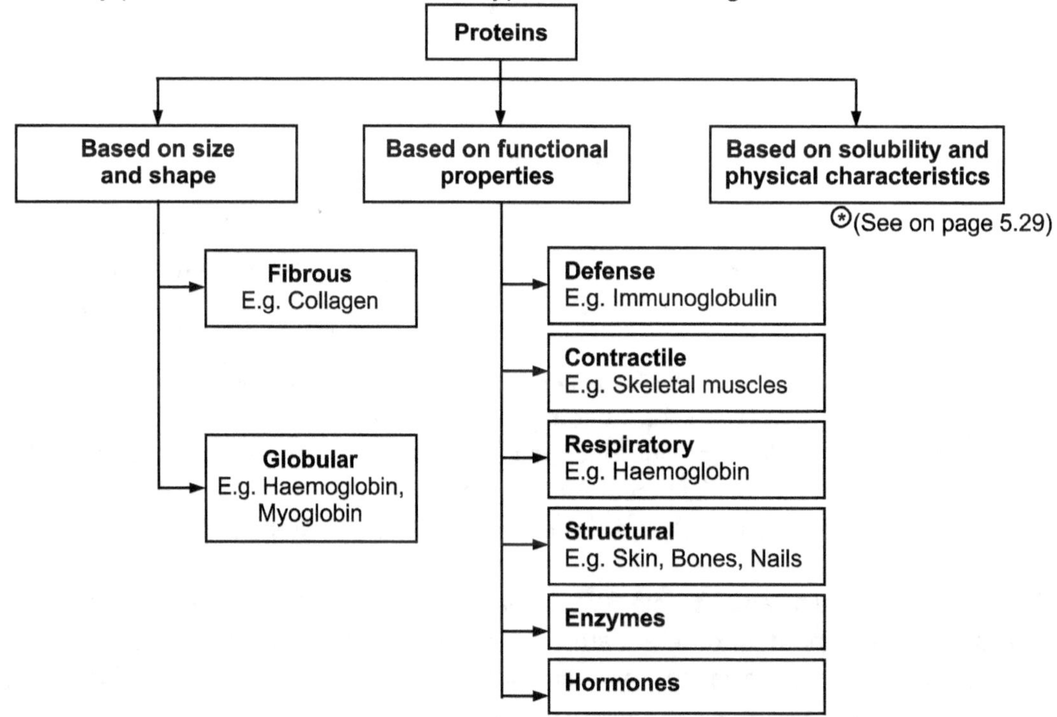

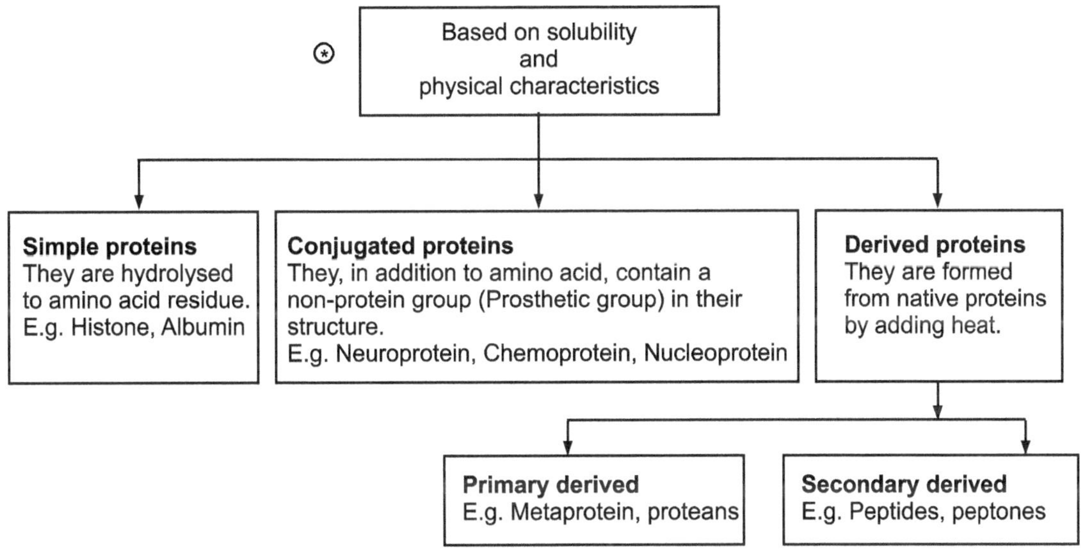

Fig. 5.17: Classification of proteins

Isolation of Proteins:

Various modern isolation techniques are used for the isolation of proteins that include cell disruption method, mechanical homogenization, solid-phase micro-extraction, supercritical-fluid extraction, pressurized-liquid extraction, microwave-assisted extraction, solid-phase extraction and surfactant-mediated techniques.

Generally, protein is extracted with trichloroacetic acid (TCA) and acetone or by using phenol or by homogenization with buffer. Plant tissue is homogenized in 10% TCA containing 2% beta mercaptoethanol using liquid nitrogen. Further the solution is kept at −20°C for overnight to form the precipitate which is subjected to centrifugation at high r.p.m for 30-40 minutes at 4°C. The precipitate is washed with cold acetone.

Analysis Methods of Proteins:

- **Biuret Method:** A violet-purplish colour is produced when cupric ions (Cu^{2+}) interact with peptide bonds under alkaline conditions. The biuret reagent is mixed with a protein solution and then allowed to stand for 15-30 minutes and then the absorbance is taken at 540 nm.

- **Lowry Method:** The lowry method combines the biuret reagent with another reagent i.e. Folin-Ciocalteau phenol reagent which reacts with tyrosine and tryptophan residues in proteins. This gives a bluish color which can be read somewhere between 500-750 nm. There is a small peak around 500 nm that can be used to determine high protein concentrations and a large peak around 750 nm that can be used to determine low protein concentrations.

- **Turbimetric Method:** Protein molecules which are normally soluble in solution are precipitated by the addition of certain chemicals, e.g., trichloroacetic acid. Protein precipitation causes the solution to become turbid and the final concentration of protein is determined by measuring the degree of turbidity.

Some other methods are like Kjeldahl method, Dye binding method, UV spectroscopy method etc.

General Chemical Tests for Proteins:

- **Biuret Reaction:** Sample solution is mixed with 10% sodium hydroxide and 0.1% copper sulphate solution. The solution becomes violet or pink colour.

  Compounds with two or more peptide bonds give a violet colour with alkaline copper sulphate solution. Proteins in the alkaline environment reduce Cu^{2+} to Cu^{+}, which forms a coordination complex with proteins, leading to a blue to light violet colour change.

- **Ninhydrin Test:** Sample solution is mixed with 0.1% freshly prepared Ninhydrin solution and then boiled to get violet or purple colour.

- **Xanthoproteic Reaction:** Sample solution is mixed with few ml of concentrated nitric acid and boiled. Then 40% sodium hydroxide is added slowly. The yellow colour of solution turns to deep orange colour. The yellow colour is due to the nitro derivatives of the aromatic amino acids present in the protein. The sodium salts of nitro derivatives are orange in colour.

- **Sulphur Test:** Sample solution is mixed with few ml of 40% NaOH and few drops of 2% lead acetate solution and then boiled. The solution forms black precipitate after cooling.

- **Sakaguchi Reaction**: Sample solution is mixed with 0.02% alpha naphthol solution, 10% sodium hydroxide solution and few drops of alkaline hypobromide solution. The solution gives intense red colour.

5.3.1 Protein Related Drugs

GELATIN

Synonyms: Collagen Hydrolysate, Denatured Collagen, Gelatina.

Source: Gelatin is mainly polypeptide with higher molecular weight protein obtained by boiling skin, tendons, ligaments, and/or bones with water. It is usually obtained from cattle bones, cattle hides and pork skins.

Biological Source: Cattle: *Bos taurus*, **Family:** Bovinae Pork: *Sus scrofa*, **Family:** Suidae

Preparation: Gelatin is prepared by hydrolysis of collage. Animal skins and bones are used as the raw materials. There are two main types of gelatin. Type-A gelatin which has isoionic point of 7-9. It is derived from collagen with exclusively acid pretreatment and it takes about 7-10 days. Whereas, Type-B gelatin has isoionic point of 4.8 to 5.2. It is prepared by an alkaline pretreatment of the collagen and it takes more time than former one.

The bones are defatted and then decalcified with organic solvent and acid respectively to give a soft sponge like material called ossein. Calcium phosphate is produced as a byproduct. The ossein is soaked in lime pits for several weeks for hydrolysis and then treated with hot water at 85°C to get solubilized gelatin from collagen. The resultant weak solution of gelatin is concentrated in a series of evaporators and chilled to form gel. Gels are spread into metal trays and allowed to set into jelly and then removed by drying at 10°, 30° and 60°C for a month. They are further bleached in sulphur dioxide to produce light coloured gelatin, which is then dried at room temperature (Fig. 5.18).

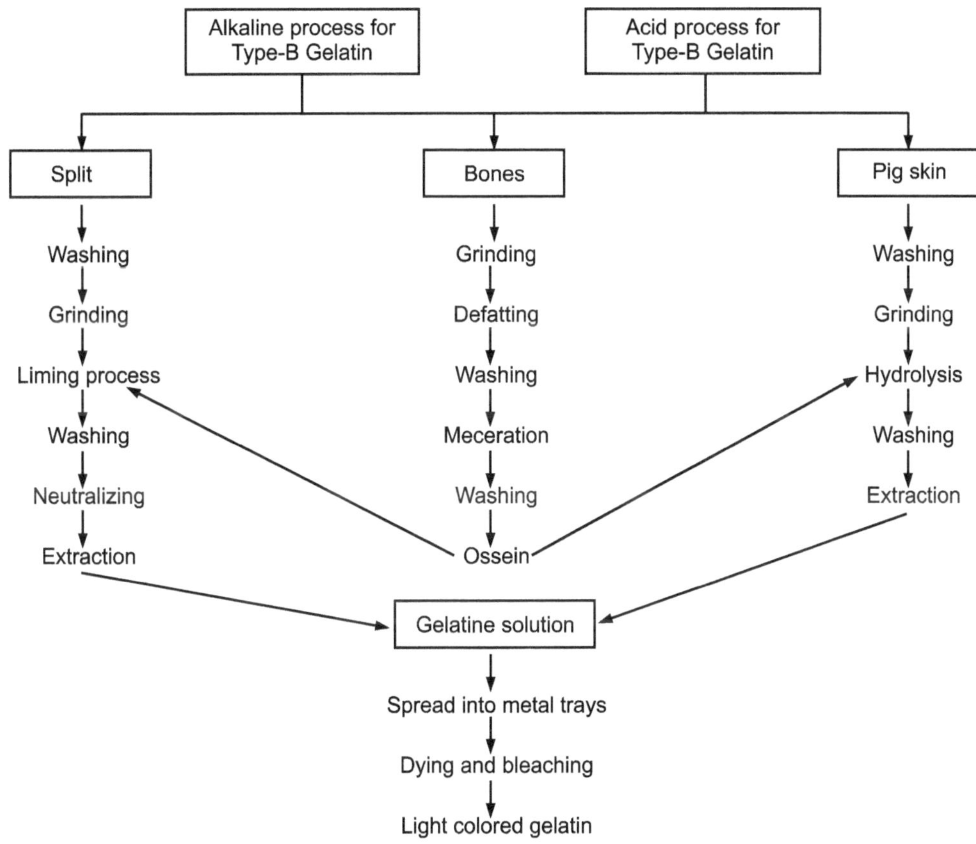

Fig. 5.18: Production of Gelatin

Physical Properties:

Appearance	:	Translucent, brittle when dried.
Colour	:	Colourless
Odour	:	None
Taste	:	Unpleasant
Solubility	:	Soluble in hot water, but forms gel when cooled. Insoluble in alcohol, ether
Stability	:	Stable in air, but in moisture condition it is degraded.
Extra feature	:	In cold water it swells and softens
Strength	:	Determined by bloom strength
		(Bloom is a test to measure the strength of gelatin. The test was originally developed and patented in 1925 by O.T. Bloom. The test determines the weight in gm, needed by a probe with a diameter of 0.5 inch to deflect the surface of the gel 4 mm without breaking it. The result is expressed in Bloom. It is usually between 30 and 300 Bloom).
Relative density	:	1.3 to 1.4
Isoionic point	:	5-9
Foaming property	:	Efficient foam stabilizer pH (1%) : 5
Moisture	:	16%

Chemical Constituents: Gelatin contains 98-99% protein by dry weight. Gelatin is unusually high in the non-essential amino acids like glycine (26%), proline (16%), hydroxyproline (14%), glutamic acid, alanine, arginine, aspartic acid, lysine, serine, baline, etc.

Chemical Tests:

1. Aqueous sample solution + Tannic acid = White precipitation
2. Aqueous sample solution + Picric acid = Yellow precipitation
3. Aqueous sample solution + Millon's reagent = White precipitation
4. Aqueous sample solution + Soda lime $\longrightarrow$ Ammonia gas evolves

Sterile Gelatin: They are of two types like absorbable gelatin sponge and absorbable gelatin film. Sterile gelatin sponges are sterile white products. They are absorbable and water-insoluble. They are prepared by warming gelatin solution to form foam and then dried and cut into small pieces. They are finally sterilized at 150°C, whereas absorbable gelatin film is light amber coloured and transparent. They are insoluble in water.

Uses: It is used in face masks, shampoos and other cosmetics; as a thickener for fruit gelatins and puddings, in candies, marshmallows, cakes, ice cream, and yogurts. It is used in preparation of bacteriological culture media. It is also used on photographic films, in vitamins as a coating and as capsules shells. Medically it is used for weight loss, treating osteoarthritis, rheumatoid arthritis and brittle bones (osteoporosis).

CASEIN

Casein is related to phosphoprotein. These proteins are commonly found in mammalian milk, making up 80% of the proteins in cow milk and between 20% and 45% of the proteins in human milk.

Isolation:

1. Specified amount of milk is kept in the flask and heated at 40°C in a water bath.
2. Few drops of glacial acetic acid are added and stirred.
3. The resultant mixture is filtered through filter paper held in a funnel and most of the liquid is gently squeezed out.
4. Casein and fat are removed from the cheesecloth, the solid is placed into a beaker and few ml of 95% ethanol is added.
5. Then it is stirred well to break up the product. The liquid is poured off and few ml of 1 : 1 ether-ethanol mixture is added to the solid.
6. It is stirred well and filtered through filer paper.
7. Solid is scraped into a weighed filter paper and then dried in the air.
8. The casein content is then calculated as follows:

$$\% \text{ Casein} = \frac{\text{gm of casein}}{\text{gm of milk}} \times 100$$

Normal Range is 3-5%.

Properties:

1. It is purified powder and yellow in colour.
2. It is found in milk as a suspension of particles called "casein micelles".
3. It is relatively hydrophobic.
4. It is poorly soluble in water and insoluble in neutral salt solution.

5. The caseins in the micelles are held together by calcium ions and hydrophobic interactions.
6. The isoelectric point of casein is 4.6.
7. It is readily dispersible in dilute alkalis and in salt solutions such as sodium oxalate and sodium acetate.
8. Melting point is 280°C.

Chemical Nature:

1. It is a phosphoprotein, which has phosphate groups attached to some of the amino acid side chains. Mostly these amino acids are serine and threonine.
2. Casein is made up of the main 3 types of proteins – alpha-casein, beta-casein and kappa-casein.
3. All casein proteins have different hydrophobic and hydrophilic regions along the protein chain.
4. Alpha-caseins are the major casein proteins. They contain 8-10 phosphate groups.
5. Beta-casein contains about 5 phosphate residues.
6. Beta-casein is more hydrophobic than alpha-caseins and kappa-casein.
7. Casein micelles consist of water, protein and salts.
8. Casein is present as a caseinate that binds primarily calcium and magnesium.

Uses: Casein is the major component of cheese. It is used as a food additive, binder for safety matches. As a food source, casein supplies amino acids, carbohydrates and the two inorganic elements calcium and phosphorus. Derivatives of Casein are used in tooth remineralization products to stabilize amorphous calcium phosphate. Casein peptides are used for high blood pressure, high cholesterol, anxiety, fatigue, epilepsy, intestinal disorders, cancer prevention and stress reduction.

5.4 PROTEOLYTIC ENZYMES

Enzymes are proteins that catalyze biochemical functions. They are required for various physiological processes. Proteolytic enzymes are also known as protease that digest proteins, i.e. breakdown of long chain of protein molecules into shorter peptides and their components such as amino acids. They act as digestive aids, blood cleansers, rebalance immune system and reduce oedema in inflamed region.

PAPAIN

Biological Source: It is obtained from green fruits of papaya, *Carica papaya*.

Family: Caricaceae

Characters:

- Commercial papain is buff to light brown powder.
- It is soluble in water and glycerol, but insoluble in most organic solvents.
- Commercial papain contains chymopapain, lysozyme, lipase, peptidase-A.
- It activates at pH 3-11.
- Its activity will retain at 70°C at pH 7.0.
- Optimum pH for papain activity is 5-7.
- Optimum temperature range is 60-70°C.

Chemical Composition:

- It is a sulfhydryl protease enzyme.
- It contains 212 amino acid residues with cysteine 25 bearing the essential active thiol groups.
- Isoeletric point at pH 8.75.
- Its molecular weight is 21,000 to 23,700 dalton.
- Its 3-D structure is identified by X-ray crystallography which shows presence of two parts, each part containing about 100 amino acid residues.
- It hydrolyses into proteins, peptides, amides and esters.

Activators: Glutathione, Cysteine, Bisulphite, Sulphide, Ammonium sulphate.

Inhibitors: Thiol reagents, Heavy metals ions like Zn^{+2}, Fe^{+2}, Ascorbic acid etc.

Uses: It is used as anti-inflammatory, anti-ulcer, wound healing, digestive aids, oedema, stabilizer etc.

Method of isolation: It has two steps: (a) Extraction of latex followed by (b) Latex to papain.

The method is as follows:

Method-I (Fig. 5.19):

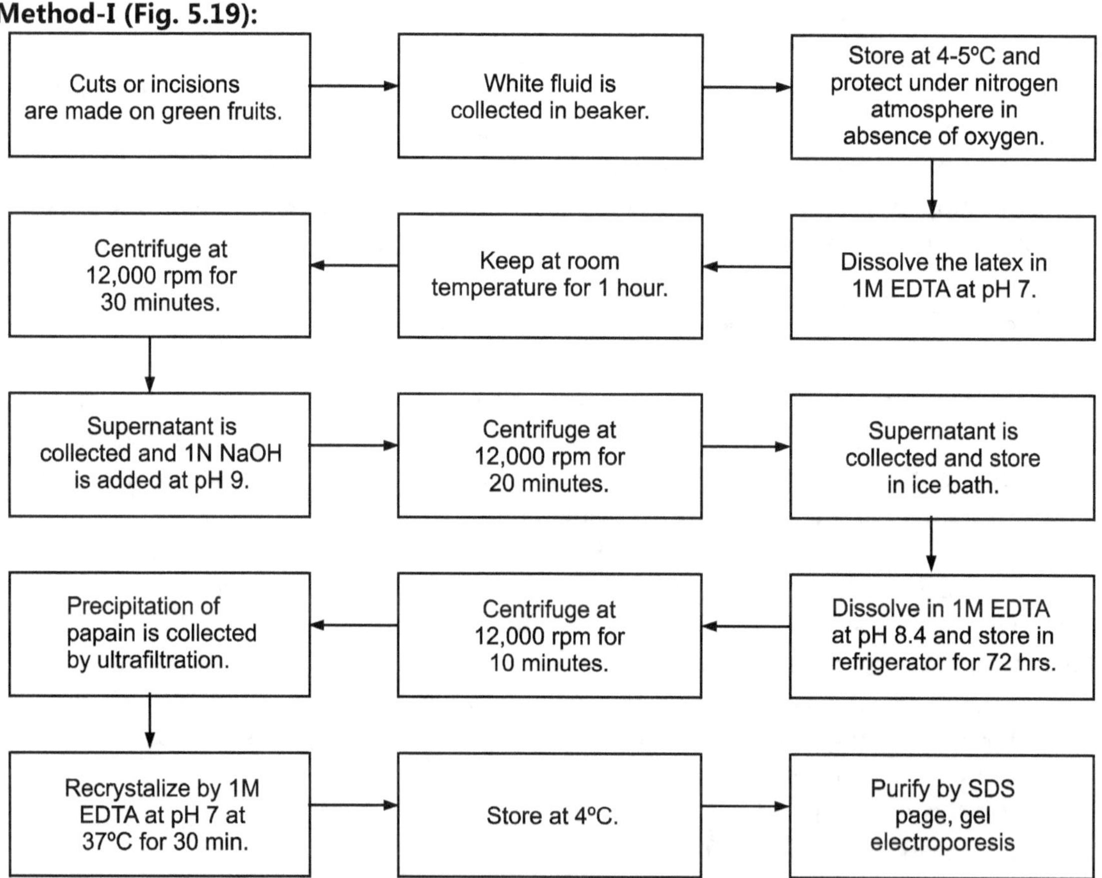

Fig. 5.19: Papain isolation from papaya fruit

Methods-II:

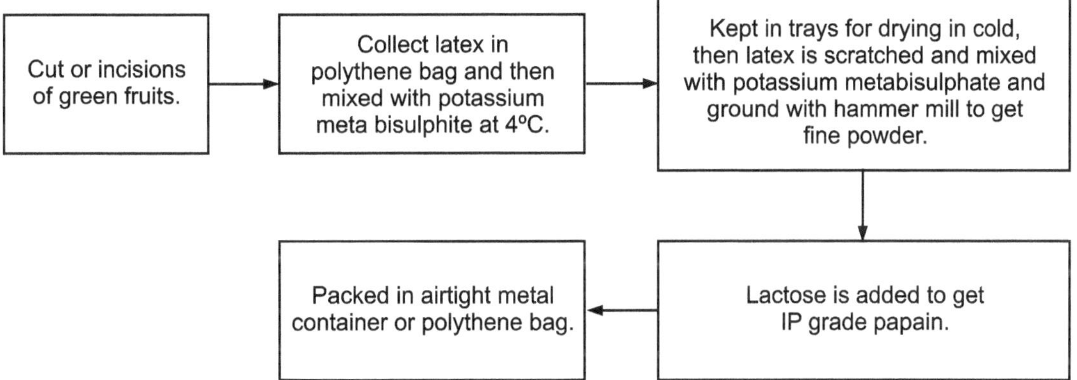

Fig. 5.20: Papain isolation method

Storage: Lyophillized powder or crystalline suspension of papain is stored in NaCl solution at near neutral pH at 4-5°C for 6 months.

BROMELAIN

Biological Source: It is obtained from stem and fruits of pine apple of *Ananus comosus*.

Family: Bromeliaceae.

Characters:

- It is sulphydryl proteolytic enzyme.
- It contains mixture of proteases and non-proteolytic enzymes like acid phosphatise, peroxidise etc.
- It is colourless.
- It is slightly soluble in water and glycerol, but insoluble in organic solvents.
- Optimum pH required is 5-8.
- Optimum temperature: 50-60°C.
- Molecular weight is 15000 to 18000 dalton.

Extraction (Fig. 5.21):

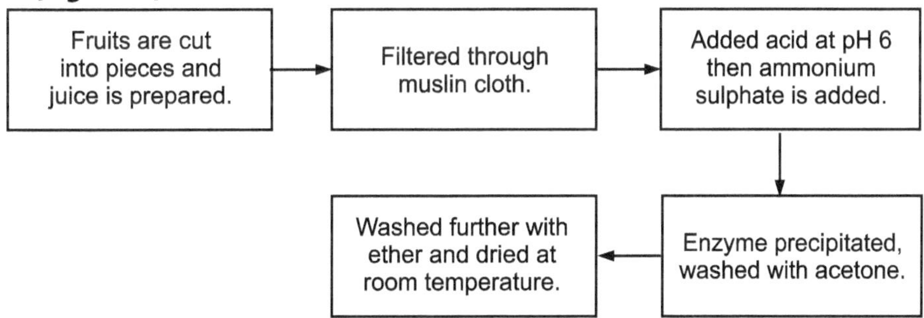

Fig. 5.21: Bromelain isolation method

Uses: It is used as digestive agent, in CVS diseases, Joint inflammation, arthritis etc.

SERRATIOPEPTIDASE

Serratiopeptidase is a proteolytic enzyme.

Biological Source: Non-pathogenic *enterobacterium Serratia marcescens* E-15. This microorganism was originally isolated in the late 1960s from silkworm *Bombyx mori*.

Family: Enterobacteriaceae.

Properties:

- It has high degree of substrate specificity.
- The molecular weight of Serrapeptase ranges from about 45 kDa – 60 kDa.
- It is a metalloprotease and contains three zinc atoms as ligands and one active site. The presence of zinc atom is essential and also enhances the proteolytic activity of Serrapeptase.
- The gene encoding Serrapeptase reveals that it is made up of 470 amino acids. The amino acid sequence is free of Sulphur containing amino acids, cysteine and methionine.
- The maximum enzyme activity of Serrapeptase is observed at pH 9.0 and at a temperature of 40°C.
- It is degraded or inactivated completely at a temperature of 55°C.
- It is an active enzyme that binds to the alpha-2 macroglobulin in biological fluids and in blood, it binds in the ratio of 1 : 1 and this binding helps to mask its antigenicity.
- The doses usually range from 10 mg to 60 mg per day.

Production: The production of Serrapeptase depends upon a secretory protein on the membrane of the host cell and it is secreted by the N-terminal signal peptide-independent pathway.

Soil and contaminated water are a rich source of a diverse variety of microorganisms. Isolated pure cultures of the bacterial strains are maintained on nutrient agar plates and stored at 4°C. *Serratia marcescens* is a Gram-negative bacterium. It grows in a wide range of temperatures (5-40°C) and pH (5.0-9.0) and secretes a variety of enzymes such as serine and thiol proteases, metalloproteases, lipases, chitinases etc.

Medium Preparation (Fig. 5.22): *Serratia marcescens* are usually cultured in trypticase soy broth. A medium containing carbon source - maltose, organic nitrogen source - peptone, inorganic nitrogen source - ammonium sulphate, dihydrogen phosphate, sodium bicarbonate, inorganic salt source - sodium acetate, glycerin and ascorbic acid is used as a production medium.

Another medium reported for production of Serrapeptase contained maltose 45 g/lit, soybean meal 65 g/lit, KH_2PO_4 8.0 g/lit, and NaCl 5.0 g/lit at a pH 7.0 which gives maximum yield. Casein medium is also used, but trypticase soy is a preferred substrate over casein as the specific activity is higher when trypticase soy is used as the substrate in the production medium.

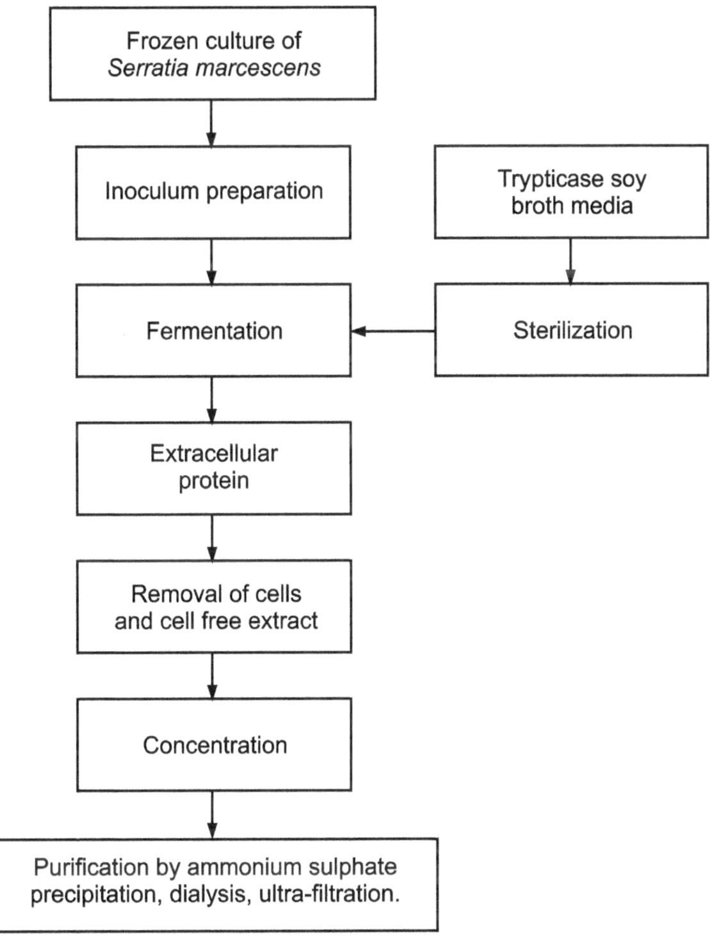

Fig. 5.22: Industrial production of Serratiopeptidase

Uses: It is used to reduce pain and swelling associated with conditions like back pain, arthritis, tension headaches and migraine headaches. It also has anti-atherosclerotic effects due to its fibrinolytic and caseinolytic properties.

UROKINASE

Biological Source: It is obtained from human urine.

Characters: They are plasminogen activator and are obtained from human renal cells. They are serine protease enzymes. Urokinase is a 411-residue protein, consisting of the domains: the serine protease domain, the kringle domain and the growth factor domain. Urokinase is synthesized as a zymogen form and is activated by proteolytic cleavage between Lys 158 and Ile 159. The two resulting chains are kept together by a disulphide bond.

Isolation (Fig. 5.23):

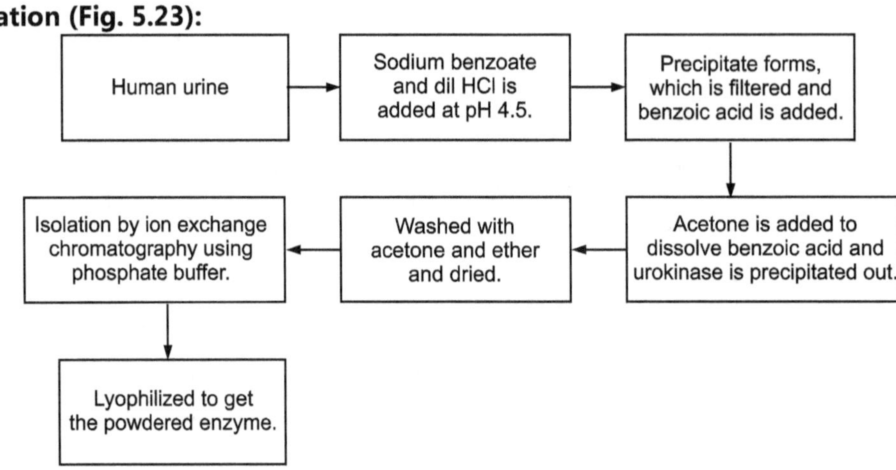

Fig. 5.23: Urokinase isolation

Uses: It is thrombolytic agent, used in treatment of severe or massive deep venous thrombosis, pulmonary embolism, myocardial infarction and dialysis cannulas. It is used intrapleurally to improve the drainage of complicated pleural effusions and empyemas.

STREPTOKINASE

Biological Source: It is obtained from the bacteria *Beta haemolytic streptococci*.

Family: Streptococcaceae.

Characters: It is white powder, soluble in water. Optimum pH range is 7-8. It is extracellular enzyme containing single chain polypeptide. Molar mass is 47 kDa. It is made up of 414 amino acid residues. The protein exhibits its maximum activity at a pH of 7.5 and its isoelectric pH is 4.7.

Isolation (Fig. 5.24):

Medium Composition: Casein solution, potassium dihydrogen phosphate, lysine, dextrose, uracil, adenine sulphate, nicotinic acid, pyridoxine, tryptophan, calcium pentothenate, thiamine-HCl, riboflavin, thioglycollic acid and some salts of trace elements.

Procedure:

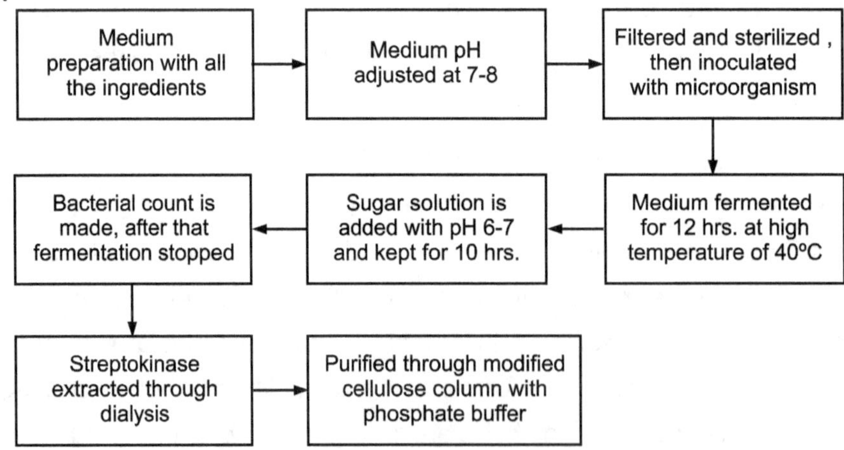

Fig. 5.24: Extraction of streptokinase

Uses: It is used as thrombolytic medication, in case of blood clot in myocardial infarction, treatment of burns, respiratory problems etc.

Storage: The enzyme is supplied as a lyophilized white powder in 50 ml infusion bottles or in 6.5 ml vials with a coloured label and is stored in room temperature of 15-30°C.

PEPSIN

Biological Source: Pepsin is the principal proteolytic enzyme of vertebrate gastric juice.

Properties:

- It is an endopeptidase enzyme.
- It is buff coloured or white coloured amorphous powder.
- It has little acidic or saline taste with slight meaty odour.
- It is soluble in water but insoluble in alcohol, ether and chloroform.
- It breaks down proteins into peptones and proteases.
- Molecular weight of Pepsin: 34.5 kDa
- Pepsin is a monomeric, two domain, mainly beta protein with a high percentage of acidic residues.
- It is produced in the stomach and is one of the main digestive enzymes in the digestive system.
- It has three-dimensional structure, of which one or more polypeptide chains twist and fold, bringing together a small number of amino acids to form the active site.
- It is an aspartic protease, using a catalytic aspartate in its active site.
- It is efficient in cleaving peptide bonds between hydrophobic and aromatic amino acids such as phenylalanine, tryptophan and tyrosine.
- Pepsinogen is the proenzyme of pepsin.
- Pepsin is most active in acidic environments between 37 °C and 42 °C.
- Its primary site of synthesis and activity is in the stomach (pH 1.5 to 2).
- Pepsin exhibits maximal activity at pH 2.0 and is inactive at pH 6.5.
- Optimal pH: 1.0-4.0
- Isoelectric Point: 1.0
- There are four reported pepsin proteins: pepsin A, pepsin B (parapepsin I), pepsin C (gastricsin), and pepsin D (an unphosphorylated version of pepsin A).

Preparation: It is prepared by using stomach linings. The mucous membrane is separated from the stomach by stripping process. Then minced stomach linings are digested with hydrochloric acid for autolysis at 37°C for 2 hours. The liquid sample contains pepsin and peptone. Then the sample is subjected to dialysis and concentrated through vacuum evaporation. The spongy pepsin is obtained.

Activator: Pepsinogen.

Inhibitor: Pepstatin is a low molecular weight compound and potent inhibitor specific for acid proteases with a Ki value of about 10^{-10} M for pepsin. Sucralfate also inhibits pepsin activity.

Specificity: Pepsin has broad specificity for peptides containing linkages with aromatic or carboxylic L-amino acids. It preferentially cleaves C-terminal to Phe and Leu and to a lesser extent Glu linkages. The enzyme does not cleave at Val, Ala, or Gly.

Uses:
- Digestion of antibodies.
- Preparation of collagen for cosmeceutical purposes.
- Assessment of digestibility of proteins in food chemistry.
- Subculture of viable mammary epithelial cells.

Storage: Pepsins should be stored at very low temperatures (between −80°C and −20°C) to prevent autolysis.

5.5 LIPIDS (WAXES, FATS, FIXED OILS)

5.5.1 Lipid

Lipids are the structural and functional building blocks of the living cells and they are made up of hydrocarbons with highly reduced form of carbon. Chemically they are heterogenous group of compounds related to fatty acids.

Examples: Fats, oils, waxes etc.

Source of Lipid: Lipids are a wide-ranging group of organic compounds found in all living organisms, including humans, plants and other animals. Lipids exist in tissues in many different physical forms. The simple lipids are often part of large aggregates in storage tissues, such as oil bodies or adipose tissue. Membranes are constituted with complex lipids and occur in a close association with such compounds as proteins and polysaccharides. In plants, lipids are stored in the form of triglycerides. The most known of these is jojoba, which stores its seed lipid as a liquid wax. Storage lipids are accumulated in one or both of the main types of seed tissue and endosperm. In oilseeds such as sunflower, linseed or rapeseed, the cotyledons of the embryo are the major sites of lipid accumulation. The endosperm of castor bean, coriander or carrot, is the main site of lipid accumulation. In tobacco, both embryo and endosperm tissues store lipids. Phospholipids are another class of lipids which are found in animal and plant cell membranes.

Properties:
1. They are hydrophobic or amphiphilic compounds.
2. They are insoluble in water, but soluble in organic solvents like chloroform.
3. When metabolized, lipids are oxidized to release large amounts of energy and thus are useful to living organisms.

Chemistry of Lipids:
1. Lipids are organic compounds formed mainly from alcohol and fatty acids combined together by ester linkage.
2. They are hydrophobic small molecules consisting of two biochemical subunits like keto acyl (Polyketides) and isoprene (C_5H_8) (Sterol lipids and Prenol lipids).
3. Triglycerides are the most commonly occurring class of lipids.
4. Triglycerides have a glycerol backbone bonded to three fatty acids.
5. Phospholipids also contain glycerol and fatty acids, plus phosphoric acid and a low-molecular-weight alcohol.
6. Common phospholipids include lecithins and cephalins.
7. The tail of fatty acid is a long hydrocarbon chain, which is hydrophobic, and the head of the molecule is a carboxyl group, which is hydrophilic in nature.

Functions:

1. Lipids are important sources of metabolic energy (ATP). They are the most energy rich of all classes of nutrients.
2. They form the structural components of cell membranes and form various messengers and signalling molecules within the body.
3. Lipids serve as biological carriers for the absorption of fat-soluble vitamins A, D, E and K.
4. Lipids are a source of essential fatty acids, which are required for optimal lipid transport and are precursors of the prostaglandin hormones.
5. Lipids function as a mechanical support for the vital body organs.
6. Lipids are a source of essential steroids, which in turn perform a wide range of important biological functions.
7. Lipids also act as lubricants for the passage of feed through pellet diet.
8. Lipids are applied in the cosmetic and nanotechnology.

Classification of Lipids:

Lipids are broadly classified into three groups. They are listed in Fig. 5.25.

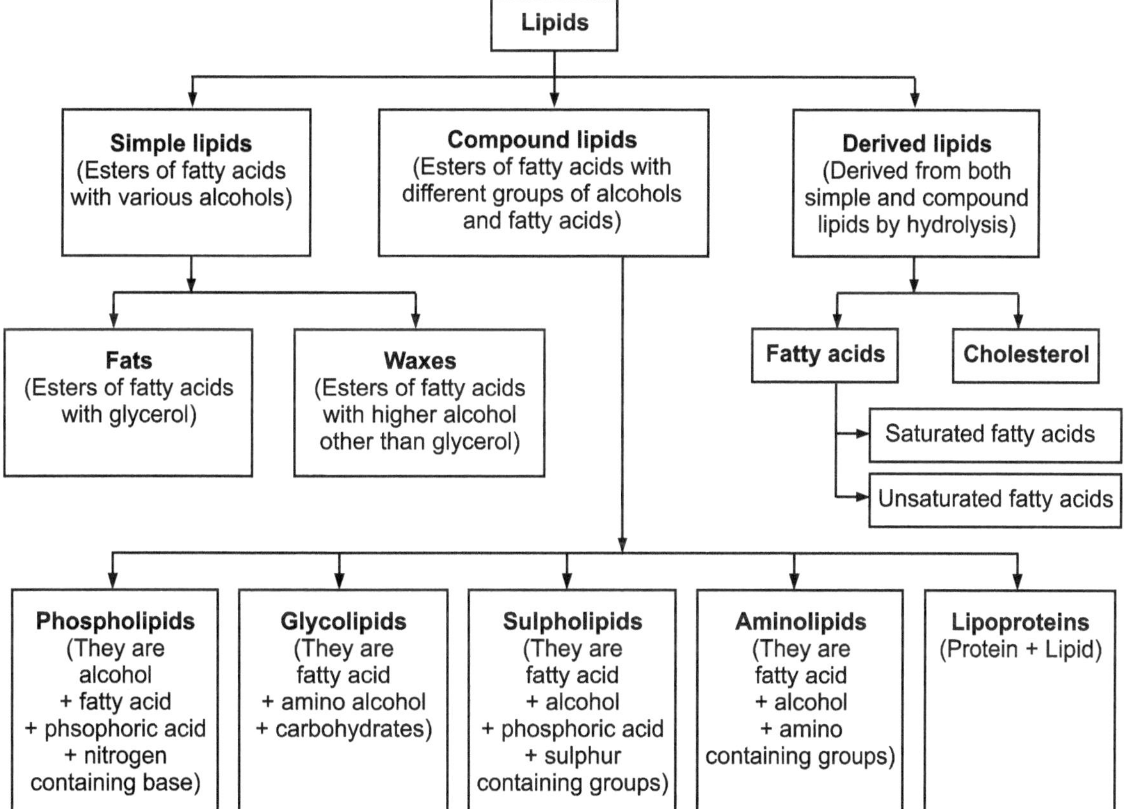

Fig. 5.25: Classification of lipids

5.5.2 Fatty Acids

They are long chain carboxylic acids and may or may not contain C-C double bonds. The hydrocarbon chain length may vary from 10-30 carbons. They are important component of lipids and are present in plants, animals and microorganisms. Generally, fatty acid is unbranched with an even number of carbon atoms, with hydrogen atoms along the length of the chain and at one end of the chain, and a carboxyl group (–COOH) at the other end. Commonly they exist in combination with the alcohol glycerol in the form of triglyceride.

The most widely distributed fatty acid is oleic acid, which is abundant in some vegetable oils like olive, palm, peanut, and sunflower seed. There are two groups of fatty acids viz. saturated and unsaturated. Unsaturated fatty acids contain one or more double bonds between carbons as in alkenes, whereas saturated fatty acids contain all bonding positions between carbons occupied by hydrogens. Saturated fats are typically solids and are derived from animals, while unsaturated fats are liquids and usually extracted from plants.

Some examples of saturated and unsaturated fatty acids:

Table 5.3

Unsaturated Fatty Acids	Chemical Structure
Oleic acid	$CH_3(CH_2)_7\ CH=CH(CH_2)_7COOH$
Linoleic acid	$CH_3(CH_4)_2CH=CHCH\ CH=CH(CH_2)_7COOH$
Palmitoleic acid	$CH_3(CH_2)_5CH=CH(CH_2)_7COOH$

Table 5.4

Saturated Fatty Acids	Chemical Structure
Myristic acid	$CH_3(CH_2)_{12}COOH$
Palmitic acid	$CH_3(CH_2)_{14}COOH$
Stearic acid	$CH_3(CH_2)_{16}COOH$

Essential Fatty Acids: Fatty acids that are required by the human body but cannot be made in sufficient quantity from other substrates, and therefore must be obtained from food are called essential fatty acids. Two essential fatty acids are linoleic acid (LA) and alpha-linolenic acid (ALA). They are widely distributed in plant oils. The human body has a limited ability to convert ALA into the longer-chain n-3 fatty acids eicosapentaenoic acid (EPA) and docosahexaenoic acid (DHA).

Waxes/Fats and Oils: Waxes are a class of organic compounds that are malleable near ambient temperatures and are synthetic and naturally occurring lipids. They melt above 45°C to give a low viscous liquid. They are insoluble in water, but soluble in organic, non-polar solvents. These are esters with long-chain carboxylic acids and long-alcohols. The esters in waxes are more resistant to saponification than glycerides of oils and fats. Waxes are synthesized by many plants and animals. The most commonly known animal wax is beeswax and others are spermaceti, wool fat etc. Plants secrete waxes into and on the surface of their cuticles to control evaporation, wettability and hydration, e.g., carnauba wax and Japan wax. Some are obtained from the mineral sources like hard paraffin, Ceresin etc.

Fats and oils are esters of the tri-alcohol, glycerol (or glycerine). Therefore, fats and oils are commonly called triglycerides, although a more accurate name is triacylglycerols. One of the reactions of triglycerides is hydrolysis of the ester groups. Fat plays an important role in human health. They are solid or semisolid in room temperature and are mainly present in animals. Chemically, they are triglycerides, trimesters of glycerol and other fatty acids. There are mainly three types of fats; saturated fats which increase blood cholesterol, mono- and polyunsaturated fats, which lowers the blood cholesterol, and the trans fats which are used to make baked products. Omega-6- and omega-3 fats are beneficial to human health. For example, edible animal fats are lard, fish oil, butter, ghee etc. They are obtained from fats in the milk and meat, as well as from under the skin of an animal. Edible plant fats are peanut, soya bean, sunflower, sesame, coconut and olive oils, and cocoa butter.

Oils are fats that are liquid at room temperature. They are obtained from various plants and fishes. They provide essential nutrients. Chemically they are triglycerides. Some of the edible oils are canola oil, corn oil, olive oil, sunflower oil etc.

Lipid extraction from Plant Tissue: Plant tissues are difficult to extract because of active lipases which hydrolyze rapidly phospholipids, glycolipids and increase the amount of free fatty acids in the extract. Hence organic solvent like isopropanol is used to inhibit these enzymes.

Nichols' Method: Plant tissues are coarsely powdered and macerated with 100 parts (w/w) of isopropanol. The mixture is filtered and then the solid is extracted again with 200 parts of chloroform and isopropanol mixture (1 : 1, v/v). The combined filtrates are evaporated, dissolved in a small volume of chloroform and methanol (2 : 1, v/v) and washed to get the lipid.

Methods of Analysis:

1. **Determination of Moisture Content:**

Moisture content of oils and fats is the loss in mass of the sample on heating at $105 \pm 1°C$ under operating conditions specified.

Procedure: Weigh in a previously dried and tared dish about 5-10 g of oil or fat which has been thoroughly mixed by stirring. Loosen the lid of the dish and heat in an oven at $105 \pm 1°C$ for 1 hour. Remove the dish from the oven and close the lid. Cool in a desiccator containing phosphorus pentoxide or equivalent dessicant and weigh. Heat in the oven for a further period of 1 hour, cool and weigh. Repeat this process until change in weight between two successive observations does not exceed 1 mg. Carry out the determination in duplicate

$$\text{Moisture and Volatile Matter} = \frac{W_1 \times 100}{W}$$

where, W_1 = Loss in gm of material on drying; W = Weight in gm of material taken

2. **Determination of Specific Gravity:**

Melt sample if necessary. Filter through a filter paper to remove any impurities and the last traces of moisture. Make sure that the sample is completely dry. Cool the sample to 30°C or ambient temperature desired for determination.

Procedure: Fill the dry pycnometer with the prepared sample in such a manner to prevent entrapment of air bubbles after removing the cap of the side arm. Insert the stopper, immerse in water bath at $30°C \pm 0.2°C$ and hold for 30 minutes. Carefully wipe off any oil that has come out of the capillary opening. Remove the bottle from the bath, clean and dry it thoroughly. Remove the cap of the side arm and quickly weigh ensuring that the temperature does not fall below 30°C.

$$\text{Specific gravity at } 30°C = \frac{A - B}{C - B}$$

where A = Weight in gm of specific gravity bottle with oil at 30°C

B = Weight in gm of specific gravity bottle at 30°C

C = Weight in gm of specific gravity bottle with water at 30°C

3. Determination of Saponification Value:

The saponification value is the number of mg of potassium hydroxide required to saponify 1 gm of oil/fat.

Principle: The oil sample is saponified by refluxing with a known excess of alcoholic potassium hydroxide solution. The alkali required for saponification is determined by titration of the excess potassium hydroxide with standard hydrochloric acid.

Significance: The saponification value is an index of mean molecular weight of the fatty acids of glycerides comprising a fat. Lower the saponification value, larger the molecular weight of fatty acids in the glycerides and vice-versa.

Procedure: Melt the sample if it is not already liquid and filter through a filter paper to remove any impurities and the last traces of moisture. Make sure that the sample is completely dry. Mix the sample thoroughly and weigh about 1.5 to 2.0 g of dry sample into a 250 ml Erlenmeyer flask. Pipette 25 ml of the alcoholic potassium hydroxide solution into the flask. Conduct a blank determination along with the sample. Connect the sample flasks and the blank flask with air condensers, keep on the water bath, and boil gently but steadily until saponification is complete, as indicated by absence of any oily matter and appearance of clear solution. Clarity may be achieved within one hour of boiling. After the flask and condenser have cooled somewhat, wash down the inside of the condenser with about 10 ml of hot ethyl alcohol neutral to phenolphthalein. Titrate the excess potassium hydroxide with 0.5 N hydrochloric acid, using about 1.0 ml phenolphthalein indicator.

$$\text{Saponification value} = \frac{56.1 \, (B - S) \, N}{W}$$

where, B = Volume in ml of standard hydrochloric acid required for the blank.

       S = Volume in ml of standard hydrochloric acid required for the sample.

      N = Normality of the standard hydrochloric acid and

      W = Weight in gm of the oil/fat taken for the test

4. Determination of Acid Value:

The acid value is defined as the number of milligrams of potassium hydroxide required to neutralize the free fatty acids present in one gm of fat. It is a relative measure of rancidity as free fatty acids are normally formed during decomposition of oil glycerides. The value is also expressed as per cent of free fatty acids calculated as oleic acid.

Principle: The acid value is determined by directly titrating the oil/fat in an alcoholic medium against standard potassium hydroxide/sodium hydroxide solution.

Significance: The value is a measure of the amount of fatty acids which have been liberated by hydrolysis from the glycerides due to the action of moisture, temperature and/or lypolytic enzyme lipase.

Procedure: Mix the oil or melted fat thoroughly before weighing. Weigh accurately about 5 to 10 g of cooled oil sample in a 250 ml conical flask and add 50 ml to 100 ml of freshly neutralized hot ethyl alcohol and about one ml of phenolphthalein indicator solution. Boil the mixture for about five minutes and titrate while hot against standard alkali solution shaking vigorously during the titration. The weight of the oil/fat taken for the estimation and the strength of the alkali used for titration shall be such that the volume of alkali required for the titration does not exceed 10 ml.

$$\text{Acid value} = \frac{56.1 \, VN}{W}$$

where, V = Volume in ml of standard potassium hydroxide or sodium hydroxide used.

N = Normality of the potassium hydroxide solution or sodium hydroxide solution;

W = Weight in g of the sample

5. Determination of Iodine Value:

The iodine value of an oil/fat is the number of gm of iodine absorbed by 100 g of the oil/fat, when determined by using Wij's solution.

Principle: The oil/fat sample taken in carbon-tetrachloride is treated with a known excess of iodine monochloride solution in glacial acetic acid (Wij's solution). The excess of iodine monochloride is treated with potassium iodide and the liberated iodine estimated by titration with sodium thiosulphate solution.

Significance: The iodine value is a measure of the amount of unsaturation (number of double bonds) in a fat.

Procedure: Weigh accurately an appropriate quantity of the dry oil/fat into a 500 ml conical flask with glass stopper, to which 25 ml of carbon tetrachloride have been added. Mix the contents well. The weight of the sample shall be such that there is an excess of 50 to 60% of Wij's solution over that actually needed. Pipette 25 ml of Wij's solution and replace the glass stopper after wetting with potassium iodine solution. Swirl for proper mixing and keep the flasks in dark for half an hour for non-drying and semi-drying oils and one hour for drying oils. Carry out a blank simultaneously. After standing, add 15 ml of potassium iodide solution, followed by 100 ml of recently boiled and cooled water, rinsing in the stopper also. Titrate liberated iodine with standardized sodium thiosulphate solution, using starch as indicator at the end until the blue colour formed disappears after thorough shaking with the stopper on. Blank sample is also conducted as per the same manner.

Calculation:

$$\text{Iodine value} = \frac{1.69 \, (B - S) \, N}{W}$$

where, B = Volume in ml of standard sodium thiosulphate solution required for the blank

S = Volume in ml of standard sodium thiosulphate solution required for the sample

N = Normality of the standard sodium thiosulphate solution.

W = Weight in g of the sample

Classification of Oils and Fats:

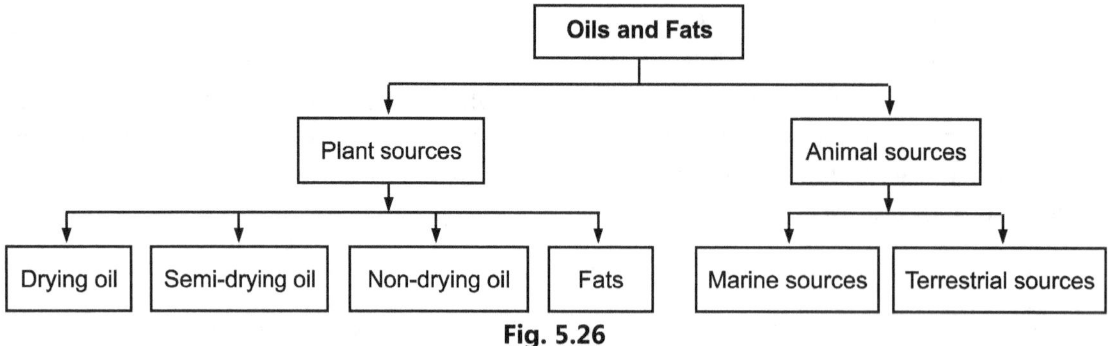

Fig. 5.26

Plant Source Oils and Fats:

Drying oil: Linseed oil, Hemp oil.

Semi drying oil: Mustard oil, Castor oil, Cottonseed oil.

Non-drying oil: Olive oil, Almond oil, Rice bran oil.

Fat: Cocoa butter, Palm oil, coconut oil.

Animal Source Oils and Fats:

Marine source oils: Cod liver oil, Shark liver oil, Spermaceti.

Marine source fats: Bone tallow.

Terrestrial source oils: Lard oil.

Terrestrial source fats: Butter, Tallow Lard.

Carbohydrate related Drugs:

CASTOR OIL

Castor oil is also known as Ricinus oil.

Biological Source: It is fixed oil, obtained from the seed of *Ricinus communis*.

Family: Euphorbiaceae.

Distribution: The castor bean is considered native to tropical Africa and is grown particularly in arid and semiarid regions. The plant is cultivated in different countries of the world. India, China, Brazil, Ethiopia, Paraguay, Vietnam and Thailand are the major castor growing countries. In India, the major cultivated zones are Andhra Pradesh, Gujarat, Karnataka and Punjab.

Production of Oil: Castor beans contain about 30-55% oil. It is extracted by two processes viz. pressing and solvent extraction. The extraction and commercialization of oils from castor seeds is carried out extensively for the oil, because there exist a range of free fatty acid contents of the oil due to geographical origin and the method of extraction. Castor oil is extracted from castor beans by cold expression method either by mechanical pressing or solvent extraction or combination of the two. In mechanical pressing, the seeds are crushed and then adjusted to low moisture content by warming in a steam-jacketed vessel. Then, the crushed seeds are loaded into a hydraulic press (1-2 tonnes) and pressed by mechanical means to extract oil. The extracted oil contains lipase enzyme and some toxic protein like ricin, are destroyed by steaming (75-85°C). The resulting oil has a light colour, low free fatty acids and other impurities. Mechanical pressing recovers only about 45% of oil from the beans and the remainder in the cake can be recovered by solvent extraction.

In solvent extraction method, the crushed seeds are extracted with any one of the solvents like heptane, hexane and petroleum ethers in a Soxhlet extractor or commercial extractor, followed by refining. Refining is essential to remove impurities such as colloidal matter, free fatty acid, colouring matter and other undesirable constituents that make oil less resistance to deterioration during storage. Before extraction, the castor beans are cleaned by hand, followed by drying in shed or hot air oven (90°C) to remove moisture. Then the seed coats are separated and finally seeds are crushed to a required uniform sieve size by mortar and pestle and the sample is placed in the thimble and inserted in the centre of the Soxhlet extractor for extraction of oil. After extraction refining of castor oil is carried out with degumming, neutralization, de-waxing, deodorization and bleaching. With this method the oil recovery is around 50-52% which is higher than mechanical process. Cold-pressed castor oil has low acid and iodine values, but slightly higher saponification value compared to solvent extracted oil.

Physical Properties of Oil:

Type	:	Fixed oil.
Colour	:	Pale yellow to colourless.
Odour	:	Soft and faint.
Taste	:	Highly unpleasant.
Solubility	:	Soluble in alcohol, organic solvents like benzene, chloroform but insoluble in other mineral oils.

Physical Standards:

Density (Wt/ml)	:	$0.945 - 0.965 \ g/cm^3$
Acid value	:	Not more than 2
Flash point	:	229.4°C
Refractive index	:	1.473 - 1.477
Saponification value	:	176 - 187
Iodine value	:	81 - 90
Acetyl value	:	Not less than 142
Viscosity	:	6.8 poises
Optical rotation	:	Between +3.5° and + 6.0°

Chemical Constituents: The oil is made up of triglycerides of 91-95% ricinoleic acid, 4-5% linoleic acid, and 1-2% palmitic and stearic acids. The viscosity mainly depends on the presence of ricinoleic acid (95%). Apart from that Oleic acid (6%), Linolenic acid (5%), stearic acid and palmitic acid are also present.

Ricinoleic acid

Chemical Tests:

1. Castor oil is missible with half its volume of light petroleum ether at 55°C.
2. An equal proportion of oil and ethanol gives clear liquid even after storage of 3-4 hours; there will be no change in clarity.

Uses:

(a) Industrial Applications: In the textile industry, castor oil is used for moisturizing and removal of grease in fabrics, and for the manufacturing of waterproof fabrics. In the steel industry, it is used in cutting oils and lubricants for steel lamination at high temperatures and it is also used in other liquids that are necessary for steel work. The automotive industry uses castor oil for the production of high performance motor oil and braking fluids, in the production of fluids for hydraulic devices, artificial leather, varnish, paint, linoleum, insulators, powder, fatty acids, enzymes as a moisturizer for stationary.

(b) Medicinal Uses: Castor oil, seeds, leaves and roots have numerous medicinal importance. Mainly the oil is used as laxative. Besides, these are utilized in peritonitis, diarrhea, dysentery, lumbago, constipation, piles, paralysis, sciatica, boils, asthma, dropsy, leprosy, arthritis, amenorrhoea backache, rheumatoid arthritis, ano-rectal problems, burning feet, period pain, sores, boils, chest, back or abdomen pain, headache, broken tooth, joint pains, pelvis pain, uterine pain, dermatitis, eczema, lactation, nodules in breasts etc. Ricinoleic acid, the active constituent of the oil, is effective against growth of various species of viruses, bacteria, yeasts and molds.

<h2 style="text-align:center">CHAULMOOGRA OIL</h2>

It is also known as Hydnocarpus oil.

Biological Source: It is a fixed oil obtained from the seeds of the plant *Taraktogenos kurzii, Hydnocarpus anthelmintica, H. pentandrus.*

Family: Flacourtriceae.

Distribution: The tree is native to South-East Asia, chiefly in Indo Malayan region, cultivated in Sri Lanka, Nigeria and Uganda. In India, it grows in tropical forests along western Ghats, along the coast in Maharashtra, Kerala, Assam and Tripura.

Description: The tree grows to a height of 12–15 m in India. The trees bear fruits in August and September. Bark is brownish, fissured; blaze pinkish. Branch lets are round, minutely velvet-hairy. Leaves are simple, alternate, usually oblong to elliptic-oblong, tip long-pointed, often falling off, base narrow. Flowers are greenish white. Berry is woody, round and black when young. Flowering takes place from January to April. The fruits are ovoid, 10 cm in diameter, with a thick woody rind. Internally they contain 10-16 black seeds embedded in the fruit pulp. A typical tree produces 20 kg of seeds/annum. The kernels make up 60–70% of the seed weight and contain 63% of pale yellow oil.

Extraction of Oil: Generally the oil is extracted from the ripe seed by cold expression method through hydraulic press. Fruits are peeled by knife and seeds are washed in water and dried in sun. Seeds are decorticated by millet, hand hammers or by decoricator. Kernels yield 43 – 48% oil in ghani. The kernel is also crushed in expeller and rotary. Extracted oil is stored in zinc barrels and exported.

Physical Properties:

Colour	:	Yellow
Odour	:	Characteristic
Taste	:	Acrid
Solubility	:	Soluble in organic solvents like chloroform, benzene, alcohol etc.
State	:	White solid below 25°C and soft.
Refractive index, at 40°C	:	1.472 - 1.476
Iodine value	:	98 - 103
Sap value	:	198 - 204
Acid value	:	Not more than 10
Density	:	0.935 - 0.960
Specific rotation	:	+46° to +60°

Chemistry: Gas liquid chromatography analysis has revealed the presence of following fatty acids like hydnocarpic acid (48-50%), chaulmoogric acid (26-30%), gorlic acid, myristic acid, palmitic acid, stearic acid, oleic acid, linoleic acid, linolenic acid etc.

$$CH = CH$$
$$CH(CH_2)_nCOOH$$
$$CH_2 - CH_2$$

where, n = 10 for Hydnocarpic acid, n = 12 for Chaulmoogric acid

Uses: Mainly the oil is useful against psoriasis, eczema and other skin disorders when applied to the skin. It is useful against T.B, leprosy, rheumatism when given intravenously. The oil is used up to 15% in medicated soap.

Substitution: The original oil is sometimes substituted with the oil obtained from *Hydnocarpus wightiana, H. alpine* which are abundantly available in Eastern and Southern parts of India.

WOOL FAT

Common Name: Lanolin, purified wool fat.

Biological Source: It is a yellow waxy substance secreted by the sebaceous glands of wool bearing animals like sheeps, *Ovis aries*.

Family: Bovidae.

Geographical Location: Commercially it is prepared in New Zealand, Australia, USA and India.

Method of Preparation: Sheep's wool contains about 45% of a fat known as suint, which must be removed. Crude lanolin is separated by washing with sulphuric acid and then purified and bleached. The product is known as anhydrous lanolin or wool fat. Further the hydrous wool fat is produced by intimately mixing wool fat with 30% of water.

Physical Properties:

Colour	:	Whitish yellow
Odour	:	Characteristic
Taste	:	Bland

Solubility	:	Insoluble in water but forms turbidity with ether and chloroform
Melting-point	:	40° to 44.4°C
Saponification value	:	92 - 106
Iodine value	:	18 - 35
Acid value	:	Less than 1

Chemical Constituents: Wool fat contains the alcohols, cholesterol and isocholesterol, together with various esters. Hydrous wool fat also contains the acids in combination with lanoceric, lanopalmitic, carnaubic, myristic, oleic, cerotic and palmitic acids. It contains 50% of water.

Cholesterol

Chemical Tests:

- 1 g of wool fat is boiled with 20 ml of alcohol and the solution is filtered and cooled, the filtrate should not be rendered turbid by the addition of a 5% alcoholic solution of silver nitrate. This indicates the absence of chlorides.
- 1 g of the fat is dissolved in 3 or 4 ml of acetic anhydride and few drops of sulphuric acid are added. An initial pink colour changes to green and then finally blue. This indicates the presence of cholesterol.
- When a 2% solution in chloroform is gently poured over the surface of concentrated sulphuric acid, it gradually develops a purple-red colouration at the junction of the liquids.
- 10 g of wool fat is heated with 50 ml of water on a water-bath. The aqueous layer on filtration should not yield glycerin on evaporation, and when boiled with potassium hydroxide should not evolve the odour of ammonia. This indicates the absence of nitrogenous organic matter.

Uses: It is used as a moisturizer to treat dry, rough, scaly, itchy skin and in minor skin irritations. It is mainly used as water absorbable ointment base. Lanolin is often used as a raw material for producing cholecalciferol using irradiation (vitamin D).

BEESWAX

Common Name: Yellow beeswax, Cera-flava.

Biological Source: It is a purified wax obtained from the honey comb of the bee species, *Apis mellifera.*

Family: Apidae.

Preparation of Beeswax: Two wax extraction methods are generally used — melting and chemical extraction. Melting is the most frequently used procedure. Wax can be melted by boiling water, by steam, or by electrical or solar power. Chemical extraction by solvents is feasible only in a laboratory, where small scale wax production is needed. Good wax solvents are gasoline and xylene. The disadvantage of this method is that all organic wax contaminants and constituents of the pupae, propolis and pollen are dissolved. Thus the quality of wax is impaired.

The combs of honey comb are broken and boiled in soft water and is kept for some time in water by enclosing in porous bag. After some time the wax oozes out from the bag and forms a cake which is collected after cooling. The foreign matters from debris are removed by scraping. The beeswax is purified by treating with dilute sulphuric acid or in hot water and thereafter bleaching of wax is carried out by treatment with hydrogen peroxide or chromic acid to get white bees wax.

Soft water is used because during the manufacturing of wax, there is often the formation of water emulsions. There are two emulsion types: in the first one, water particles are dispersed into wax, and in the second one, wax particles are dispersed into water. These emulsions are built with the help of emulsifiers. Proteins and dextrines are emulsifiers, contained in honey, pollen and salts of wax fatty acids with sodium and potassium. The second type of emulsion is caused by the salts of wax fatty acids with calcium, copper and iron cations. Hard water contains cations that are diffused out of the vessels and used for wax production.

Physical Properties: Beeswax consists primarily of a mixture of esters of fatty acids and fatty alcohols, paraffinic hydrocarbons and free fatty acids. Two types of beeswax are marketed — yellow beeswax and white beeswax. Yellow beeswax is light-brown solid, brittle in nature when cold and presents a characteristic odour of honey. White beeswax is a white or yellowish white solid having a characteristic, but faint, odour of honey. Yellow beeswax is smooth and soft to touch but breaks with granular fracture. It is insoluble in water, but soluble in hot alcohol and other organic solvents. In hot water it melts in liquid form and can be made any required shape and design after cooling. They are partially soluble in cold carbon disulfide and completely soluble in the same solution at temperatures of 30° and above. Beeswax has a specific gravity of about 0.95.

Melting range	:	60 - 65°C
Acid value	:	17 - 24
Peroxide value	:	Not more than 5
Saponification value	:	87 - 104
Ester value	:	72 - 79

The composition of beeswax depends to some extent on the subspecies of the bees, the age of the wax and the climatic circumstances of its production, and hence the physical properties are also varied.

Chemical Properties:

Beeswax consists of five main groups of components:

1. Free fatty acids, most of them are saturated and have chain length of C_{24}- C_{32}.
2. Free primary fatty alcohols with a chain length of C_{28}- C_{38}.

3. Linear wax monoesters and hydroxymonoesters (35-45%) with chain lengths generally C_{40}-C_{48}. The esters are derived almost exclusively from palmitic acid, 15-hydroxypalmitic acid and oleic acid.

4. Complex wax esters (15-27%) containing 15-hydroxypalmitic acid or diols, which, through their hydroxyl group, are linked to another fatty-acid molecule.

5. In addition to such diesters, tri and higher esters are also found.

The main constituents of beeswax are myricin (80%), cerotic acid, melissic acid and 15% hydrocarbons.

Uses: Beeswax is used as a component in dietary food supplements (soft gelatin capsules and tablets), glazings and coatings, chewing gum, water-based flavoured drinks, and as a carrier for food additives (including flavours and colours) and cosmetics (Lipsticks, face creams). Beeswax is suitable stabilizer for keeping oil-based capsule contents in suspension as well as in tablet formulations. Beeswax is blended with other oils and is used as a glazing agent for confectionery (including chocolate), in small products of fine bakery ware coated with chocolate, in snacks, nuts, coffee beans, dietary food supplements and in certain fresh fruits.

Adulterants: Beeswax is adulterated with paraffin, microcrystalline wax, Jan wax, carnauba wax, tallow and stearic acid. They are identified by saponification values and as well as solubility and melting point which is about 10-20°C lower than other waxes. Beeswax will not give turbidity when boiled with sodium hydroxide and cooled, but other waxes will form turbidity.

5.6 MARINE DRUGS

It is a branch of Pharmacognosy which deals with the isolation and identification of bioactive molecules from marine organism. That means study of chemicals that derived from marine sources.

Sources: Bioactive molecules obtained from microbes, sponges, seaweeds and other marine organisms.

Reason for Less Popularity of Marine Products:

1. Source of material and their identification is not familiar.
2. The quality or characters depend on environmental changes, factors, and food availability.
3. Collection is difficult unlike in land products.
4. Lack of literature, therefore identification is difficult.
5. Constant supply is not guaranteed and this depends on collection of the materials.
6. Cost is high and therefore chances of adulteration are possible.
7. Variations in constituents' i.e. chemical constituents of drugs which can be due to biotic and abiotic or external factors.

5.6.1 Factors Affecting Distribution and Occurrence of Marine Drugs

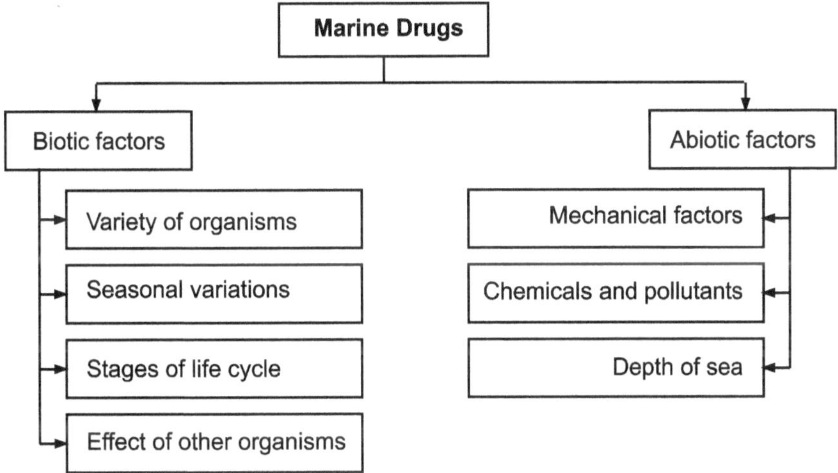

Fig. 5.27

1. **Variety of organisms:** The species varies with respect to the kingdom, phyla, genus etc. Organisms should belong to same genus i.e. phenotypically and genotypically similar with gererations, different species may develop and hence giving variety. E.g. Extreme variation in Carrageenan (Red algae).

2. **Seasonal variations:** Depending on the seasonal changes, it may affect the body enzyme system, biochemical reaction varies, and therefore composition varies in the organism. E.g. Benetic algae, Caulerpa is the most popular edible algae in the Phillipins which becomes poisonous during rainy season because of agitation, California sea weed was found to have greater antibacterial activity during fall of spring.

3. **Stages of life cycle:** A tentative correlation between toxicity and reproductive cycle was established for some puffer fish. Studies on male and female fish at different stages of maturation show different levels of toxicity along with seasonal variations. E.g. During reproductive season, the king crabs (*Tachypleus tridentalis*) become toxic.

4. **Effect of other organisms**: When other toxic organisms are taken as food, they may also develop certain toxins which are not harmful to them but harmful to others. E.g. Sand crabs which become toxic because of shellfish poisoning. Enemies in environment may develop toxins in the host for their self defense.

Abiotic Factors:

1. **Mechanical factor:** Due to agitation in rainy season the Benthis algae, Caullerpa which is edible become poisonous. An injury to plant thalus causes extrusion of Caulerpin.

2. **Chemical and pollutants:** A major problem which affects both superficial animals and also deep sea animals. These may be toxic and may lead to extinction of organism. Organism may produce chemical changes or organism, may produce artificial compounds not originally present in organism, but produce due to other factors like industrial waste water, pesticides, human waste sewage, oils i.e. hydrocarbons etc.

3. **Depth of sea:** Effect of depth of the toxicity of marine organism vary mainly due to changes in bathymetry (changes in temperature, salinity, pH and nutrient composition). Changes in depth are also parallel by change in species dominance, e.g.: three species of gulf puffer, encountered in Florida west coast water, have different toxicities and can be separated bathymetrically.

Extraction and Purification of Marine Constituents:

1. **Extraction:** The marine source must be dried and powdered because the solvent enters cell effectively and homogenization by particular solvent like methanol, water and alcohol is done. Salt does not dissolve in the solvent, thus desalting takes place. In maceration process, fungal growth takes place rapidly.

2. **Concentration:** Concentration of the extracts is generally done by evaporating the solvent at high temperature or by vacuum flash evaporation at low temperature.

3. **Desalting:** Membrane filtration differentiates on molecular size of salts and the compounds present. Hence it is not suitable. Salting out by gel filtration using Sephadex biogel is suitable polymeric compound containing pores depends upon molecular size and of gravitational pull it moves up and down. E.g. Isolation and purification of drugs from marine source - Algae material. The algae *Gracilaria edulis* was collected from mandaform, coast in south eastern Indian Peninsula.

Extraction and Isolation: Algae is washed with fresh water. It is extracted with hexane for 120 hours at room temperature, filtered and the solvent is removed on a rotaevaporator to yield a dark green extract. The extract is chromatographed over silica gel (by column adsorption) and the elution is carried out with solvents of increasing polarity using hexane, benzene and ethyl acetate. Removal of solvent from hexane, benzene (9 : 3) afforded a residue in each case. All the residues are further purified separately by repeated column chromatography and finally recrystallised from benzene.

1. Residue from hexane-benzene (9 : 1) fraction gave poriferacta 3,5 diene-7 one.
2. Benzene: ethylacetate (19 : 1) elutes afforded dionacterol.
3. Benzene: ethylacetate (44 : 1) elutes afforded cholesterol.

Table 5.5 : Marine anticancer natural products with established mechanism of action

Organism	Compound	Chemistry	Mechanism of action
Ascidian (*Cion intestinalis*)	Aplidine	Depsipeptide	Oxidation and inactivation of low molecular weight protein tyrosine phosphatase activity.
	Fucoxanthinol	Carotenoid	Induction of apoptosis and decrease in Bcl-2 protein.
Bryozoan (Moss animal)	Bryostatin-I	Macrolide	Apoptosis induction enhanced by PKCe over expression.
Mollusk (*Tonicella lineata*)	Kahalalide F	Depsipeptide	ErbB3 protein and PI3K-Akt pathway involved innecrosis induction.
Sea Hare (*Aplysia californica*)	Aplyronine	Macrolide	Binding to hydrophobic cleft in actin molecule involving trimethylserine moiety.

Organism	Compound	Chemistry	Mechanism of action
Yellow Sponge (*Aplysina fistularis*)	Aaptamine	Alkaloid	Induction of p21 gene and G2/M cell cycle arrest.
	Agosterol A	Steroid	Azido agosterol A binding to MRp1 abolished by ICL5 and ICI7 domain mutations.
Tube worm (*Riftia pachyptila*)	Cephalostatin	Steroid	Bcl-2 hyperphosphorylation independent of M-phase arrest and DNA damage.

Table 5.6 : Marine anticancer natural products currently in market or in clinical phases

Chemical constituents	Source	Application area	Status
Arac-c Marine	Marine sponge	Anticancer	Market
Squalamine lactate	Shark	Anticancer	Phase-II
Aplidin	Sea squirt	Anticancer	Phase-II
Bryostatin-I	Bryozoan	Anticancer	Phase-I

5.6.2 Cardiovascular Active Agents from Marine Sources

Recent development in marine pharmacology has explored biomedicinal potential of cardioactive marine agents such as antianginal, antiarrhythmic, antihypertensive, cardiotonic activities are encountered in Marine Cardiovascular agents (MCAs). Mechanism of actions of MCAs is delineated for rationalizing the roles of their structural uniqueness in drug action are as follows:

(a) **Antianginal MCAs:** They should have vasodilatory effect and are useful in coronary heart disease. Ca^{++} channel antagonists block the L-type Ca^{++} channels specifically present in heart and vascular smooth muscles. They are potent arteriolar vasodilators so effective in antianginal therapy.

(b) **Antiarrhythmic MCAs:** Antiarrhythmics modify and restore normal cardiac rhythm. Arrhythmias are due to disorder of electrical impulse formation by disturbances in impulse condition through the myocardium. They act by blocking Na^+, K^+, Ca^{++} ion channels. Voltage gated Na^+ channel blockers reduce the excitability of nodal regions of heart. They prevent Ca^{++} mediated depolarization in SA node and Purkinje fibres.

(c) **Antihypertensive MCAs:** The compounds act by lowering the sympathetic tone or vasopressor activity. They also inhibit biosynthesis of octapeptide, mediated by angiotensin converting enzyme in nephron. They block release of nitric oxide and ET1 factor from active endothelium.

(d) **Cardiotonic:** They have therapeutical value in congestive heart failure (CHF) or myocardial infarction. They increase the contractile force of the heart and have positive ionotropic properties. They improve cardiac output and oxygen consumption per min, thus cardiac efficacy is improved.

(e) **Marine pollution:** Increasing quantities of industrial waste, agricultural chemicals, untreated sewage, radioactive discharges, oil, plastics, and a huge variety of other pollutants are dumped directly in the sea – or slowly make their way there via rivers, run off and atmospheric deposition. Once released into the environment recovering them is very difficult and they could continue to cause harm for years or even decades. The effect of these pollutants on marine organisms is difficult to measure. In large quantities they may cause immediate death. However, in most cases they are believed to weaken the animals, gradually causing hormonal imbalances, a lowering of disease resistance, brain damage and various neurological disorders, cancer, liver troubles, lowering or a total loss of fertility, thickening of shells, and many other abnormalities and chronic health problems.

(f) Minute quantities of toxins in the sea are picked up by marine plankton, which are then eaten by fish and squid and these in turn are eaten by top predators, such as whales, dolphins and sharks. In this way, high concentrations of toxins build up in the body of animals at the top of the food chain. This build-up increases with age and may be passed on from one generation to another. For example, a lactating female whale may deliver high concentrations of toxins to her calf through her milk.

(g) Marine animals may accumulate and use a variety of toxins from prey organisms and from symbiotic microorganisms for their own purposes. Thus, toxic animals are particularly abundant in the oceans. The toxins vary from small molecules to high molecular weight proteins and display unique chemical and biological features of scientific interest. Many of these substances can serve as useful research tools or molecular models for the design of new drugs and pesticides.

Some chemical constituents from marine sources that are used in various therapeutic activities are given in Table 5.7.

Table 5.7: Marine sources of drugs for various therapeutic activities

CVS agents		
Organism	**Chemical compound**	**Uses**
Laminaria angustata	Laminine	Hypotensive agent
Eptatretus stoutii	Eptatretin	Potent cardiac stimulant
Antitumour agents		
Bugula neritina	Bryostatin	Stimulate haemopoitic cell
Dolabella auricularia	Dolastatin	Active Antineoplastic agent
Anthelmintic agents		
Chondria armata	Domoic acid	Anthelmintic activity
Digenia simplex	Alpha-Kainic acid	Anthelmintic activity
Anticoagulant agents		
Chondrus crispus	Carrageenans	Anticoagulant
Iridaea laminarioides	Galaxtan Sulphuric acid	Anticoagulant
Antimicrobial agents		
Cephalosporium acremonium	Cephalosporin	Antibiotic
Thelepsus setosul	Thelpin	Antimicrobial agent
Antiinflammatory agents		
Sinularia flexibilis	Flexibilide	Antiinflammatory
Flustra foliaceal	Flustramine- A	Muscle relaxant

Marine Toxins: Marine toxins are chemicals and bacteria that can contaminate certain types of seafood. Eating the seafood may result in food poisoning. The seafood may look, smell, and taste normal. There are five common types of marine toxins, and they all cause different symptoms. Food poisoning through marine toxins is rare. Marine toxin poisoning occurs most often in the summer.

Examples: *Anacystis cyanea* - As fast death factor; Mainotoxin from *Gambierdiscus toxicus* organism shows ionotropic effect.

EXERCISE

Long Essays:
1. Explain bast fibre. Note on Cotton and Jute fibres.
2. Explain Hallucinogens and Teratogens with examples.
3. Explain natural allergens with examples.
4. Define Carbohydrates. Classify them with examples. Give their general chemical test. Note on Acacia.
5. Explain detail about Agar and Tragacanth.
6. Explain detail about Honey.
7. Define Proteins. Classify them with examples. Explain their chemical nature and biochemical importance. Give the method of analysis of Proteins.
8. Explain Gelatin and Casein.
9. Explain proteolytic enzyme with detail study of Papain and Bromelain.
10. Explain Pepsin and Streptokinase.
11. Define lipids. Classify them with examples. Give their chemistry and function. Explain various methods of analysis of fats and oils.
12. Explain Castor oil and Chaulmoogra oil.
13. Explain wool fat and Bees wax.
14. Explain various marine sources of drugs for therapeutic applications.

Short Essays:
1. Explain various types of fibres. Differentiate animal and plant fibres.
2. Explain about cotton.
3. Explain about Hemp.
4. Explain about natural allergens.
5. Give the source, method of preparation and adulterants of Acacia gum.
6. Explain chemistry and method of production of Tragacanth gum and Agar.
7. Explain Teratogenic plants.
8. Explain source, properties, chemical tests and adulterants of Honey.
9. Explain plant containing Hallucination.
10. Explain sources and method of preparation of jute.
11. Explain colour reactions of Carbohydrate and Protein.
12. Explain chemical tests of Acacia, Agar, Gelatin and Tragacanth.
13. Explain Casein.
14. Explain Serratiopeptidase.
15. Explain method of production and uses of Streptokinase and Urokinase.
16. Explain method of production and uses of Papain and Bromelain.
17. Explain source and properties of Pepsin.

18. Explain acid value, saponification value and iodine value.
19. Explain Chaulmoogra oil.
20. Explain the method of production, physical properties and uses of Castor oil.
21. Explain source, physical, chemical properties and chemical tests of Wool fat.
22. Explain source, method of preparation, chemical properties, uses and adulterants of Beeswax.
23. Explain various methods of analysis of Proteins and fats.
24. Explain drugs used in CVS and anticancer activities from marine sources.
25. Explain various factors affecting distribution and occurrence of marine drugs.

Multiple Choice Questions (MCQs):

1. Bast fibres are separated from stem by ......
    (a) Peeling   (b) Mulching
    (c) Cutting   (d) Retting
2. Dietary fibres are used for ......
    (a) Laxative   (b) Astringent
    (c) Antioxidant   (d) Anti-tussive
3. Example of bast fibre from seed is ......
    (a) Soya   (b) Flax
    (c) Bamboo   (d) Palm
4. Example of bast fibre from grass is ......
    (a) Coir   (b) Bamboo
    (c) Agave   (d) Hemp
5. Pulping process is used to remove the ......
    (a) Mineral   (b) Lignin
    (c) Cellulose   (d) None
6. "Asbestos" is an example of ......
    (a) Animal fibre   (b) Wood fibre
    (c) Mineral fibre   (d) Synthetic fibre
7. Cuoxam solution contains ......
    (a) Ammoniacal copper sulphate   (b) Ammoniacal copper nitrate
    (c) Ammoniacal copper oxide   (d) Alkaline copper oxide
8. Millon's reagent reacts with animal fibre to give ...... precipitate.
    (a) Violet   (b) Yellow
    (c) Red   (d) White
9. Cotton fibres are separated from seeds by ......
    (a) Retting   (b) Plucking
    (c) Peeling   (d) Ginning
10. Length of fibre between 20 mm to 24 mm is known as ......
    (a) Short staple cotton   (b) Long staple cotton
    (c) Medium staple cotton   (d) None of these
11. Hemp contains ......
    (a) High cellulose and low protein   (b) High cellulose and low lignin
    (c) High lignin and low cellulose   (d) High lignin and low protein

12. Photodynamic agents are required ...... for their action with ....
    (a) CO_2 (b) O_2
    (c) H_2 (d) N_2
13. Aflatoxin is produced by ......
    (a) *Aspergillus versicolor*   (b) *A. purpurea*
    (c) *A. flavus*   (d) *A. purpurea*
14. *Claviceps purpurea* causes ......
    (a) Ochratoxin   (b) Stearigmatocystin
    (c) Ergotoxin   (d) None of these
15. Glyceraldehyde is an example of ......
    (a) Pentose   (b) Biose
    (c) Triose   (d) Tetrose
16. Hemicellulose is an example of ......
    (a) Pentose   (b) Biose
    (c) Tetrose   (d) Triose
17. Fabric is prepared from ......
    (a) Chitin   (b) Cellulose
    (c) Hemicellulose   (d) None of these
18. Benedict's test for carbohydrates gives ...... precipitate.
    (a) Violet colour   (b) Purple colour
    (c) Brown colour   (d) Reddish
19. The reagent mixture of copper acetate and acetic acid is known as ......
    (a) Benedict's reagent   (b) Barfoed reagent
    (c) Bial's reagent   (d) Selwanoff's reagent
20. Chemical test that is used to differentiate aldohexoses from ketohexoses is ......
    (a) Bial's test   (b) Barfoed's test
    (c) Seliwanoff's test   (d) Fehling's test
21. Composition of Bial's reagent is ......
    (a) Orcinol, HCl and $FeCl_3$ (b) Resorcinol, HCl
    (c) Sodium citrate, Sodium carbonate   (d) Sodium citrate, $CuSO_4$
22. *Anogeissus latifolia* is used as adulterant of ......
    (a) Agar   (b) Tragacanth
    (c) Acacia   (d) Gelatin
23. Red colour of red algae is due to ......
    (a) Mucilage   (b) Phycoerythrin
    (c) Gelidium   (d) None of these
24. Agar reacts with Ruthenium red and gives ......
    (a) Yellow colour   (b) White colour
    (c) No reaction   (d) Red colour
25. Bassorin is ......
    (a) Water soluble   (b) Alcohol soluble
    (c) Alcohol insoluble   (d) Water insoluble
26. Aqueous solution of Tragacanth reacts with Guaicol and few drops of H_2O_2 and gives ...... precipitate.
    (a) Red colour   (b) Brown colour
    (c) No colour   (d) White colour

27. Citral gum is used as adulterant of ......
    (a) Acacia   (b) Agar
    (c) Gelatin   (d) Tragacanth
28. Sterculia gum is used as adulterant of ......
    (a) Gelatin   (b) Agar
    (c) Tragacanth   (d) Acacia
29. The major amino acid present in Honey is ......
    (a) Leucine   (b) Proline
    (c) Aspartic acid   (d) Glycine
30. Fiehe's test is carried out to detect adulterant of Honey with ......
    (a) Inverted sugar   (b) Cane sugar
    (c) Glucose   (d) Commercial sugar
31. "Aniline chloride test" is performed to detect adulteration of honey with ......
    (a) Inverted sugar   (b) Cane sugar
    (c) Glucose   (d) Commercial sugar
32. Chemoprotein is an example of ......
    (a) Simple protein   (b) Derived protein
    (c) Conjugated protein   (d) None of these
33. Reagent used in turbidity method for detection of protein is ......
    (a) $FeCl_3$ (b) $CuSO_4$
    (c) Trichloroacetic acid   (d) Folin ciocalteau Phenol
34. Alpha naphthol is a reagent used in ......
    (a) Xanthoproteic reaction   (b) Sakaguchi's test
    (c) Salkavoski's test   (d) Remond's test
35. Type-A gelatine has isoionic point ......
    (a) 7-9   (b) 4-5
    (c) 9-12   (d) 1-4
36. Type-B gelatine has isoionic point ......
    (a) 7-9   (b) 4-5
    (c) 9-12   (d) 1-4
37. Light colour gelatine is obtained by bleaching in ......
    (a) H_2S (b) H_2O_2
    (c) SO_2 (d) Lead acetate
38. Moisture content in gelatine is ......
    (a) 17%   (b) 6%
    (c) 16%   (d) 7%
39. Gelatine solution reacts with soda lime and forms ......
    (a) White precipitate   (b) Yellow precipitate
    (c) Gel   (d) Ammonia gas precipitate
40. Isoelectric point of Casein is ......
    (a) 3.6   (b) 7.6
    (c) 5.6   (d) 4.6
41. Phosphate group present in alpha casein is ......
    (a) 10-15   (b) 8-10
    (c) 6-8   (d) 3-7

42. Isoelectric point of papain is ......
    (a) 4.7   (b) 8.7
    (c) 1.7   (d) 5.7
43. Activator of Papain is ......
    (a) Cysteine   (b) Thiol
    (c) Ascorbic acid   (d) Metal ions
44. Serratiopeptidase is obtained from ......
    (a) *Serratia marcescens*   (b) *S. rubidae*
    (c) *S. odoriferae*   (d) *S. plymuthica*
45. Serratia is ......
    (a) Round shape bacteria   (b) Rod shape bacteria
    (c) Round shape virus   (d) Rod shape virus
46. Maximum enzyme activity of Serratiopeptidase is at ......
    (a) pH 7   (b) pH 9
    (c) pH 5   (d) pH 12
47. Suitable medium for Serratiopeptidase culture is ......
    (a) Casein   (b) Yeast
    (c) Agar broth   (d) Trypticase soy
48. Urokinase has ......
    (a) 400 residue proteins   (b) 311 residue proteins
    (c) 300 residue proteins   (d) 411 residue proteins
49. Amino acid residue present in Streptokinse is ......
    (a) 314   (b) 514
    (c) 414   (d) 214
50. Molecular weight of pepsin is ......
    (a) 30.5 kDa   (b) 44.5 kDa
    (c) 34.5 kDa   (d) 25 kDa
51. Proenzyme of pepsin is ......
    (a) Kymopepsin   (b) Kimopepsin
    (c) Sarapepsinogen   (d) Pepsinogen
52. Inhibitor of pepsin is ......
    (a) Pepstatin   (b) Sucrafate
    (c) Pepsinogen   (d) (a) and (b) both
53. Cephalins are ......
    (a) Glycolipid   (b) Phospholipid
    (c) Sulpholipid   (d) Triglyceride
54. Alpha-linolenic acid is converted into human body as ......
    (a) Linoleic acid   (b) Linolic acid
    (c) Docosahexaenoic acid   (d) Triglyceride
55. Nichol's method is used to isolate ......
    (a) Lipid from plant   (b) Protein from animal
    (c) Lipid from animal   (d) Protein from plant
56. Wij's solution is used for determination of ......
    (a) Saponification value   (b) Acid value
    (c) Iodine value   (d) Ester value

57. Composition of Wij's solution is ......
    (a) Iodine monochoride in glacial acetic acid
    (b) KI in glacial acetic acid
    (c) KIO_3 in glacial acetic acid
    (d) KCl in glacial acetic acid
58. Family of castor oil is ......
    (a) Ranunculaceae   (b) Euphobiaceae
    (c) Leguminosae   (d) Flacourtriceae
59. Oleic acid present in castor oil is ......
    (a) 95%   (b) 5%
    (c) 6%   (d) 49%
60. Refractive index of Chaulmoogra oil is ......
    (a) 1.472 - 1.476   (b) 1.270 - 1.276
    (c) 2.172 - 2.176   (d) 0.742 - 0.746
61. Percentage content of Chaulmoogric acid in Chaulmoogra oil is ......
    (a) 48-50   (b) 26-30
    (c) 62-68   (d) 18-22
62. Substituent used in Chaulmoogra oil is ......
    (a) *Hydnocarpus anthelmintica*   (b) *H. alpine*
    (c) *H. wightiana*   (d) (b) and (c) both
63. Specific gravity of Beeswax is ......
    (a) 0.45   (b) 0.95
    (c) 0.25   (d) 0.55
64. Percentage content of Myricin in beeswax is ......
    (a) 15   (b) 40
    (c) 80   (d) 95
65. Anticancer drug from marine source is ......
    (a) Aplyronine   (b) Domoic acid
    (c) Laminine   (d) Thelpin
66. Antimicrobial agent from marine source is ......
    (a) Aplyronine   (b) Domoic acid
    (c) Laminine   (d) Thelpin

ANSWERS

1. (d)	2. (a)	3. (a)	4. (b)	5. (b)	6. (c)	7. (c)	8. (c)	9. (d)
10. (c)	11. (b)	12. (b)	13. (c)	14. (c)	15. (c)	16. (a)	17. (b)	18. (d)
19. (b)	20. (c)	21. (a)	22. (c)	23. (n)	24. (d)	25. (d)	26. (c)	27. (d)
28. (c)	29. (b)	30. (a)	31. (d)	32. (c)	33. (c)	34.(b)	35. (a)	36. (b)
37. (c)	38. (c)	39. (d)	40. (d)	41. (b)	42. (b)	43. (a)	44. (a)	45. (b)
46. (b)	47. (d)	48. (d)	49. (c)	50. (c)	51. (d)	52. (d)	53. (b)	54. (b)
55. (a)	56. (c)	57. (a)	58. (b)	59. (c)	60. (a)	61. (b)	62. (d)	63. (b)
64. (c)	65. (a)	66. (d)						

✹✹✹

BIBLIOGRAPHY

1. Biren Shah. Textbook of Pharmacognosy and Phytochemistry. Published by Elsevier, India, 2010.
2. Cock I.E. Pharmacognosy Communications: The Scope of Pharmacognosy. 2011; 1(1): 1–3.
3. Indian Pharmacopoeia. Published by The Controller of Publications, Under Govt. of India Ministry of health and Family Welfare, Delhi. 1996, Vol: II. pp. A104–A107.
4. Kokate C.K., Purohit A.P., Gokhale S.B. Text book of Pharmacognosy. Published by Nirali Prakashan. 2010.
5. Sayeed Ahmad. Introduction to Pharmacognosy. I.K. International Publishing House Pvt. Ltd. 2012.
6. Trease and Evans. Pharmacognosy. Sixteenth Edition. Elsevier Publication.
7. Tyler, V.C., Brady, L.R., and Robers, J.E. Pharmacognasy., 11th to 14th Editions.
8. Vikas Anand Saharan, M.K., Moond, P.C., Chouhan and Manish K., Gupta. A Textbook of Pharmacognosy. Riddhi International exporter and distributor. 2008.
9. Wallis. T.E. Textbook of Pharmacognosy, 5th edition, J. and A., Churchill Limited, U.K.
10. Blumenthal M., Brusse W.R., Goldberg A., Gruenwald J., Hall T., Riggins C.W., Rister R.S. The Complete German Commission E Monographs. Therapeutic Guide to Herbal Medicines. The American Botanical Council, Austin, T.X. 1998.
11. Burness communications. Adapting agriculture to climate change: new global search to save endanger crop wild relatives. Web site: http://www.sciencedaily. com/releases/2010/12/101209201938.htm
12. Das DK. Introductory Soil Science. Kalyani Publishers, Ludhiana, Punjab. 2015.
13. Kokate CK, Purohit AP, Gokhale SB. Pharmacognosy 54th Edition. Nirali Prakashan, Pune. 2017.
14. Roberts J.E., Tyler V.E. Tyler's Herbs of Choice. The Therapeutic Use of Phytomedicinals. 1997. The Haworth Press, New York.
15. WHO. Guidelines on Good Agricultural and Collection Practices (GACP) for Medicinal Plants. 2004. World Health Organization, Geneva.
16. Trenkel M.E. Slow and Controlled-Release and Stabilized Fertilizers: An Option for Enhancing Nutrient Efficiency in Agriculture. Second edition, IFA, Paris, France.
17. Carrel, Alexis and Montrose T. Burrows "Cultivation of Tissues in Vitro and its Technique"; Journal of Experimental Medicine.
18. Gupta P.K. Element of Biotechnology. Rastogi Publications. 1994.
19. Hartmann and Kester's Plant Propagation, Principles and Practices 8th Edition.
20. Kalia AN. Text book of Industrial Pharmacognosy, CBS publishers and Distributors Pvt. Ltd, 1st Edition, 2005.
21. Lorraine Mineo. Plant Tissue Culture Techniques. Chapter 9. 1990.
22. Singh B.D. Biotechnology. Kalyani Publishers, 2010. 4th Edition.
23. Siya S.Top 6 Types of Tissue Culture | Biotechnology. 2016.

24. A.O.A.C 17th edn, 2000, Official method 920.212 Specific gravity (Apparent) of Oils, Pycnometer method/I.S.I. Hand book of Food analysis (Part XIII) 1984, page 72.

25. A.O.A.C 17th edn, 2000, Official method 921.08 – Index of refraction of oils and fats/I.S.I Handbook of Food analysis (Part XIII) – 1984, page 70.

26. A.O.A.C. 17th edn, 2000, Official method 920. 159 –Iodine absorption number of oils and fats/I.S.I. Handbook of Food Analysis (Part XIII) – 1984 page 76.

27. Bender D.A., "Benders' Dictionary of Nutrition and Food Technology". 8th Edition. Woodhead Publishing. Oxford, 2006.

28. Carper J. The Food Pharmacy. New York, NY: Bantam Books; 1989, 242–245.

29. Dunn BM. "Overview of pepsin-like aspartic peptidases". Current Protocols in Protein Science. 2001; Chapter 21: Unit 21.3.

30. Evans W.C. Trease and Evans' Pharmacognosy. 14th ed. London: WB Saunders; 1996, 185–186.

31. Heinrich M. Fundamentals of Pharmacognosy and Phytotherapy. Production, Standardisation and Quality control, Elsevier publication, London, 2004: 144–159.

32. I.S.I. Hand book of Food Analysis (Part XIII) – 1984, page 62.

33. I.S 1448 – 1970 Methods of test for petroleum and its products (P: 21) Flash Point

34. (Closed) by Pensky Martin apparatus.

35. I.S.I. Hand book of Food Analysis (Part XIII) – 1984 page 75/I.S. 548 (Part 1) – 1964, Methods of sampling and test for Oils and Fats.

36. I.S.I. Handbook of Food Analysis (Part XIII) – 1984, page 68/I.S : 548 (Part 1) – 1964, Methods of Sampling and test for Oils and Fats page 33.

37. I.S.I. Handbook of Food Analysis (Part XIII) – 1984, page 67/A.O.A.C 17th edn, 2000, Official method 933.08, Residue (unsaponifiable) of oils and fats.

38. I.S.I. Handbook of Food Analysis (Part XIII) – 1984, page 67/IUPAC 2.201 (1979)/I.S: 548 (Part 1) – 1964, Methods of Sampling and Testfor Oils and Fats.

39. I.S.I. Handbook of Food Analysis (Part XIII) – 1984 page 81)/A.O.A.C 17th edn, 2000. Official method 925.41 Acids (volatile) in oils and fats.

40. Joshi S.G. Medicinal plants: Family Apiaceae. 1st ed. Delhi: Oxford and IBH Publishing Co.; 2000.

41. Kokate C.K., Purohit A.P., Gokhale S.B. 2005. Pharmacognosy, 31st edition Nirali Prakshan.

42. Oosterhuis D.M., Jornstedth. Morphology and Anatomy of Cotton Plant. Cotton: Origin, History, Technology and Production, edited by Wayne C. Smith ISBN 0-471-18045-9. 1999.

43. Reynolds J.E., ed. The Extra Pharmacopoeia: Martindale. 31st ed. London: Royal Pharmaceutical Society; 1996, 1734.

44. Wielinga W.C., Maehall A.G. Galactomannans. In: Philips G.O., Williams P.A., editors. Handbook of hydrocolloids. New York: Woodhead Publ Ltd; 2000. pp. 137–153.

45. Bidlack, Wayne R. Phytochemicals as Bioactive Agents. Lancaster, PA: Technomic Publishers, 2000.
46. Chopra RN, Chopra IC,Handa KL ,Indigenous Drugs of India, 2nd edn. Academic Publishers, New Delhi, 1982.
47. Cuellar NG. Conversations in complementary and alternative medicine: insights and perspectives from leading practitioners. Boston: Jones and Bartlett. 2006.
48. Evans, W. C. Trease and Evans Pharmacognosy, 16th ed.; Elsevier: New York, 2009.
49. Farington E.A., Clinical Materia Medica, B.Jain Pulishers New Delhi, 1975.
50. Haehl R, Henry CJ. Samuel Hahnemann; his life and work, based on recently discovered state papers, documents, letters, etc. 1922.
51. James Duke. Handbook of Medicinal Herbs. CRC Publication, 2nd edition, 2006.
52. Jean Bruneton. Pharmacognosy, Phytochemistry and Medicinal Plants. Lavoisier Publication, 2nd edition, 1999.
53. Kirtikar KR, Basu BD. Indian Medicinal Plants, Vol. 1-4. Allahabad, India, 1933.
54. Kokate, C. K.; Gokhale, S. B.; Purohit, A. P. A textbook of Pharmacognosy, 29th ed.; Nirali Prakashan: Pune, 2009.
55. Mandal PP, Mandal B. A text book of Homeopathic Pharmacy. New Central Book Agency, Kolkata, 2009.
56. Peter KV. Handbook of Herbs and Spices. Woodhead Publishing Ltd., 2012.
57. Rangari VD. Pharmacognosy and Phytochemistry. Career Publication, Vol 1, 2nd edition, 2009.
58. Rosenthal, Gerald A., and May R. Berenbaum. Herbivores, Their Interactions with Secondary Plant Metabolites. San Diego, CA: Academic Press, 1991.
59. Shah B.N. Textbook of pharmacognosy and phytochemistry. 1st ed. New Delhi: Reed Elsevier India Pvt. Ltd; 2010.Tadeusz Aniszewski. Alkaloids – Secrets of life. Elsevier Publishers, The Netherland. 2007.
60. Tyler V.E., Brady L.R., Robbers J.E. Pharmacognosy, 9th Edition - Leo and Fabiger. Philadelphia, 1988.P. 856.
61. Wallis T.E. Textbook of Pharmacognosy. CBS Publisher, 5th Edition, 2004.
62. Whorton JC. The History of Alternative Medicine in America. Oxford University Press, Nature Cures. 2004.

****